Health, Society and Medicine

AN INTRODUCTION TO COMMUNITY MEDICINE

BEING THE THIRD EDITION OF

AN INTRODUCTION TO SOCIAL MEDICINE

BY THOMAS McKEOWN & C. R. LOWE

ROY M. ACHESON
MA, DM, ScD, FRCP, FFCM, FFOM
Professor of Community Medicine
University of Cambridge

SPENCER HAGARD
MA, MB, ChB, PhD, FFCM, DPH
District Medical Officer
Cambridge Health Authority and
Associate Lecturer
University Department of
Community Medicine, Cambridge

BLACKWELL SCIENTIFIC PUBLICATIONS
OXFORD LONDON EDINBURGH
BOSTON PALO ALTO MELBOURNE

Editorial offices:
Osney Mead, Oxford, OX2 0EL
8 John Street, London, WC1N 2ES
23 Ainslie Place, Edinburgh, EH3 6AJ
52 Beacon Street, Boston
Massachusetts 02108, USA
744 Cowper Street, Palo Alto
California 94301, USA
107 Barry Street, Carlton
Victoria 3053, Australia

First published 1966
Reprinted 1968
Second edition 1974
Reprinted 1977
Third Edition 1984

Set by DMB (Typesetting), Oxford and printed and bound in Great Britain by Redwood Burn Limited, Trowbridge, Wiltshire

DISTRIBUTORS

USA
Blackwell Mosby Book Distributors
11830 Westline Industrial Drive
St Louis, Missouri 63141

Canada
Blackwell Mosby Book Distributors
120 Melford Drive, Scarborough
Ontario M1B 2X4

Australia
Blackwell Scientific Book Distributors
31 Advantage Road, Highett
Victoria 3190

British Library
Cataloguing in Publication Data

Acheson, Roy M.
Health, society and medicine:
an introduction to
community medicine.—3rd ed.
1. Community health services
2. Public health
I. Title II. Hagard, Spencer
III. McKeown, Thomas. Introduction
to Social Medicine.
362.1′0425 RA425

ISBN 0-632-00965-9

Contents

Introduction

Although we have changed the title, this is the third edition of Thomas McKeown's and C. R. Lowe's *An Introduction to Social Medicine.* It is about twenty years since the first manuscript was being drafted, and ten since it was revised to make the second edition.

During the interim years, in Britain at least, social medicine has become an historic concept, and community medicine has been born. They share a great deal of common ground; indeed the biggest difference between them is probably that while social medicine was essentially an academic discipline without a service component, British community medicine, like surgery and obstetrics, is a practical specialty of medicine with a formal career structure. It inherited the body of knowledge, and epidemiology and statistics of social medicine, which are described in the introduction to the first edition (pp. xi-xiv); it also inherited the philosophies and practices of public health. Therefore in preparing this edition a good deal of updating has been necessary. We have also changed some of the emphases. Our approach to preventive medicine and the protection of the individual from ill-health is developed in part from the late Professor Anthony Payne's conceptualization of the genotype and its environment (figure 1.1) and in part from a belief in the need to stress the importance of the role society plays in influencing the behaviour of its individuals. Payne classifies the 'agent' as an integral part of the environment and not separate from it. The society of modern man is, however, the most important of all the components of his environment. Acceptance of this background has led us to classify protection of health under two headings which, to avoid confusion, we have called primary and secondary *protection*. For purposes of comparison we have included Leavell's three-stage classification of *prevention* which, unlike ours, is based on the natural history of disease.

These changes have necessitated the introduction of two new chapters, Chapters 1 and 8, and a rearrangement of the presentation of the existing chapters in part 2. Also included are new chapters on the role of clinical medicine and planning health. The chapters on international comparisons of incidence of disease and health services have been omitted as separate entities, but some of the material in them has been retained elsewhere in the book. We have been able to keep unchanged some two-thirds of the original text, and hope that, despite the change in title which reflects changing times and a slightly different emphasis, the flavour of the book is not lost.

The book is primarily directed towards medical students, but we hope it will also be of value to a much wider readership including other health professionals and the members of health authorities, and community health councils.

Cambridge 1984

R. M. Acheson.
S. M. Hagard.

Acknowledgements

It is a pleasure to express our indebtedness to the following: Professor Thomas McKeown for allowing us to include as Chapter 7, parts of his book *The Role of Medicine*, Basil Blackwell, Oxford; Professor C. R. Lowe for revising Chapter 19; Dr D. R. R. Williams, University Lecturer in the Department of Community Medicine, Cambridge University for rewriting Chapter 14; Professor John Fox of the Office of Population Censuses and Surveys for providing us with unpublished SMRs; Heather Ashton, Robert Stepney and the Tavistock Press for their permission to publish figure 17.3 in modified form; Miss Linda Craft for redrawing the majority of the diagrams, and Mrs J. L. Robinson of the Information Unit of the Cambridge Health Authority. One of us (RMA) was awarded a Scholarship in Residence from the Rockefeller Foundation which enabled him to work on the text at Bellagio, Lake Como, Italy.

Introduction to the First Edition

In most branches of biology and medicine the nature of the subject matter is accurately reflected in the title. Anatomy is concerned with structure, physiology with function and obstetrics with childbearing; and whatever differences of opinion there may be about methods of instruction, teachers can usually take it for granted that they are talking about the same thing. This is an assumption which the writer on social medicine cannot make, and it is essential at the outset to clarify the use of the term.

In contemporary usage social medicine has two meanings, one broad and ill-defined, the other more restricted and precise. In the broad sense, social medicine is an expression of the humanitarian tradition in medicine, and people frequently read into it any interpretation consistent with their own experience and interests. Thus it may be identified with humane care of patients, prevention of disease, health education, the work of local health authorities, finance of medical services; indeed with almost any subject in the extensive field of health and welfare. But in the more restricted sense in which we shall be using the term, social medicine is concerned with a body of knowledge and methods of obtaining knowledge appropriate to a discipline.

This discipline may be said to comprise (*a*) *epidemiology and* (*b*) *the study of the medical needs of society.*

These subjects were a relatively late development in medicine. Until the nineteenth century medical service comprised little more than the care of patients who sought the assistance of the doctor. It was the threat of infection which finally led to recognition of the need for another approach. Diseases such as smallpox, cholera and typhoid could not be treated effectively in individual patients; but they could be prevented by measures directed to the community as a whole.

The new developments in the second half of the nineteenth century had two important features. One was investigation of disease by epidemiological methods; the other an interest in the medical needs of society, for example in protection against smallpox, in control of the physical environment and in provision of fever hospitals. These features were adopted, not because our predecessors were exceptionally perceptive, but because they offered the only feasible approach to the predominant problem of infection. It was not a coincidence that public medical services were introduced at the time when epidemiological methods were first widely applied to the study of disease.

In technically advanced countries the problem of infection is today much smaller, but the two features of social medicine are as necessary as ever. Indeed their full significance is only beginning to be realized. In almost all branches of medicine investigation based on groups rather than on individuals is an indispensable complement to the traditional methods of laboratory and clinical research. And acceptance of national responsibility for medical services, far from resolving the problems of medical care, has revealed the paucity of data required for their solution.

It is convenient to consider the use of epidemiological methods in medicine in relation to two main themes: human disease; and human biology.

Epidemiological methods were first employed extensively to investigate the causes and distribution of infections, and until about the middle of the present century this was almost their sole use. The same methods have now been applied with considerable success to a wide range of disease problems other than infections. They include cancer, coronary artery disease, mental illness, congenital malformations and accidents.

Epidemiological research in human biology was a later development and is even now not fully exploited. Yet it is no less important and can frequently be combined with advantage with the study of disease. For example an understanding of the nature of hypertensive disease requires knowledge of the distribution of arterial pressure in the general population. Moreover the sources from which information concerning disease in human populations is derived are frequently the same sources which provide essential data for human biology. It is profitable to associate the study of congenital malformations with examination of pre-natal growth, and to link investigation of cancer of the breast with observations on the menopause. It is for these reasons that social medical research is concerned with the application of epidemiological methods to biological themes such as normal growth, development and behaviour, as well as to the study of disease for which they were first employed.

The reasons for including the study of the medical needs of society in the concept of social medicine are two-fold. First, investigation of medical institutions—hospitals, general practice, preventive medicine, medical education, etc.—also relies heavily on epidemiological methods. And second, from the point of view of tradition and experience the department of social medicine is able to make a substantial contribution to this important development.

The university department of social medicine is not primarily a 'clinical' or 'laboratory' department, although its research and teaching sometimes require clinical attachments and laboratory facilities. Its main interest is the application of numerical methods in medical research and practice, and it is becoming the focus in medical schools of the computing and related facilities needed for the handling of extensive data.

In addition to the work we have outlined, departments of social medicine frequently take responsibility for medical statistics and sometimes for other subjects such as human genetics. It is imporant to emphasize that these are independent disciplines, and the reasons for associating them with social medicine are essentially practical. Medical statistics and social medicine require the same kinds of facilities, and to some extent the same staff. In human genetics the relationship turns largely on the nature of the work done. Where this is biochemical or cytological (for example) there is no reason to associate it with social medicine, since the facilities needed are mainly laboratory or clinical. But where the main line of interest is population genetics, it may require the same sources of data and equipment as social medicine, and there may then be close links between the subjects, sometimes within a single department.

It follows from what has been said that research in social medicine may be concerned with any medical problem in which epidemiological methods are useful. There are few in which they are not; but as in other subjects, the research work of an individual, or even of a department, is necessarily more restricted than the teaching commitments. A department of physiology which teaches the whole subject may limit its research to one division such as reproduction or carbohydrate metabolism. Similarly a department of social medicine, which provides instruction in a wide field that may include medical statistics and human genetics, usually limits its research to a subject determined by the training and interests of its staff. This subject may be a branch of human biology, such as growth and development; or a disease such as cancer or chronic bronchitis; or some problem related to medical institutions, such as the organization of hospitals or of medical practice. In each case the research is characterized by its epidemiological basis.

This account of the basis of the work of a department of social medcine, and of its research activities, is a necessary introduction to its teaching. For although the department is concerned with the application of epidemiological methods to human biology and to human disease, and with the study of the medical needs of society, its responsibilities in undergraduate medical education are not the same for each. In human biology and human disease the main responsibility rests with preclinical and clinical teachers, and the contribution of the teacher in social medicine is limited to discussion, usually by joint teaching, of subjects to which epidemiology has contributed significantly. The theme for which the department is chiefly responsible is the medical needs of society.

This instruction may be said to be concerned broadly with *appraisal of the medical problems of society and the means at our disposal for solving them*. It is needed because the role of medicine in society is immensely complex, and cannot be understood without some knowledge of the problems of sickness and death, of the wide range of methods which contribute to health, and of the services through which our resources are mobilized.

Birmingham 1966 T. McKeown
C. R. Lowe

1

Health and Society

1

The Genotype and its Environment

In the year 1818 Shelley left England for the last time, accompanied by his wife, his two children, Byron's mistress, Byron's child and two nursemaids. A year later his wife gave birth to a third child. By the time of Shelley's death 4 years later, three of the four children were dead. Mortality of this order was not restricted to the children of poets with a predilection for foreign travel. It was an accurate reflection of prevailing death rates, a situation vividly portrayed in nineteenth century novels.

History does not record the precise diseases to which the children succumbed, nor would the terms in which the illnesses would have been described be likely to convey much meaning to the contemporary medical scientist. However, it can be stated without question that they arose from interactions between the environment and the childrens' genotypes.

Life starts at conception when the spermatozoon fertilizes the ovum to form a gamete. The gamete immediately begins to assimilate material from its environment and to grow (figure 1.1). Details of this interaction

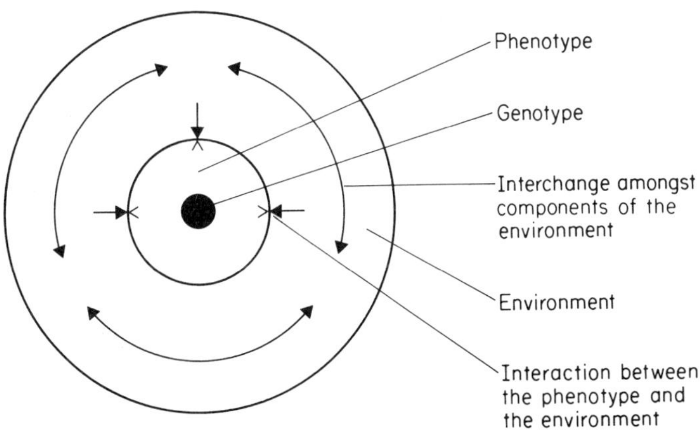

Figure 1.1. The dynamics of the human ecosystem.

from which the phenotype develops depend upon the genotype, upon the environment and upon the reaction between them. Nearly always the uterine environment is well regulated and constant and provides optimal conditions for health and development of the fetus but this is not necessarily the case. The mother herself may provide an environment which is hostile to her child because the two genotypes are incompatible. For example, if she has the Rhesus factor on her erythrocytes and her child does not, antibody formation will be stimulated in the fetus and so it will destroy its own erythrocytes. Environmental factors to which the

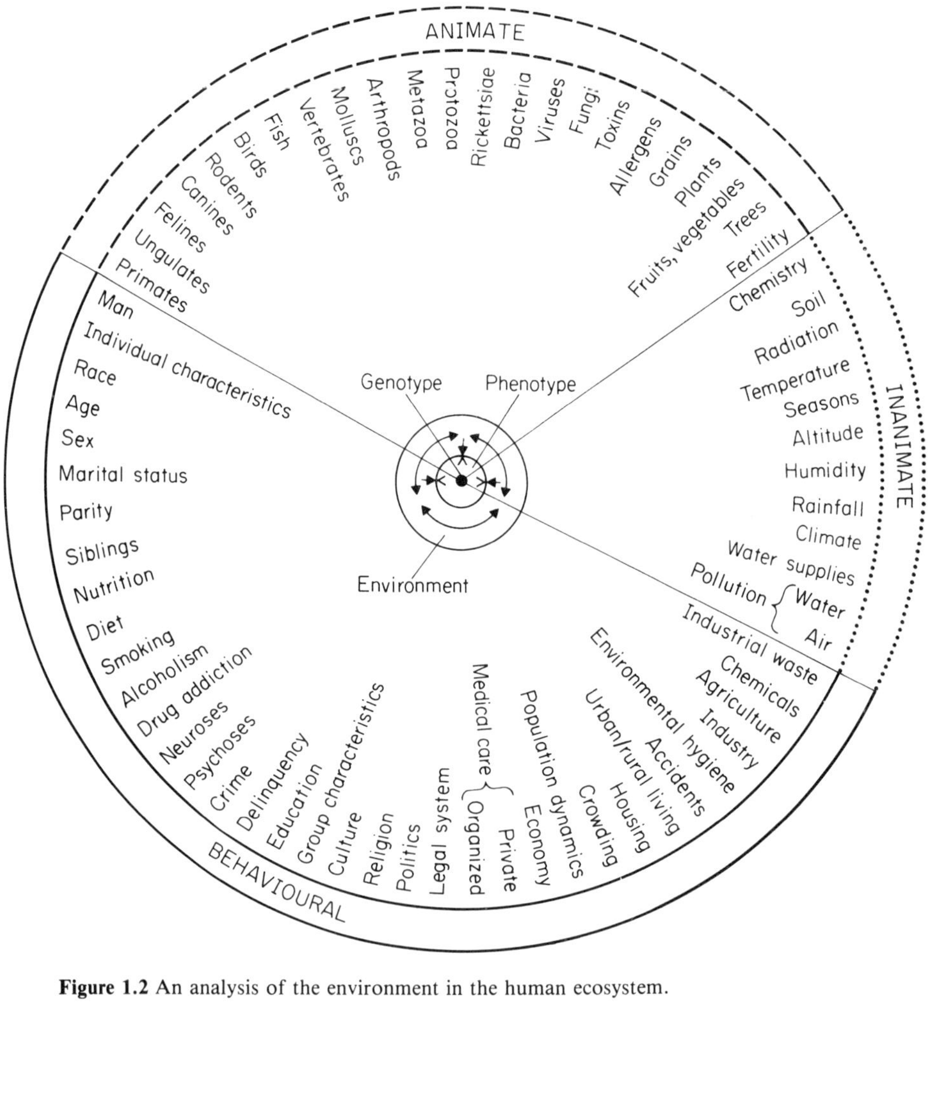

Figure 1.2 An analysis of the environment in the human ecosystem.

mother herself is exposed, such as her use of tobacco or drugs, for example thalidomide, or her exposure to infections such as rubella may also affect the development and therefore the health of the unborn baby. This can happen without evident change in the mother's own health. Once it is born, the baby becomes directly exposed to and becomes part of the general environment in which it will live for the rest of its life (the human ecosystem) and its health and ability to survive will depend on how successfully it reacts to the diverse components of that environment. Although complex, these can be broadly classified into animate, inanimate and behavioural as illustrated in figure 1.2. The behavioural—man himself and his society—comprises the most important components. The rest of the animate environment includes such diverse other organisms as mosquitoes, household pets, bacteria, fruit and poisonous fungi. The inanimate environment includes, for instance, water and solar radiation and the weather. The primary principle of protecting people from disease is to keep apart healthy individuals and the environmental factors which cause sickness, be they a louse, bacterially contaminated water or excessive exposure to the sun.

The importance of mankind as a component of his own environment lies with his intelligence and the fact that he is a social animal. His society, whether it is relatively simple or highly sophisticated is composed of families and is greater than the sum of its parts. Individuals form it, but the groups and institutions which they construct have a collective will and impose an influence on many other individuals. There are innumerable ways in which this happens, but an example applicable to all human societies is the making and enforcing of laws, both of which are social processes; any member of a well ordered society who breaks a law will be sought out and if found guilty held to account for his action and punished. The law has contributed enormously to the prevention of disease by enforcing modification of the inanimate and animate components of the environment—for example in the protection of drinking water from microbial contamination; regulation of the combustion of fuel in the control of atmospheric pollution; and in the behavioural components of the environment—for example in the control of consumption of alcohol by motor vehicle drivers.

Society can also influence its members in other ways, some of them subtle. Matters too trivial for the law, for instance whether or when a neck tie is appropriate for men, or the wearing of trousers by women, have influenced society at large in Britain, and cultures elsewhere. At different times norms for both have been firmly established only to be changed. The changing of behaviour in this way may have a significant influence on health. For example, the widespread and increasing fashion of exposing their scantily clad (or naked) bodies to long periods of solar radiation is having a pronounced effect on the incidence of skin cancers among Australians and North Americans. The origins of a great deal of sickness can be traced to fashion, or in other words to socially determined behaviour.

Within society, groups can establish their own norms. Between 1950 and the present time the hair-styles and clothing of some adolescents and young adults have also changed constantly and dramatically. Such examples of personal appearance may again seem a triviality but it is in this way that violent motorcycle gangs develop their identity by wearing sinister black uniforms. In this instance, and in many others, we are unaware of the origins of such behaviour. Those young men and women of today who wear their hair as green coxcombs are no more able to provide an explanation for this practice than were those of a decade or so ago able to explain why they liked it down to their shoulders. For similarly inexplicable reasons, it was society that accepted the smoking of cigarettes as a fashionable practice, first among rich men, then poor men and finally among women; it is society that is now beginning to make people of either sex who smoke feel self-conscious and expect them to apologize. Similarly social values determine to a considerable extent the kind of food we eat, whether we take exercise and even whether we allow our children to watch television programmes which may be emotionally damaging to them.

Society also determines the means which will be employed to generate wealth and how that wealth is to be distributed. Social postures of this nature usually develop over a considerable period of time and are rarely susceptible to swift change, except at the cost of social dislocation. Their effects are therefore profound and longlasting. Since they determine the extent and nature of employment and its coincidental consequences (such as the industrial pollution of whole communities) their influence on health is considerable. And, since the distribution of wealth determines the standards of housing, clothing, nutrition and recreation, it too can be expected to influence health significantly.

The origins of disease are thus to be found in the patterns of human society and of people's lives. Because the primary principle of protection from disease—keeping separate healthy individuals from the environmental factors which cause sickness—is only applicable to the animate and inanimate components of the environment it cannot be expected to be effective against all diseases. If the diseases which *primary protection* cannot influence are to be controlled, the behavioural components of the environment need to be changed; protection obtained in this way is designated secondary. Such *secondary protection* can be brought about in many ways, ranging from individual persuasion which may be rapid, through the modification of a social norm like smoking which takes time, to the restructuring of employment opportunities and the redistribution of wealth which are dependent on changing political values. We shall develop these points further in Chapter 8.

Further Reading

Dubos R. (1959) *Mirage of Health.* George Allen and Unwin Ltd., London.

2

Assessment of Improvement in Health

The improvement in health which has occurred since the death of Shelley in 1822 is well illustrated by the increase in expectation of life (table 2.1). In 1693 Halley prepared the first 'life tables' (for Breslau) which show per 1000 individuals born alive the numbers expected to live to different ages. At that time approximately half would survive to age 10. Similar data are available for England and Wales since 1838, when half could expect to live to 40. By 1980 rather more than half of the boys could expect to live to 70, and of the girls to 75.

To assess the extent and causes of improvement in health more precisely it is necessary to clarify objectives and define indices of achievement. This is more difficult in medicine than in most other public activities. A broadcasting system should entertain and inform; a postal service should deliver mail quickly and reliably; but it is not possible to state medical objectives which are equally clear and acceptable. Few people would quarrel with the view that it is desirable to prevent illness and premature death; but some would feel that these aims are not ambitious enough, that it is also necessary to prolong the normal life span and promote positive health. Unfortunately these objectives are not yet within reach; and for the purpose of assessing past achievement the only ones that can be accepted without reservation are prevention of sickness, disability and premature death and alleviation of the suffering caused by illness. In relation to these aims the most suitable indices are sickness and death rates.

Sickness (or morbidity) is not so easy to measure and it should be said at once that even today the data are limited, and that there is no reliable information before the present century. The reason is clear: many non-fatal illnesses never come to medical attention, and some which do come from populations at risk which are difficult to identify. Frequently there are also formidable problems of diagnosis and classification. Until recently knowledge of morbidity was almost restricted to a group of 'notifiable diseases', such as smallpox, tuberculosis and diphtheria, with two things in common: they usually present in recognizable form; and their occurrence is of considerable practical importance to public medical authorities.

Table 2.1. Expectation of life at different periods

	Number surviving out of 1,000 live born males				
Age	1693*	1838-54†	1891-1900†	1920-22†	1970-72†
0	1,000	1,000	1,000	1,000	1,000
5	582	724	750	870	977
10	531	690	734	857	975
15	505	673	725	849	973
20	481	652	712	837	969
30	426	595	673	805	960
40	356	532	616	763	947
50	275	456	531	699	909
60	191	356	410	588	802
70	110	223	247	395	567
80		80	82	150	243

* Halley's life tables (Breslau).
† From English life tables.

Because knowledge of sickness is so deficient, assessment of the improvement in health must be based chiefly on information about death; this is available for England and Wales since 1838, when births, deaths and cause of death were first registered nationally. In Sweden birth and death rates were recorded earlier, but cause of death was not included until the late nineteenth century.

National statistics leave no doubt that mortality declined rapidly, at least from about 1870. But they also suggest that a significant improvement in health had begun to take place at least a century earlier. This conclusion is based, not on the trend of mortality, which as we have seen was unknown before 1838, but on the growth of population, to which we must now turn our attention.

The population of England and Wales has apart from 1941 been recorded by a decennial census since 1801. There were two earlier estimates, however, one based on a count of families for the Doomsday Book in 1086, and the other on an estimate of the number of hearths in

1695. The growth of population since the eleventh century is shown in figure 2.1 which like many subsequent figures shows rates plotted against a logarithmic scale. When this technique is used, a straight line is shown as long as the rate of change is constant, and when the rate of change alters, the slope will alter. (This will be discussed again later in this Chapter). In the first 6 centuries despite the Black Death (or bubonic plague) of 1348 which may have reduced the population by as much as two-thirds, it appears to have rather more than trebled from 1½ million in 1086 to 5½ in 1695. The rate of increase then accelerated twice so that it had again trebled in the next 150 years (to 1851), more than doubled in the following 100 years (to 1951) and in 1981 was still increasing. Reasons

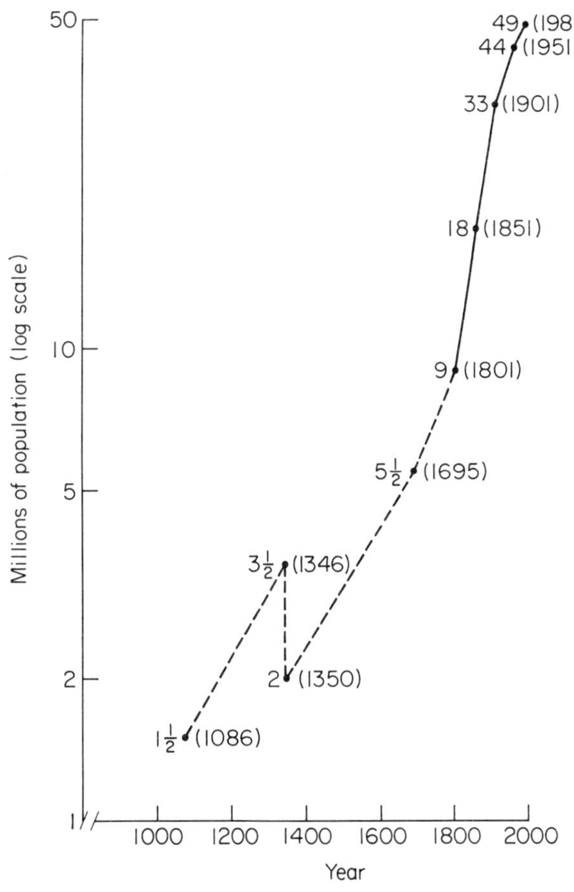

Figure 2.1. Growth of population of England and Wales. The fall in the middle of the fourteenth century is due to the Black Death. Figures in brackets denote dates.

will be given later for believing that this increase has resulted from a decline of mortality and that it is the most reliable indication of the period during which health in Britain improved significantly.

Finding explanations of the improvement presents very different problems before and after registration of death became mandatory. After 1838 it is possible to base conclusions on the trend of mortality and as time has gone on, to an increasing extent on the contribution of different causes of death to its decline. Before 1838 we must rely on judgement based on later experience about which we can be reasonably confident. For this reason we shall consider first the change in health since registration.

The Improvement of Health since Registration of Births and Deaths

Figure 2.2 gives in simplified form the levels of birth rate, death rate and population as we believe them to have been before registration, and as we know them to have been since. We are concerned here with the latter period.

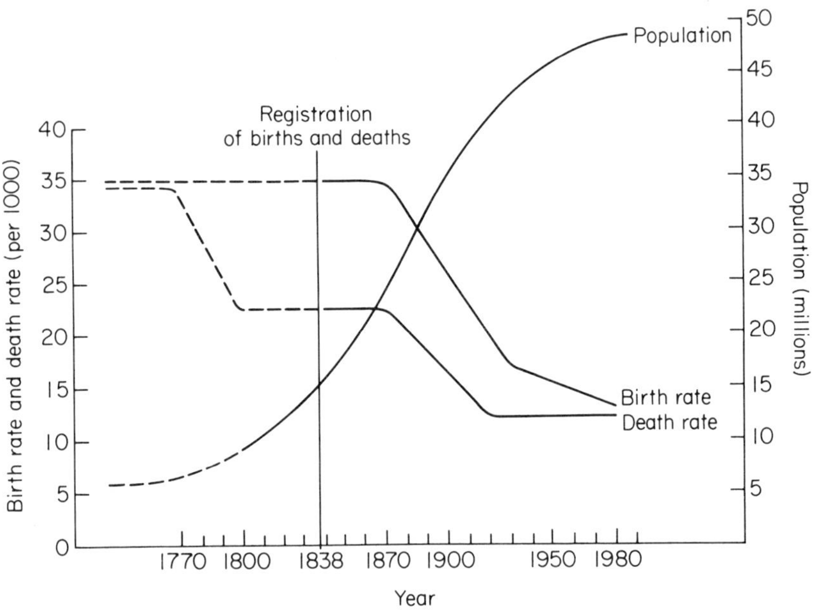

Figure 2.2. Population, birth rate and death rate: England and Wales.

The figure shows that mortality remained fairly constant between 1838 and 1870 and then began to decline. The continuous growth of population since 1838 is explained by the fact that an excess of births over deaths had been established by that date and has continued until recent years. A decline of the birth rate from about 1880 considerably reduced this excess, but because of the further reduction of mortality still has not eliminated it.

To explain the continued growth of population it is necessary to account for the reduction of mortality, and it seems clear that until 1950 this was almost entirely due to a decrease in deaths from infectious disease although over the past few decades migration (a problem with which we shall not be concerned here) has also had a role to play. Figure 2.3 shows clearly the separate death rates due to infectious and non-infectious causes. The latter undoubtedly include some deaths from infection (such as heart disease caused by rheumatic fever or syphilis) and this probably explains in part at least the slight reduction in mortality attributed to non-infectious causes in the nineteenth century.

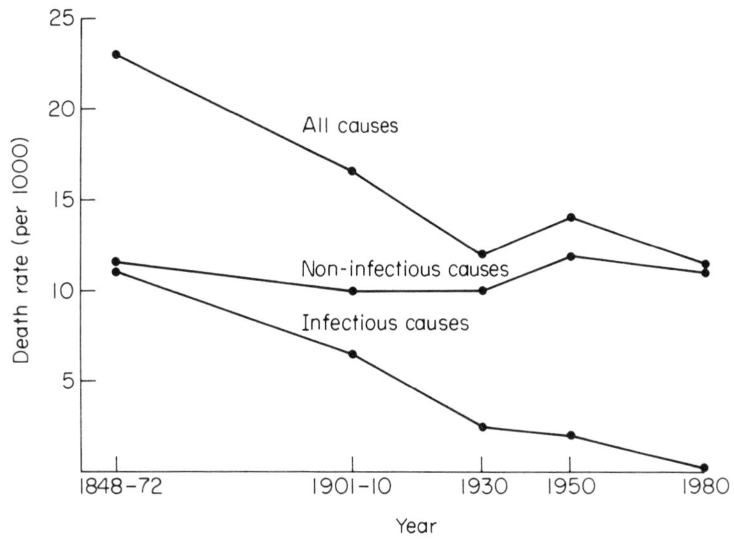

Figure 2.3. Mean annual death rate (males) in various categories: England and Wales.

For a closer examination of the diseases which contributed to the decline of mortality we shall consider first the period from 1838 to 1900.

Interpretation is more difficult in the twentieth century, when personal medical services were introduced and effective methods of preventing disease in the individual became available and then, mainly after 1935, of treating it.

1838–1900

Although cause of death was registered from 1838 procedures were not consistent until the mid century and our examination therefore begins at 1851. Table 2.2 compares mean annual mortality rates due to certain communicable diseases in the decades 1851-60 and 1891-1900. Five diseases or groups of diseases accounted almost entirely for the decline of mortality in this period: tuberculosis for nearly half; typhus, typhoid and continued fever for about a fifth; scarlet fever for a fifth; cholera, dysentery and diarrhoea for nearly a tenth; and smallpox for a twentieth. The explanation for the reduction of mortality from each of these diseases appears to be as follows.

Tuberculosis

Mortality from tuberculosis was falling in the fifth decade of the nineteenth century, at least 30 years earlier than in the case of the other major infections (figures 2.4 and 2.5). There is no reliable information

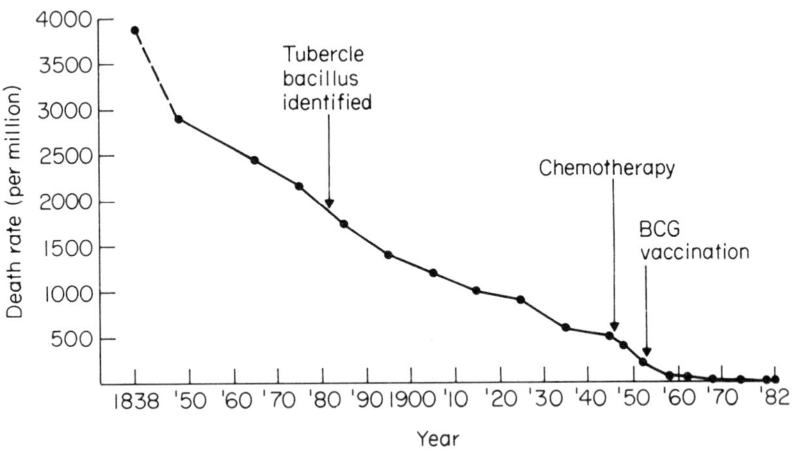

Figure 2.4. Respiratory tuberculosis—mean annual death rate: England and Wales. Arithmetic scale.

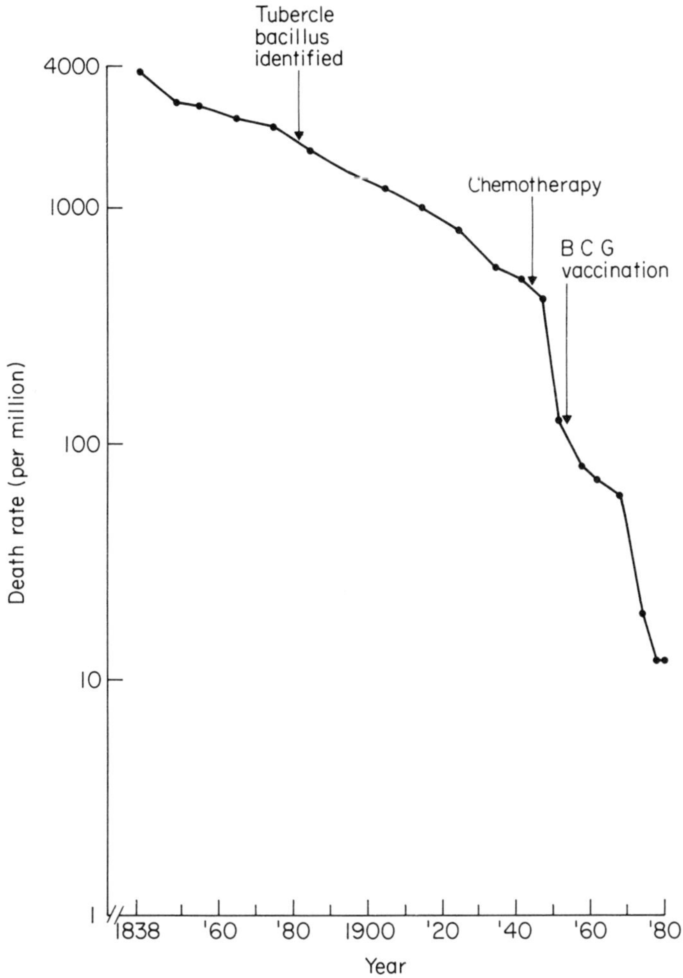

Figure 2.5. Respiratory tuberculosis—mean annual death rate: England and Wales. Logarithmic scale.

about its level or trend before registration, although there is no serious doubt that the disease was common in the previous three centuries. We have already seen the use of logarithms in the drawing of graphs concerned with time trends in figure 2.1. Figures 2.4 and 2.5 show the same mortality data presented in two different ways. In figure 2.4 the death rate for tuberculosis is plotted against an arithmetic scale which gives the impression of a rapid fall between 1838 and 1850, and subsequently a

Table 2.2. Mean annual mortality rates per million living (standardized*) due to certain communicable diseases in decennia 1851-60 and 1891-1900

Cause	1851-60 (a)	1891-1900 (b)	Difference (a − b)	Difference per cent of total difference $\frac{(a-b)\,100}{3{,}085}$
Tuberculosis—respiratory	2,772	1,418	1,354	43.9 } 47.2
Tuberculosis—other forms	706	603	103	3.3 }
Typhus, enteric fever, simple continued fever	891	184	707	22.9
Scarlet fever	779	152	627	20.3
Diarrhoea, dysentery, cholera	990	715	275	8.9
Smallpox	202	13	189	6.1
Whooping cough	433	363	70	2.3
Measles	357	398	−41	−1.3
Diphtheria	99	254	−155	−5.0
Other causes	13,980	14,024	−44	−1.4
Total	21,209	18,124	3,085	100

* Standardized to age and sex distribution of 1901 population.

steady one for the next century, tailing off over the last 25 years. The use of a logarithmic scale for mortality data in figure 2.5 gives a very different impression. Thus between 1838 and the end of the second world war when Waksman discovered streptomycin the rate of decline in mortality from tuberculosis had been constant, a fact which cannot reasonably be attributed to medical practice. Thereafter however, there has been an acceleration in the rate of fall of mortality rates which is not evident in the arithmetic plot shown in figure 2.4. Associations of this kind do not prove cause and effect, but they are helpful in examining the possible influences of scientific discoveries and procedures developed for prevention and cure.

It is useful to consider possible reasons for the decline of mortality from infectious disease under three headings.

1. Medical measures, that is the treatment of disease in the individual, and procedures provided to individuals for its prevention.
2. A 'spontaneous' change in the character of infectious disease, due to a shift in the balance between the virulence of an infective organism and the resistance of the host. The relationship between an infective organism and its host is a changing one, which reflects the influence on both of the genotype and its interaction with the environment. However the stability of this relationship differs greatly for different organisms; for example it is much more stable for the tubercle bacillus than for the haemolytic streptococcus.
3. Changes in the environment of man. Under this heading are included all environmental influences with the exception of medical measures (as defined in 1).

The interpretation of trends is always difficult. Nevertheless, although one must assume that Koch's demonstration that tuberculosis is spread by an infectious organism had some effect on death rates, figures 2.4 and 2.5 suggest that this was not dramatic in general, and that medical measures made little contribution to the course of tuberculosis before the twentieth century. In the case of an infectious disease it is never possible to be confident that there has been no change in the balance between the virulence of the organism and the resistance of the host, but there is little evidence of such variation in the tubercle bacillus in the period in which it has been observed. Man's resistance is a more difficult matter; but the fact that the population of Britain had been heavily exposed to the infection for many centuries makes it unlikely that genetic selection was the main reason for the favourable trend in the nineteenth century, since the effect of selection tends to be greatest at first exposure of a population.

Having argued that medical measures, modification of the organism, or of response to it, are not likely to be major influences, we are left with changes in the environment as probably the most important influence in determining the trend of mortality from tuberculosis in the nineteenth century.

The environment as it relates to disease will be considered in some detail in subsequent chapters. It is sufficient at this juncture to say that as far as the transmission of tuberculosis is concerned, the most important component of the environment is the society of man himself. The food people eat, the houses in which they live, the extent and equity with which goods are distributed and the way in which society is organized depends on the wealth, technical expertise and above all, the social values of the community or nation concerned. During the second part of the nineteenth century in Britain these were modified by a series of Parliamentary Acts. Among these the Factories Acts banned children from the industrial labour force and reduced to a controlled level the hours which men and women were allowed to work in industry (and consequently raised productivity) and the Public Health Acts laid down other aspects of environmental control. These together with reduction in overcrowding and improved housing are believed to have contributed significantly to the fall in the death rate from tuberculosis. Among other things which accompanied the increase in the standard of living was a general improvement in the diet.

Evidence in this respect is the increase in tuberculosis mortality in both World Wars which is most reasonably attributed to a deterioration of nutrition, a conclusion reached by Hart and Payling Wright in their study of tuberculosis and social conditions in England.

Typhus, enteric, and simple continued fever

Because they were not separated in national statistics before 1871, these diseases are grouped together. The data are given separately for the last three decades; in this period mortality from enteric fever was reduced by about half and mortality from the other two almost disappeared.

Interpretation of trends of typhus, a louse-borne disease, is complicated by the fact that its prevalence varied greatly at different periods, and it is impossible to say to what extent that was attributable to environmental change. Nevertheless, it is generally agreed that the disappearance of the disease from the British Isles, many years before identification of the body louse as the vector, was due largely to an improved standard of living. But although a good deal is now known about the nature of the disease and the way in which it is spread, it is still difficult to assess the relative importance of various aspects of the environment affected by the standard of living. It seems probable, however, that the two main influences were: improved hygienic standards, particularly in respect of water supply and personal cleanliness and the regular donning of new clothes, which prevented infection by reducing contact with the louse; and perhaps better diet, which affected the response to infection. The first of these influences would have begun to operate by about 1880 and the second somewhat earlier.

There is little difficulty in interpretation of the behaviour of typhoid fever. The spread of the disease is due to defective sanitary arrangements, and the rapid reduction of mortality during the last third of the nineteenth century can be attributed confidently to the specific measures, particularly safer water supplies, introduced at that time.

Scarlet fever

Views concerning interpretation of the decline of mortality from scarlet fever (figure 2.6) are probably more consistent than in the case of any other infectious disease. No specific measures of prevention or treatment were available in the nineteenth century, and the only possible explanations are environmental improvement or a change in the nature of the disease. Scarlet fever has exhibited cycles of severity followed by periods when the disease has taken a milder form. These changes have been attributed to variation in the virulence of the haemolytic streptococcus. Mortality trends shown in figure 2.6 provide support for this view. Since the mid-nineteenth century when data became available, although the general trend has been downwards, there have been three periods of a decade, one at the turn of the century, one from the end of the First World War through the nineteen-twenties, and the third at the end of the Second World War when this fall has been arrested. The figure also shows a relationship between the second of these and the introduction first of sulphonamides and then penicillin. Although over 10,000 cases are notified annually, the disease is rarely serious in Britain today and causes

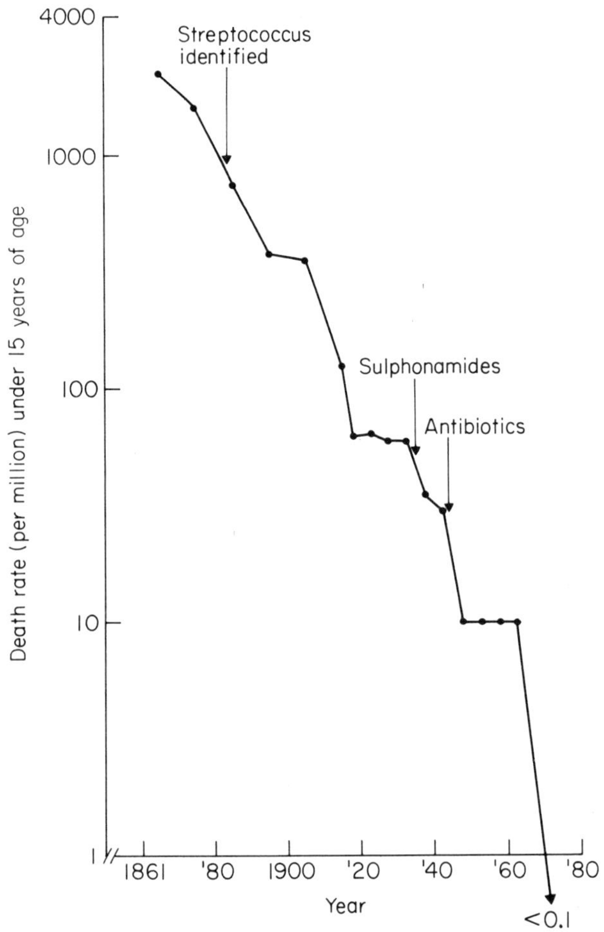

Figure 2.6. Scarlet fever—mean annual death rate in children under 15: England and Wales. Logarithmic scale.

less than half a dozen deaths a year. Like *Mycobacterium tuberculosis*, the haemolytic streptococcus is usually transmitted by droplet infection so that reduction in overcrowding also had a part to play in reducing spread, as did improved nutrition in increasing resistance.

Cholera, dysentery, and diarrhoea

These infections were grouped together in national statistics before 1871, but severe epidemics of cholera can nevertheless be distinguished in the records because of their abruptness and high case of fatality rate. Unlike diarrhoea and dysentery, cholera was never endemic in the British Isles, and was introduced from abroad at least 5 times during the nineteenth century, but apparently not before. It is therefore not possible to speak of the reasons for its disappearance with quite the same confidence as in the case of the other causes of death.

But with this reservation, there is little doubt about the main reasons for the rapid reduction of mortality from bowel infections in the late nineteenth century. These diseases are spread by water infected from sewage, or contaminated food, and their decline began in the 1870s when substantial improvements were made in hygienic conditions. There are no grounds for thinking that either therapy or (with a possible reservation in the case of cholera) modification of the nature of the disease made any impact. The reduction of mortality may therefore be attributed to the decline of intestinal infection resulting from improved hygiene which in turn was a consequence of social action through legislation. For the same reason mortality from typhoid, which was grouped with typhus, fell.

Smallpox

Since the contribution of smallpox to the reduction of mortality in this period was small, the reasons for it are less important in the interpretation of the causes of the total decline. This is a disease in which a specific medical measure—vaccination—appears to have made control possible. The fact that smallpox, prevalent for several centuries, declined rapidly from the time when vaccination was introduced suggested that this was probably the main reason for its decline, and the subsequent successful campaign by the World Health Organization to use this method for eliminating it from all countries has borne this out.

Let us now summarize our conclusions. In order of their relative importance the influences responsible for the decline of mortality in the second half of the nineteenth century were (1) a rising standard of living, of which the most significant features were probably improved diet and reduction of overcrowding, responsible mainly for the decline of tuberculosis and perhaps sequelae of streptococcal infections, (2) the hygienic changes introduced by sanitary reformers which insured that drinking water was not contaminated by sewage and so brought about the decline of typhoid, cholera, dysentery, and diarrhoea, and (3) changes in the virulence of the infectious agent which may have accounted for the decline of mortality from scarlet fever and some other conditions. The effect of specific medical measures was restricted to smallpox but did not greatly effect the total death rate.

Since 1900

Twentieth century data show that the continued decline of the death rate after 1900 continued mainly to be due to a decrease in deaths from infectious disease. Between 1901 and 1947 the age adjusted mortality rate from all causes fell by a half. Nearly a third of this reduction was due to a decrease of mortality from a group of diseases traditionally recognized as infectious fevers, including measles, scarlet fever, whooping cough, smallpox and diphtheria, tuberculosis, typhoid, paratyphoid, dysentery, influenza and syphilis. A further third of the reduction was due to lower mortality from certain groups of diseases which may also be regarded as infectious, since they are caused mainly by pathogenic microorganisms communicable from person to person. These include diarrhoea and enteritis, convulsions in infancy (usually associated with infection) and the respiratory infections, bronchitis and pneumonia. Although bronchitis in the elderly may in some cases be due primarily to causes other than infections, pathogenic organisms usually contribute significantly to the progress of the disease.

On this evidence, about two-thirds of the reduction in mortality during the first half of the century is attributable to the decline of deaths from infectious disease. Moreover this is probably an underestimate of their contribution, because several other diseases (such as rheumatic heart disease and nephritis) are sequelae to infections.

A most striking feature of the trend of mortality since 1900 has been the decline of infant mortality, that is, of children alive at birth but dying during the first year of life (figure 2.7). It was remarkable that despite the improvements referred to above during the second half of the nineteenth century this age group was not affected and at the turn of the century about 150 of every 1,000 children born alive in England and Wales still died within a year of birth. Reasons for this can only be conjectural, but one must assume that changes in the microenvironment of the new born baby did not change as rapidly as those of older children and adults. The traditions of mothercraft with their bearing on feeding, health and sani-

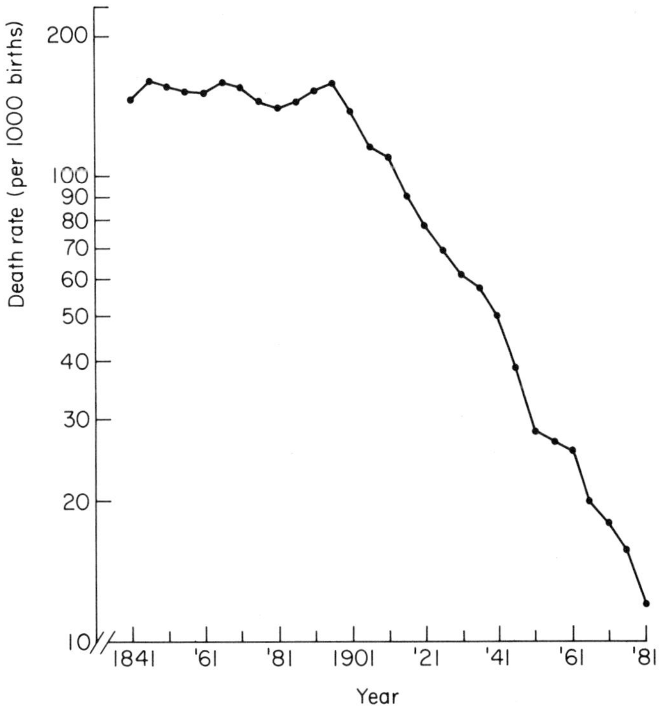

Figure 2.7. Infant mortality rate: England and Wales. Logarithmic scale.

tary practices strike deep into culture and it was generally accepted, if not expected, that as many as half of the numerous babies born into a family would die in early childhood. Fifty years later infant mortality was reduced to 30, and it is now 12. As the figure shows, the rate of decline has in general accelerated since the Second World War.

Assessment of reasons for the decline of infant mortality during the twentieth century (and still more of mortality at all ages), would require a close investigation of different causes of death. Several developments have made this task more complicated than it was in the nineteenth century. In the first place there has been a great extension of medical and related social services. The personal medical services concerned with maternity and child welfare and school health were developed progressively from 1906. The relative importance of the varied measures—cheap and safe scientifically constituted infant foods, routine examination of children, advice about health and treatment—embraced by these services is still uncertain, but there can be little doubt that together they have contributed significantly to the saving of infant and child life. Over the same period the standard of living continued to rise and was supported by social services. Further advances were made in the control of the environment, launched effectively in the second half of the nineteenth century. And, finally, specific measures for preventing and treating disease in the individual began to fulfil the promise of clinical medicine.

There is indeed some justification for the view that without a much more careful investigation it is impossible to express any worthwhile opinion about the relative importance of the influences that have contributed to the improvement in health during the twentieth century. The problem is less difficult if we consider the period since 1838 as a whole. A substantial part of the total reduction of mortality occurred during the nineteenth century, and we are on firm ground in attributing it to the rising standard of living and to the implementation through the law of measures derived from medico-scientific research leading to improved hygiene. They have continued to advance since 1900, and unquestionably have contributed powerfully to the further improvement of health since that time. The value of the personal health services, and of the specific therapies which have been notably enhanced over the past 40 years, cannot be denied. However the main influences responsible for the decline of mortality—our best index of improved health—since deaths were first registered in 1838 have been, first social, a rising standard of living and improved hygiene, and second, specific preventive and therapeutic measures.

The Improvement of Health Before Registration of Births and Deaths

We must now consider the more difficult problem of interpretation in the period before 1838 when the national birth rate, death rate and causes of death were unknown. It is one of the ironies of history that the improvement in health appears to have begun at least 70 years before reliable data are available to put the reasons for it beyond dispute.

As figure 2.1 indicates, from the nadir of the mid-fourteenth century when a stricken population was recovering from the Black Death—and its size then is a matter of considerable conjecture—the rate of increase has been exponential, but so far as can be determined from available figures was at its most rapid during the nineteenth century and has been decelerating throughout this century.

Various explanations have been put forward for the prolonged increase in population size. One is a decline in mortality. Some economic historians suggest that, at least in the late eighteenth and nineteenth centuries, there was an increase in the birth rate. They believe that the economic and social changes associated with the Industrial Revolution led to earlier marriage, a rising birth rate and larger families. Whether or not age at marriage changed, decreasing mortality in populations living a marginal existence would be accompanied by an increasing expectation of life and with it an increase in the fertile period of life. No doubt this was important during the centuries following the Black Death, but its importance will have diminished as the modal expectation of life of women came to exceed the age of the menopause.

Reasons for the decline of the death rate can be discussed under three headings: medical measures (prevention or treatment of disease in the individual); a 'spontaneous' decline of mortality; and improvement in the environment.

Medical measures

Until recently the decline of mortality in the eighteenth century was believed to be due to medical advances, the explanation proposed by Griffith in his book *Population Problems of the Age of Malthus.* He based this conclusion on medical developments at that time: they included expansion of hospital, dispensary and midwifery services; changes in medical education; and advances in physiology and morbid anatomy.

Serious objections have now been raised to Griffith's interpretation on the grounds that the medical measures then available are very unlikely to have had a significant effect on national mortality trends. Indeed since they had little influence in the second half of the nineteenth century, it would seem reasonable to assume that they were no more effective a hundred years earlier, when knowledge of disease processes was even more incomplete. Nevertheless it has been suggested that there was a measure which might have been important namely inoculation by infected material as a protection against smallpox, this was variolation, first used on the Royal children in 1722, and then vaccination a procedure introduced by Edward Jenner in 1796. This measure gained popularity so rapidly that it is difficult to believe that it did not have an influence, albeit, perhaps, a small one, on the death rate. There are however no grounds for thinking that any other medical measure made a significant contribution to its reduction in the eighteenth century.

A spontaneous decline of mortality

If medical measures are excluded there remain two possible explanations for the eighteenth century reduction of the death rate, a spontaneous decline of mortality from infections and changes in the environment. In the post-registration period, it was possible to identify the diseases which contributed to the decline of mortality and then to consider each disease separately. The same procedure cannot be used before 1838, and we must rely on our judgement, assisted by knowledge derived from the nineteenth and twentieth centuries.

As we have seen the relation between infectious organisms and their hosts is variable, and over any considerable period deaths from some infections would be expected to increase and from others to decrease or remain relatively constant. It is therefore quite possible that mortality from one or more infections may have declined spontaneously (that is without recognized medical or other intervention) in the eighteenth century, as in the example of scarlet fever at a later period. However the question is whether this explanation can be accepted for the large reduction of mortality and rise of population which occurred before 1838.

While spontaneous fluctuation of deaths from infections may have influenced the death rate over short periods in the eighteenth century, it is unlikely to have contributed substantially to the large decline of mortality and steady growth of population which occurred between 1700 and 1838.

Improvement in the environment

The conclusion that neither specific medical measures nor a spontaneous decline of infectious diseases accounts to any great extent for the decline of mortality and expansion of population in the eighteenth and early nineteenth centuries makes it necessary to consider the third possibility, that there was a significant improvement in the environment. We can be fairly confident that it was not in hygienic conditions, which if they changed, probably changed for the worse with industrialization and the growth of towns in the early nineteenth century, and can hardly have improved substantially before the passing of the 1848 Public Health Act, and probably not before the eighth decade, when mortality from intestinal infections began to decline.

There is however an important feature of the environment in respect of which there is impressive evidence of improvement, namely food supplies. Food production in England and Wales increased greatly during the eighteenth and nineteenth centuries; it was sufficient, at times more than sufficient, to feed the rapidly expanding population and it was not until the later part of this period that it was supplemented significantly by imported food. This improvement resulted from advances in agriculture which spread throughout Europe from the end of the seventeenth century. Initially these changes were not of a technological kind; they comprised essentially an extension of traditional methods such as conservation of fertility, enclosure, crop rotation, winter feeding and extension of land under cultivation. These measures, with the introduction of root crops and improved transport, brought about a change from exploitive to productive agriculture, and it was not until the nineteenth century that they were supported to any extent by chemical and other technological methods.

Thus an increase in food supplies may have been the main reason for the decline of mortality and growth of population before the mid nineteenth century. Such a conclusion rests on three considerations: first, that other possible explanations are found inadequate; second, that there was undoubtedly a great increase in home grown food; and third, that in the circumstances which existed prior to the Agricultural Revolution, an improvement in food supplies was a necessary condition for a substantial and prolonged expansion of population. The basis for the last point is a belief that prior to the eighteenth century the growth of population would have been restricted by a high level of mortality attributable to insufficient food.

This is essentially the interpretation of Malthus who in 1789 published his *Essay on the Principle of Population.* His main thesis was that food production can never keep pace with natural fertility so that population growth is inevitably checked by famine and epidemic disease: 'The power of the population is so superior to the power in the earth to produce subsistence for man, that premature death must in some shape or other visit the human race. The vices of mankind are active and able ministers of depopulation. They are the precursors in the great army of destruction and often finish the dreadful work themselves. But should they fail in this war of extermination, sickly seasons, epidemics, pestilence and plague advance in terrific array. Should success be incomplete, gigantic inevitable famine stalks in the rear, and with one almighty blow levels the population with the food of the world.'

Since Malthus's time there has been a five-fold increase in the population of England and Wales and standard of living has much more than kept pace with the increase. The disasters he predicted have not occurred because our production of machine-made goods made it possible to buy enough food from abroad to meet the needs of an expanding population. But the Malthusian principle remains valid. In India about 25 million died of famine in the last quarter of the nineteenth century the equivalent of the total population of England and Wales at that time, and 5 million died in the disastrous Bengal famine in 1945.

Reasons for Improvement in Health

It is now possible to bring together our views concerning the modern improvement in health. It probably began in the eighteenth century and was reflected in a decline of mortality which has continued, with interruptions, until the present time.

A moving force was an increase in food supplies which resulted from the Agricultural Revolution that spread throughout Europe after 1700. From about 1870 this influence was powerfully supported by improved hygiene, particularly in respect of water supplies, and sewage disposal; and at the turn of the century there was additional support from applications of the discovery of bacteria used in antisepsis, and the development of immunization. And in the twentieth century, further advance followed the introduction of therapeutic measures, mainly after 1935, the year when the sulphonamides were first used.

Together these influences were responsible for an acceleration in the expansion of population. But in time, and on an evolutionary scale a fairly short time, the advance in health would have been reversed, as other advances during man's history were reversed, by expanding numbers, if birth rates had not also declined. In England and Wales for example, if the birth rate had remained at its eighteenth century level, the population today would be nearly three times as great, with profound consequences for welfare and health. From a historical viewpoint, therefore, the limitation of population growth by control of family size was an indispensable condition for improvement, without which all other influences would in time have become ineffective.

This interpretation of the modern advance in health and rise and eventual control of population puts the emphasis on the following: increased food supplies from the early eighteenth century; limitation of numbers and removal of adverse influences in the environment by improved hygiene from the late nineteenth century; and specific medical measures (immunization, therapy and surgery) from the second quarter of the twentieth century. The improvement in human health was largely due to a change in reproductive behaviour and to modification of the environment by provision of food and protection from physical hazards. It should however be noted that two of the major influences were not introduced in order to improve health; the reasons for increasing food supplies and limiting numbers were only indirectly related to this objective.

But while the contribution of specific medical measures attributable to medical science and technology was relatively small, the contribution of science and technology as a whole was large. It is hard to judge how much the initial and very considerable increase in food supplies in the eighteenth century owed to science and technology. But from the nineteenth century the improvements were advanced further by scientific agriculture and by the rising standard of living which resulted from the Industrial Revolution. It is unlikely that scientific methods played any considerable part in birth control in the late nineteenth and early twentieth centuries, the advances in understanding which led people to limit the size of their families were closely related to the rising standard of living. And finally, although hygienic measures were introduced without knowledge of microorganisms, the control of communicable disease was greatly extended by the developments in microbiology which followed the work of Pasteur and Koch.

Hence, while the major influences responsible for the modern improvement in health were not due initially to science and technology, they were all subsequently indebted to science. Science extended the relatively simple methods which led to the first advances in agriculture, in hygiene and in birth control. It also provided a basis of understanding which ensured that the advances were not lost, as others (for example Roman hygiene) had been lost at earlier periods of man's history.

Further Reading

Burnet M. (1953) *Natural History of Infectious Disease.* Cambridge University Press, Cambridge.

Creighton C. (1965) *A History of Epidemics in Britain*. Frank Cass & Co. Ltd., London.

D'Arcy Hart P. and Payling Wright G. (1939) *Tuberculosis and Social Conditions in England*. National Association for the Prevention of Tuberculosis, London.

Glass D. V. and Eversley D. E. C. (eds.) (1965) *Population in History*. Edward Arnold Ltd., London.

Greenwood M. (1935) *Epidemics and Crowd Diseases*. Williams and Norgate, London.

Griffith G. T. (1967) *Population Problems of the Age of Malthus*, 2nd edition. Frank Cass & Co. Ltd., London.

McKeown T., Brown R. G. and Record R. G. (1972) An interpretation of the modern rise of population in Europe. *Population Studies*. **XXVII**, 345.

Malthus T. R. (1960) *Essay on the Principle of Population*. Everyman's Library, J. M. Dent & Sons Ltd., London.

3

Effect of the Decline of the Death Rate on Medical Problems

Consequences of Improved Health

Introduction

Since the time of Kepler and Harvey medical thought has been dominated by the belief that improvements in health must rely largely on an engineering analysis, based on understanding the structure and function of the body and of the relationship of these to disease processes. This approach was derived from a physical model, in which a living organism was conceived in mechanical terms. If its structure and function were fully understood it might be taken apart and reassembled. In medicine this concept led to the belief that an understanding of disease processes and of the body's response to them would make it possible to intervene therapeutically, mainly by surgical, chemical or technological methods such as irradiation or the laser.

The consequences of this view of the medical task are far more conspicuous in medicine today than they were in the seventeenth century, largely because the resources of the physical and chemical sciences are so much greater. Medical education begins with the study of the structure and function of the body, continues with examination of disease processes and ends with clinical instruction on highly selected sick people; medical service and education are dominated by the image of the acute hospital where the technological resources are concentrated; and medical science reflects the mechanistic concept, for example in the attention given to the molecular basis of inheritance and the immunological response to transplanted organs. Thus the question is not whether the engineering approach is predominant in medicine, which would hardly be disputed, but whether it is deficient as a conceptualization of the problems of human health.

Our examination in Chapter 2 of reasons for past improvement in health suggests that the traditional conceptualization is in fact deficient. We concluded that the major contributions to the improvement were social in origin such as limitation of family size, improved agricultural methods leading to an increase in food supplies and the introduction of legislation to improve water supply and sewage, and so create a healthier physical environment. The contribution of specific preventive and therapeutic measures is relatively recent.

This conclusion is in accord with experience of requirements for the health of living things other than man. In domestication of animals, their numbers and distribution are controlled; they are provided with more and better food; and they are protected so far as possible from environmental hazards, including parasites, predators and extremes of weather. Hence improvements in livestock, like improvements in the health of man, have resulted primarily from measures directed to populations rather than to individuals.

However, in technologically advanced countries the advances of the past two centuries have inevitably had a profound effect on the character of medical problems and it is conceivable that the major influences on health may no longer be the same. The common causes of sickness, disability and death have changed, primarily in response to the influences considered in Chapter 1, but also as a secondary consequence of a different age distribution of the population.

Changes in causes of sickness and death

The predominant influence has been the decline of mortality from infectious disease; some diseases such as tuberculosis and typhoid are now much less common, while for example smallpox and the bubonic plague have virtually disappeared. This decline made certain conditions relatively more prominent for example congenital malformations although their incidence was no greater than in the past.

The effects of the reduction of deaths from infections have been profound, and it is questionable whether we shall ever again see a change for the better in the spectrum of disease and disability as great as that which has occurred in the past century. Indeed the twentieth century may come to be recognized as a watershed, separating the infectious diseases which were formerly predominant from the residual problems when infections are reduced to small proportions.

We have been able to consolidate the discoveries of the nineteenth century by providing primary protection. With important exceptions such as some forms of respiratory disease, and some cancers, primary protection has little to offer in the solution of these residual problems. Instead we must depend on secondary protection, which in its nature is much less easy to implement and in any event less efficient.

The change in age distribution

The age distribution of the populations of developed countries has changed in response to two influences, the trend of mortality within age groups and, to a lesser extent, the decline of the birth rate. Figure 3.1 compares the age distribution of the population of England and Wales in 1981 with that in 1841.

(a) *The trend of mortality within age groups*

Since deaths from infectious disease were most common in early life, the trend of mortality during the past century has been different at different ages. In 1980 the death rate was 53.6 per cent of that in 1841-50 (table

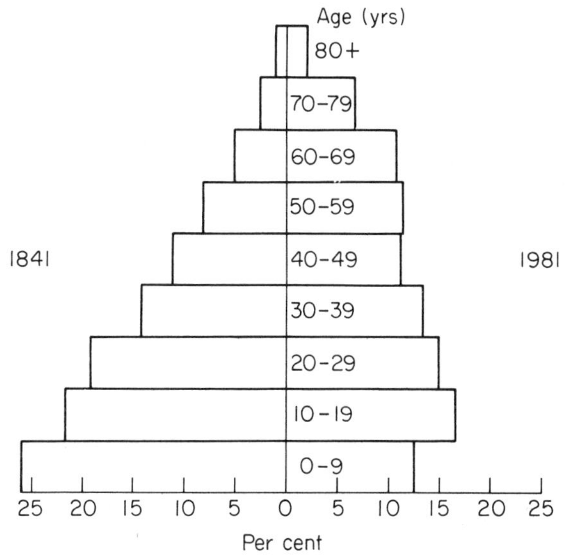

Figure 3.1. Age distribution of the population of England and Wales in 1841 and 1981.

3.1). The reduction was very great in early life, substantial in middle life and moderate in late life.

Table 3.1. Change in death rates between 1841-50 and 1980 (England and Wales)

Age	1980 rate as percentage of 1841-50 rate
0	8.0
1-4	Not known
5-14	1.4
15-44	7.2
45-64	40.9
65 and over	65.9
All ages (crude)	53.6

(b) *The decline of the birth rate*

The birth rate has declined (from 35.5 per 1,000 population in 1871-75 to 13.3 in 1980), and at first sight it might appear that this influence also would have contributed to the higher age of the present day population. However, it is the change in the number of births rather than in the birth rate which affects age distribution, and since the annual number of births is approximately the same in England and Wales today as in the middle of the last century, it is unlikely to have had much influence on the difference in the age distributions of the population shown in figure 3.1. Pre-natal death rates and death rates in early life do.

The various categories of pre-natal death have all been changing as table 3.2 shows; however, the frequency of legal terminations of pregnancy has risen rapidly since the grounds for it were liberalized in 1968. In 1970, 84,000 were reported, giving a rate of 70 per 1,000 conceptions; a decade later the number reported had increased by more than half to become 130,000 and the rate per 1,000 conceptions had risen to 140. Over the past 50 years, and almost certainly for much longer, the stillbirth rate has been falling. It was recorded in 1928 when it was 40 per thousand total births; by 1970 when there were 10,340 stillbirths, the rate had quartered, and a decade later in 1980 that number had been more than halved to 4,800, giving an estimated rate of 5 per 1,000 conceptions. The estimates of illegal abortions are the least reliable since even today their number is unknown, and the rates of 50 for 1838-54 and of 10 and 5 for recent times are merely guesses. The estimated rates indicate clearly however that the increase in the prenatal death rate is due to the increase in legal termination of pregnancy. A few of these can be attributed to terminations because of the diagnosis of congenital malformations early in pregnancy, or exposure of the fetus to a teratological influence such as rubella virus, but the vast majority will have been performed because of the risks to the mothers' physical and psychological health.

On these estimates, the proportion of conceptions which terminate prenatally is now of the order of 30 per cent. So far as can be judged from the limited data, this proportion did not appear to have altered substantially from the mid nineteenth century until 10 or 15 years ago but subsequently has been rising. In summary, therefore, since the changes in the abortion law in 1968 there has been a rapid increase in legal terminations, a fall in the number of stillbirths and, almost certainly, as we have seen, a decrease in illegal terminations.

Table 3.2. Estimates of prenatal deaths in 1838-54, 1970 and 1980

	Deaths per 1,000 conceptions		
	1838-54	1970	1980
Spontaneous abortions	140	140	140
Legal terminations of pregnancy	nil	70	140
Illegal terminations of pregnancy	50	10	5
Stilbirths	40	10	5
Total	230	230	290

At the present time different countries are at very different stages of the so-called demographic cycle. They can be grouped into five broad categories according to their mortality and natality experience.

(a) Countries in which both birth rate and death rate are still high and malnutrition and infectious disease remain the leading causes of death (parts of Africa, South East Asia and Latin America).

(b) Countries in which the birth rate is still high but the death rate is now falling (India and parts of Latin America).

(c) Countries in which the birth rate is declining and the death rate is falling very rapidly (Ceylon, Taiwan and Mauritius).

(d) China where the birth rate is declining very rapidly and the death rate, having also fallen rapidly for 30 years is continuing to do so.
(e) Countries in which both birth rate and death rate are low, cardiovascular and malignant disease are the leading causes of death and infection is no longer important (the countries of Northern Europe, North America, Japan, and parts of Latin America).

With the exception of Japan, as the countries in the last category passed through the preceding phases of the demographic cycle, their progression from high to low mortality occurred over 2 centuries. Many countries of the world are now crowding this experience into 2 generations. As we have seen in Britain the fall in mortality was well under way before public environmental and personal health services were introduced and long before the advent of effective and specific prevention and treatment of the major infections. The accumulated knowledge and experience of the western world is being applied to less developed countries with dramatic results. For example, the crude mortality rate in Japan immediately before the war was 17.4 per thousand (the level of mortality in England and Wales in the last decade of the nineteenth century); by 1970 it had fallen to 6.9 (in the same year the mortality of our much older population was 11.7). In China it was 20 in 1949 and 7 in 1981.

Problems at Different Ages

Birth to age 14

The very large reduction of mortality in the prereproductive age group since 1838-54 (table 3.1) is as we have seen attributable predominantly to a decline in deaths from infectious disease. This decline has occurred throughout childhood, but was most marked in the first year of life when mortality was formerly greatest. The infant mortality rate (number of deaths under 1 year per thousand liveborn children) fell from 150 in 1901 to 12 in 1980.

The decline of infections has increased the relative importance of some other causes of death which in the same period have shown little or no improvement; it has also altered the balance between deaths due to prenatal and postnatal causes. Table 3.3 gives for 1980 perinatal death rates by cause. It should be noted that more than half of infant deaths now occur within a week of birth, and because the common causes of

Table 3.3. Perinatal mortality rates (per 1,000 live and stillbirths) and infant mortality rates (per 1,000 live births) by cause (England and Wales 1980)

ICD No and Cause of death		Perinatal mortality rate	Infant mortality rate
ICD 740-759 Congenital anomalies		2.9	3.2
ICD 761-763 Obstetric complications affecting fetus or newborn		3.8	0.45
ICD 769 Respiratory distress syndrome		1.1	1.2
ICD E800-E899 Accidents and violence		0.05	0.3
ICD 320-322 Meningitis		0.17	0.1
ICD 480-486 Pneumonia		0.39	0.7
All causes:	Males	14.22	13.31
	Females	12.41	10.70

stillbirths and early postnatal deaths are the same the concept of the *perinatal death rate*—the number of stillbirths and deaths in the first week after birth expressed per 1,000 total births—has been introduced. Perinatal deaths are due to influences operating before (mainly) or during birth, and as table 3.3 shows obstetric factors are now the commonest cause of perinatal deaths, and congenital anomalies the commonest cause of infant mortality. In 1980 infectious diseases only caused 7 per cent of infant deaths; not only is this in contrast with the past in England and Wales, but also with developing countries today where infections, particularly diarrhoea and respiratory disease, cause over 95 per cent of infant deaths.

Table 3.4 analyses deaths between the end of the first year and age 14. In this period mortality is low and the most common causes of death—formerly the infections—are now accidents and violence and neoplasms. It should be noted that table 3.4 gives annual death rates per 1,000 living; that is to say it gives the risk of dying in a single year for all those in the age group. For an individual aged 1 year the risks of death before the 15th birthday would therefore be roughly 14 times greater than those estimated in table 3.4.

Our conclusions concerning mortality between conception and age 14 can be summarized as follows. There are approximately 305 deaths per 1,000 conceptions in this age period, of which about 285 are abortions, 5 are stillbirths and 15 deaths between birth and age 14. Of the latter, about 8 occur within the first week after delivery.

Table 3.4. Annual age specific death rates (per 1,000 living) from principal causes (England and Wales 1980)

Age 1-14 years			Age 15-44 years		
Accidents and violence	0.09		Accidents and violence	0.35	
Neoplasms	0.05		Neoplasms	0.25	
Congenital malformations	0.04		Ischaemic heart disease	0.11	
Respiratory infections	0.03		Cerebrovascular disease	0.04	0.19
Other infectious diseases	0.01		Other circulatory diseases	0.04	
Other causes	0.07		Respiratory infections	0.03	
			Other infectious diseases	0.01	
			Other causes	0.16	
All causes	0.29		All causes	0.99	

Age 45-64 years			Age 65 years and over		
Ischaemic heart disease	3.00		Ischaemic heart disease	16.05	
Cerebrovascular disease	0.49	4.27	Cerebrovascular disease	8.54	32.22
Other circulatory diseases	0.78		Other circulatory diseases	7.63	
Neoplasms	3.35		Neoplasms	11.88	
Respiratory infections	0.27		Respiratory infections	6.38	
Other infectious diseases	0.05		Other infectious diseases	0.14	
Accidents and violence	0.67		Accidents and violence	1.06	
Other causes	1.11		Other causes	8.52	
All causes	9.72			60.20	

To complete assessment of the medical problems in the prenatal and prereproductive periods we must consider handicaps and sickness in childhood. There are no means of assessing fully the extent of either of these problems but numbers of children in special schools provide an indication of the frequency of severe handicap. In England and Wales approximately 10 per 1,000 school children are so handicapped that they require special teaching. The commonest types of handicap are educational subnormality (which accounts for more than half of the total), limitations of sight and hearing and a variety of other physical abnormalities due to conditions such as congenital malformations, cerebral palsy and infectious disease. Handicaps due to infections are now much less common than formerly; but there is no evidence of a significant reduction in the incidence of congenital handicaps such as mental handicap, which now account for a large majority of those affected. But the prevalence of these conditions in the population has increased because the proportion of handicapped people who survive to maturity and even to late ages is today much greater than formerly, more as a result of an improved standard of living and better hygiene, rather than because of direct medical intervention. It follows that the problems of congenital handicap are no longer mainly restricted to childhood; indeed the majority of those living with the commonest abnormality—mental handicap—are adults.

It is even more difficult to assess accurately the frequency and causes of sickness in childhood. A steady decrease in the demand for paediatric hospital beds suggests that in parallel with the decline of mortality there has been a reduction of morbidity from infections due in part to a fall in incidence but also to the availability of effective antibiotics. Nevertheless infectious disease in childhood remains a considerable problem and is the most common reason for consulting a general practitioner about the health of children. There are also large problems associated with non-fatal accidents and violence. However, a considerable part of the problem of sickness, particularly serious sickness, like the problems of handicap and death, has been determined by the time of birth, and is associated with causes such as malformations, immaturity and birth trauma.

Apart from the reference to mental subnormality, this discussion of problems in early life has been restricted to physical causes of mortality and disability. There are other problems. For instance mental illness also presents in all age groups, and since these can be considered more meaningfully together, they will be discussed at the end of this section. Finally society is expressing concern about physical abuse of small children by their parents, but no accurate statistics of morbidity or mortality from this cause are available.

Ages 15–44

Mortality in the age group 15-44 has fallen sharply and is now less than one-tenth of the level in 1841-50 (table 3.1). As in the younger age group, the improvement has been due to a reduction of deaths from infectious disease. A hundred years ago tuberculosis was the most common cause of death and infections were responsible for more than half of the mortality. Today the common causes of death are accidents and violence, neoplasms and cardiovascular disease (table 3.4). Together these causes account for three-quarters of the total mortality while infectious diseases are responsible for only about one-tenth.

Since ages 15-44 represent approximately the reproductive age group we must refer briefly to death of women in childbirth. From the beginning of this century maternal mortality remained fairly constant until 1934, since when it has declined from 4.6 deaths per 1,000 total births to 0.12 in 1979. This change was due largely to the control of puerperal infections by chemotherapy and the effective use of blood transfusion. Nevertheless there is little doubt that a considerable proportion of the maternal deaths that remain—a recent investigation suggested about one-third—are potentially avoidable.

Ages 45-64

Between 1841-50 and 1980 mortality at ages 45-64 declined by over half (table 3.1). This again is accounted for mainly by the behaviour of the infections: in 1848-72 the death rate attributed to the specified infectious diseases of which the most common were tuberculosis and pneumonia was 8.0 of a total death rate of 22.3 per 1,000; in 1980 it was 1.1 of a total of 11.8. Because of the vagaries of the earlier classification it is difficult to interpret the trends of other causes of death, but cancer appears to have increased in frequency and cerebrovascular disease has decreased.

The common causes of death at ages 45-64 are now those shown in table 3.4. The most important in order of frequency are neoplasms, ischaemic heart disease, accidents and violence, cerebrovascular disease, and respiratory infections (especially bronchitis). In this age group the so-called degenerative diseases begin to predominate.

It is again difficult to assess fully the extent of sickness and disability. Before age 65, indeed before 69, the disabilities commonly associated with ageing—defects of hearing, vision, mobility, etc.—are relatively uncommon. The usual causes of short term sickness and disability are accidents, respiratory infection and some musculoskeletal conditions; and of prolonged disability they are bronchitis, mental illness and arthritis.

Ages 65 and over

For those aged 65 and over, mortality has declined since 1841-50 by about a third (table 3.1). In this age group, because of the unsatisfactory classification of causes of death in earlier times, it is difficult to speak confidently about reasons for this change. (What should perhaps be noted at this point is that the relation between the decrease in death rates shown in table 3.2 and the increase in expectation of life over the same period is deceptive. For example, between 1838-54 and 1970 expectation of life of males increased by 12.5 years at age 15, 4.4 at age 45 and 1.2 at age 65. These increases are smaller than might have been expected in view of the substantial reduction of mortality in the corresponding age groups.)

The common causes of death at 65 and over (table 3.4) are the same as in the previous age group although their order of importance is a little different, ischaemic heart disease and neoplasms rank first and second, but cerebrovascular disease ranks third. The common illnesses which bring patients to general practitioners are arthritis and rheumatism, respiratory disease (especially chronic bronchitis), accidents and cardiovascular disease. From age 69 the frequency of physical and mental disabilities increases rapidly and a large proportion of hospital beds is occupied by the aged who are either physically or mentally ill.

Mental illness

Assessment of the problems associated with mental illness encounters the familiar difficulties of recording accurately and meaningfully conditions which cause sickness and disability rather than death and these are exacerbated by lack of agreement about the nature and application of diagnostic criteria. There are no data which make it possible to examine experience of mental illness over a prolonged period, and for recent years conclusions must be based mainly on the results of special investigations, and on the useful observations on patients in psychiatric hospitals in England and Wales, published by HMSO since 1953.

With due regard for the limited evidence, there are two conclusions concerning the trend of mental illness which are not in doubt. The first is that with one important exception, the pattern of mental illness has not been modified by the decline of infectious disease to anything like the same extent as the pattern of physical illness, for the obvious reason that few psychiatric disorders are of infective origin. An exception is in the case of syphilis affecting the central nervous system which was once a common cause of admission to psychiatric hospital, but has now virtually disappeared.

The second trend which is evident is an increase in the proportion of psychiatric patients at older ages. To a considerable extent this is explained by the changed age structure of the population as a whole (figure 3.1); since mental illness is more common in old than in young people, its age distribution must change in an ageing population. But it is also probat that the improvement in expectation of life during the past century has been greater for psychiatric patients, as for other handicapped groups such as the mentally handicapped, than for the population as a whole because, when conditions for survival are unfavourable, as they were until recently, the survival of the handicapped is likely to be more affected than that of the rest of the population.

Thirdly, with the help of modern psychotropic drugs which have a high degree of effectiveness in depression and in some patients with schizophrenia it has become modern practice to maintain admission to mental hospitals at a minimum.

From the limited evidence it is difficult to be confident about the trend of the total volume of psychiatric illness. The data for psychiatric hospitals in England show that between 1954 and 1969 the number of inpatients per 100,000 population fell 31 per cent and during the seventies fell a further 27 per cent. The proportion of long stay patients over the same period decreased also so that by 1970 only half of all resident patients had been in hospital for more than 3 years. For 15 years from 1954 the number of admissions, about half of which were readmissions, rose so that by 1970 they were 150 per cent higher than in the mid nineteen fifties. Subsequently the overall admission rate has remained constant, although the first admission rate has fallen by 18 per cent from 137 to 111 per thousand population. These trends will be considered in more detail in relation to psychiatric services, but here it may be said that while in the first place active treatment and the development of psychotropic drugs increased the frequency of admission to hospital they are now enabling new cases of relatively serious mental illness to undergo all their treatment in the community. Similarly, patients who formerly would have spent their lives in hospital have been discharged, with the result that the total number of hospital patients has been drastically reduced. The net effect of the multiple influences—changing age structure of the population, more active treatment and changes in economic, social and other conditions—on psychiatric problems as a whole is unknown.

The Character of Contemporary Health Problems

In assessing the character of the residual health problems of technologically advanced countries it is important to distinguish between genetic and other diseases. The term genetic disease is properly used in reference to conditions due to disorders of genes or to recognizable abnormalities of chromosomes. All other diseases and disabilities, while influenced by various degrees of genetic predisposition, are not attributable to any identified genic or chromosomal disorder, and whether and when they are manifested is determined largely by the environment to which the individual is exposed.

Prenatal life

Natural selection has restricted to a low frequency diseases primarily due to disorders of genes, whether manifested before, at or after birth. A much larger number of conditions are attributable to abnormalities of chromosomes arising mainly at fertilization, but most of these are eliminated as spontaneous abortions. Hence most prenatal deaths and congenital abnormalities present at birth, whether recognized or unrecognized, are due to the hazards associated with implantation and embryonic and fetal development. In a few cases these hazards come from outside the uterus, as in the examples of malformations caused by drugs such as thalidomide or a virus infection of the mother such as rubella; but in most they are determined by intrauterine conditions which are far less susceptible to control. It is therefore not surprising that in a period when there has been a large reduction of postnatal mortality, there has been only a modest decrease in stillbirth rates, and apparently no change in the annual incidence of congenital malformations or mental handicap. For although prenatal deaths and congenital disabilities are susceptible to the influence of natural selection, the environmental conditions which lead to them are relatively constant and difficult to control.

Prereproductive and reproductive life

In assessment of the character of the residual health problems these two periods may be considered together. Since natural selection has restricted the frequency of conditions arising from disorders of genes, and most of those due to chromosomal abnormalities are eliminated before birth, the proportion of individuals affected at birth or later by genetic disease is small, probably well below 1 per cent. The large majority of diseases and disabilities presenting in the prereproductive and reproductive periods are therefore due to environmental influences, operating before birth in the case of congenital conditions and after birth in the case of abnormalities determined postnatally.

Postnatal influences are much more accessible than those which are prenatal, and as noted in Chapter 2, improvement in health has been due largely to their control—by provision of more food and removal of hazards from the physical environment. However even in the most advanced countries the control of such hazards is far from complete. Moreover a new class of environmental risks has been added, the self-imposed risks of harmful behaviour such as smoking, excessive or unbalanced diet and deficient exercise. These influences will be considered more fully in Chapter 10, but here it should be noted that they already play an important part in determining the health problems in the reproductive and postreproductive periods.

Postreproductive life

In conditions manifested after the end of the fertile period the effects of natural selection are reduced or absent. Hence while the frequency of genetic disease and disability due to disorders of genes or chromosomes is very low, genotypes causing a strong predisposition to abnormality are relatively more common in late life than at lower ages. Nevertheless there is no reason to doubt that a considerable proportion of the diseases presenting in the postreproductive period are primarily due to environmental influences which may have operated over many years, even as early as childhood. These influences include those which stem from the general environment such as deficient food, atmospheric pollution, accidents, and harmful behaviour such as smoking and lack of exercise.

Ethical Issues associated with Contemporary Health Problems

The advances of the past two centuries have resulted in a considerable extension of life for handicapped as well as for normal people. To a large extent this prolongation is due to general influences such as better food and hygiene which any humane society would wish to develop and provide for all; but it has also become possible to extend by treatment the lives of patients who are permanently disabled, and this raises the general issue of the ethics of medical intervention in such cases. The issue is most frequently discussed in relation to the elderly, but it arises even more poignantly in respect of those who are severely handicapped from birth and who may survive for many years as a result of treatment. The discussion which follows will be concerned with congenitally malformed children who epitomize the extent and nature of the problem of survival made possible by medical intervention.

About 3 in every 100 children are born with recognizable physical abnormalities, which may vary from a trivial blemish of the skin to a serious condition of the heart or brain. Most of these malformations raise no large medical or ethical issues, either because they present no threat to the quality or duration of life, or because they are so lethal that effective medical intervention is almost inconceivable. The proportion of malformed children whose lives can be substantially prolonged by treatment is certainly not more than 1 in 6 and probably less than 1 in 10.

Against this background the problem of the malformed raises three issues: prevention by contraception; elimination by abortion; and treatment from birth. Within that part of the future which it is realistic to discuss, it seems very unlikely that the conception of malformations will be preventable to any appreciable extent by genetic engineering or by recognition of parents likely to have an affected child and decide therefore to remain childless. Identification of the seriously malformed embryo or fetus early in pregnancy is now sometimes possible among mothers with access to advanced diagnostic methods. It may become more so, in which case the recommendation of abortion would probably be regarded by most, though not all, doctors as the procedure of choice. But in general, the problem of the malformed is essentially the problem as it presents from birth.

There is no dispute concerning the treatment of most malformed children. No one is likely to question the desirability of closing a cleft palate, or of surgery in congenital heart disease where operation offers the prospect of normal life to patients who would die early if untreated. The problem arises where the outcome of treatment is the survival of a child with a serious physical or mental handicap, and this occurs particularly in relation to the malformations of the central nervous system.

In such cases the desirability of treatment must be examined with two considerations in view: the quality of life which is prolonged by medical intervention; and the price paid in care of the handicapped, particularly by close relatives, but also by the community at large through provision of social, educational and medical services.

It is at this point that controversy begins and it is important to distinguish between those whose principles allow no account to be taken of quality of life or cost of care—they hold that life should be prolonged wherever possible without regard for the consequences—and those whose conscience allows no such escape from the dilemma presented by some of the most serious malformations. This distinction can be illustrated by reference to the abnormality of anencephalus, characterized by gross maldevelopment of the brain and death before or within a few hours of birth. Logically, anyone who thinks that no account should be taken of the consequences, should agree that it would be a proper goal of medical research and practice to provide a vegetable existence for the anencephalic, without regard for the cost to public services and the distress of close relatives, particularly the parents. But those who cannot accept this extreme interpretation of humanism must face the formidable problem of deciding in respect of other malformed births with what degree of handicap and at what price to the community they would consider it undesirable to intervene to prolong life.

In relation to these issues, the malformation of spina bifida is something of a test case. The condition is the result of failure of the spinal cord to close during prenatal development. By closing the lesion the surgeon is able to prolong the lives of children who without treatment would die soon after birth. Some of these children will be paralyzed and incontinent for the rest of their lives, and some will be mentally retarded as well. Moreover, in most of those who are paralyzed the paralysis is irreversible.

Since the patient cannot represent himself, and a careful weighing of the complex medical, ethical and other issues is almost impossible for the distraught parents unaided, the balance of responsibility for the decision in such cases must lie heavily with medical specialists, namely the obstetrician, paediatrician and neurosurgeon. Unless they take the uncompromising view that all lives must be saved, they have to decide whether to intervene in relation to the criteria referred to above: the quality of the life prolonged; and the cost of survival to the community.

As judged by the demand for special educational arrangements and health and social services, the cost to the community of surgical intervention in all operable cases of spina bifida would be very great, and in time, no doubt, medical decisions will have to be influenced by considerations of this kind. These judgements will be most difficult when something like a normal life can be achieved at very high cost. In the case of spina bifida, however, the issue is simplified by the fact that what is achieved at high cost is often not a normal life but a cruelly handicapped one. A life indeed of such quality that many doctors think it wrong to prolong it even if no price were paid by the community in supportive services.

This raises what is perhaps the central problem posed by the treatment of congenital deformities, and indeed of the seriously handicapped in general: on what basis can a judgement be made that the quality of life will be such that it should not be prolonged? One test is for a parent to ask: would I wish myself to live, or to have my own child survive from birth with such a handicap? When confronted by the prospect of lifelong paralysis from spina bifida, some doctors have no doubt about their answer. Yet no child who has survived treatment for spina bifida and has been asked has been reported to have expressed regret at his survival. The social and ethical implications of issues such as this are so profound that wise doctors no longer attempt to resolve them without extensive discussion with lay and professional colleagues, as well of course with relatives.

Further Reading

Burnet M. (1971) *Genes, Dreams and Realities*. Medical and Technical Publishing Co. Ltd., Aylesbury, Bucks.

Dubos R. (1959) *Mirage of Health*. George Allen and Unwin Ltd., London.

Dubos R. (1968) *Man, Medicine, and Environment*. Pall Mall Press Ltd., London.

McLachlan G. (ed.) (1972) *Patient, Doctor, Society: A Symposium of Introspections.* Oxford University Press for the Nuffield Provincial Hospitals Trust, London.

Symposium: The Cost of Life. *Proc. Roy. Soc. Med. Lond.* **60** (1967), 1195-1246.

Symposium on *Ethics in Medical Progress.* Ciba Foundation, J. & A. Churchill Ltd., London (1966).

4

Effect of the Decline of the Birth Rate and Death Rate on the Genetic Constitution of the Population

Full many a gem of purest ray serene,
The dark unfathomed cares of ocean bear,
Full many a flower is born to blush unseen,
And waste its sweetness on the desert air.

In this chapter we shall consider whether the improvements in health of the past two centuries have been achieved at the price of an increase in the proportion of genetically handicapped individuals. This is a complex issue on which opinion is sharply divided. Some people believe that genetic equilibrium is being seriously disturbed, and that unless appropriate measures are taken genetic deterioration is inevitable. Others consider that such fears are exaggerated, and that in any case the measures proposed are for one reason or another likely to be unacceptable or ineffective. Although these differences of opinion are not wholly of scientific origin, the fact that experienced observers have arrived at quite different conclusions reflects both the complexity of the problem and the inconclusive nature of much of the evidence.

The belief that genetic equilibrium is being disturbed is derived from two considerations. First, because of the improvement in health, many people who formerly would have died at an early age now survive and reproduce. Some of them pass to their children genes associated with disease and disability. This, it is suggested, must increase the frequency of harmful genes. Second, measured intelligence is consistently a little higher in school children from small than from large families. This has been interpreted to mean that conception tends to be controlled more rigorously by the intelligent than by the less intelligent, and it is concluded that this too must have had an undesirable effect on the genetic constitution of the population.

Among objections which have been raised to these interpretations two are so fundamental that if they are accepted there is little need for further discussion. We shall therefore examine them at the outset.

• First the conclusion about the consequences of improved survival has been criticized on the grounds that a gene which is undesirable in one environment is not necessarily so in another. For example genes which are harmful in wild animals may be advantageous after domestication, since fitness must be redefined in relation to the new environment. Similarly, it is suggested, changes in gene equilibrium which result from modification of man's environment are not necessarily undesirable.

However, this objection does not take account of the complexity of the problem in man. If an increase in gene frequency is a secondary consequence of a more or less permanent change in the character of the environment, for example of a shift from rural to urban life, or improvement in diet, no ill-effects need to be anticipated so long as the change is maintained. The population of Western Europe may be more susceptible to cholera and typhoid now than in the mid nineteenth century but this does not matter if primary protection is provided by controlling the source of infection. The circumstances are quite different if increased gene frequency is a direct result of medical therapy; a disease such as diabetes, which is compatible with survival and reproduction, may have unpleasant features for those afflicted. Moreover, because resources are limited the services required to care for affected people are provided at the expense of alternative uses of medical effort.

• Second the negative correlation between fertility and intelligence is also said to be misinterpreted. A similar correlation exists between fertility and other variables such as stature and longevity which show no evidence of a decline; indeed both have been increasing. In the *Biology of Mental Defect*, Penrose gives reasons for thinking that in such cases differential fertility may be a natural biological process, consistent with genetic equilibrium. The same explanation has been suggested for the differential birth rate with respect to intelligence.

However, while genetic stability is consistent with differential fertility, there is no reason to doubt that it can be disturbed by selective restrictions in breeding. Extreme variation of weight and length have been produced in farm animals by selective breeding, and it is possible that the differential use of contraception has influenced human intelligence.

Hence we conclude that if improved health has increased the frequency of genes associated with disease, to the extent that this has raised the incidence of diseases which in their nature are unpleasant or require medical treatment it must be regarded as undesirable. And if the negative correlation between intelligence and sibship size does not permit us to conclude that intelligence is declining, the concept of genetic stability does not dismiss the possibility. Thus we cannot on *a priori* grounds accept the view that a change in the genetic constitution of human populations could not have occurred, or that such a change would be unimportant. Both suggestions result from pressing the analogy with animal populations without sufficient regard for the unique circumstances associated with the growth of the human population since the eighteenth century. Although the reduction of the death rate was attributable largely to environmental changes which might be regarded as analogous to domestication, the extent that it was due to medical therapy can be described fairly as very small. Furthermore the introduction of effective measures of birth control may have superimposed on the pattern of natural fertility a new pattern not determined primarily by the activity of the ovary and the testis. It is at least possible that this change has had some genetic significance. Certainly it would have social significance, for even if no genetic influence were involved we could not regard it as unimportant if family limitation were practised most intensively by those who could create the most favourable environment for their children.

The Effect of the Decline of Mortality

It would be easier to assess the possibility that improvements in health are disturbing genetic equilibrium if we could be more confident about the mechanisms which maintain it. On the face of it, genes which prejudice survival or fertility should in time disappear from the gene pool and in view of the length of man's history it may be asked why a condition such as haemophilia still exists. It is due to a sex linked recessive gene, which is constantly being destroyed because the fertility of those affected is low. Yet the incidence of haemophila appears to remain fairly constant at about 1 per 15,000 of population. Two possible explanations are known.

Genes lost may be replaced by mutation. The mutation rates in man which have been estimated are low, but they are enough to affect substantially the frequency of rare conditions, such as haemophilia and achondroplasia.

A second explanation for the persistence of harmful genes is the phenomenon of heterosis. It is best known in plants, whose hybrids commonly exhibit vigour which may be absent or less conspicuous in the pure strains. Evidence of the same kind is available in animals, including man.

The basis of heterosis can be illustrated by reference to a condition such as sickle cell anaemia. Those seriously affected, the homozygotes, have a pair of genes associated with an abnormal type of haemoglobin. But individuals with the unpaired abnormal gene, the heterozygotes, who are affected mildly if at all appear to have a selective advantage, possibly through being more resistant to malaria, over both homozygotes and normal individuals without the gene. Thus the reduction of genes from the loss of homozygotes may be offset by the increase from the improved survival of heterozygotes.

But although mechanisms of this kind tend to maintain genetic stability, there can be little doubt that the improvement in health since the eighteenth century has raised the frequency of some genes related to disease. For as we have seen the increased expectation of life has been due mainly, until the present century wholly, to a decline of mortality from infectious disease. In the past, in order to reproduce, an individual had to survive and remain fertile after extensive early exposure to a wide range of infections. This must have been among the most powerful influences in natural selection, and its substantial reduction in technologically advanced countries must have produced a population genetically less fit with respect to certain infections. But whether this change should be regarded as undesirable depends on the nature of the influences which have brought it about. In Chapter 2 it was concluded that they were as follows.

Improvement in diet

This was considered to be the most important influence on the decline of mortality and growth of population in the eighteenth and early nineteenth centuries. It was probably the main reason for the decline of tuberculosis, and the population may be genetically more susceptible to this disease now than formerly. But whether this is undesirable depends upon the possibility of a reversal of the conditions under which the susceptible have survived and reproduced. Specifically, since improved diet and a rising standard of living have been the most significant influences the question is whether they are likely ever again to be reduced. It is ironic that in a nuclear age an unequivocal answer cannot be given, but if the improved living standard proves to be a permanent feature in countries where it has been achieved, the modification of the genetic constitution of the population which has resulted may not be unfavourable.

Better hygiene

Hygiene was judged in importance to be second only to food supplies. As we have indicated the population is probably now genetically more susceptible to cholera, typhoid and other intestinal infections than two centuries ago, and the question is again whether the means responsible for this change are permanent. It seems reasonable to believe they are, for the methods which ensure a clean water supply (for example) are not costly and are specific in their effects on disease. Hence in a developed country there is little reason to be concerned about increased susceptibility to diseases which are preventable by hygienic measures.

Spontaneous change in the character of disease

Scarlet fever and influenza are outstanding examples of diseases whose epidemiology and natural history are to a considerable extent independent of both medical measures and environmental changes, and due to modifications of the infective organisms and their relationship with the human genotype. Mortality from both diseases has varied greatly during the present century, and the genetic susceptibility of the population may also have varied. But this variation appears to be independent of human intervention and is a cause rather than a consequence of improved health.

Specific medical measures

In the nineteenth century smallpox was the only disease significantly affected by specific medical measures and until recently their contribution to the total decline of mortality from infections to the present time has been smaller than that of other influences. It is hardly possible to predict the long term consequences of immunization on genetic susceptibility to infectious disease. Since many people have survived and reproduced who formerly would have died in childhood it is certainly possible that the number of susceptibles has increased. But vaccination and immunization procedures provide substantial protection which may compensate for any genetic change which has resulted from them. Treatment has been relatively less important, and is unlikely to have had much effect on the genetic basis of susceptibility.

Broadly, if infectious disease can be prevented, provided the measures are inherent in changing living conditions, or, if they are not inherent, are not too costly, an increase in the incidence of susceptibles is probably of little consequence. In the case of most infections from which mortality has declined during the past two centuries these conditions have been met. At the same time it must be admitted that long term predictions are hazardous, unless the source of infection is effectively controlled. It is conceivable that an organism such as the tubercle bacillus may adapt by mutation and become more virulent.

The probabilities for non-infectious diseases are somewhat different. Some have responded to the same environmental influences which led to the decline of infections and the significance of genetic change is similar. For example, an increase in the proportion of children who require a higher level of nutrition might be unimportant, because the improved diet can probably be maintained. But an increase in the frequency of disease which is unpleasant or requires continued therapy would certainly be undesirable.

There is little evidence that therapy has so far altered the frequencies of genes associated with disease or disability. In a common condition such as insulin dependent diabetes, where the effect of treatment on survival and reproduction has been striking, the genetic basis of the disease is far from clear. And in the few uncommon conditions, such as haemophilia and fibrocystic disease of the pancreas, where the genetic background is fairly clear, the increase in life expectations has as yet had little effect on reproduction.

The Effect of Contraception

Although the birth rate in England and Wales undoubtedly fluctuated in earlier centuries in association with changes of mortality and possibly through such influences as age at marriage and expectation of life in women, it was not until the late nineteenth century that it began to show the effect of intentional restriction of family size. There is little evidence of birth control in the English demographic literature of the seventeenth century, and it is doubtful whether deliberate abstinence has had much influence on population growth.

The observation that measured intelligence is a little higher in children from small than from large families suggests that contraception may have altered the pattern of differential fertility. Whether it has done so is not clear. The negative correlation between intelligence and sibship size might be wholly due to biological causes; but we cannot exclude the possibility that to some extent it also reflects the influence of contraception. Since the evidence is inconclusive we must try to give a common sense answer. And common sense suggests that it is likely that intelligent people made early and efficient use of contraceptives, as they must have made early and efficient use of other amenities provided by the sanitary revolution.

However, the interpretation of this conclusion is complicated by the fact that to an unknown extent intelligence reflected in both test performance and reproductive behaviour is environmentally determined. The higher scores by children from small families, or the greater use of contraceptives by intelligent parents, might be due to their favourable environments rather than to their superior genes. If this is so the restricted reproduction may have little or no influence on the transmission of genes which determine intelligence.

The available evidence gives no answer to the very theoretical question whether, in a uniform environment in which contraceptives were readily available, variation in fertility in relation to intelligence would be greater than could be attributed to biological influences alone. But it seems reasonable to suppose that it would, since the level of intelligence below which people are capable of practising contraception is probably higher than the level below which they are invariably infertile. That is to say there are fertile individuals of low intelligence who are incapable of limiting the size of their families. Their frequency is unknown, and the effect of their reproduction on the pattern of differential fertility would be determined to some extent by the practice of other fertile people. In a society in which small families have considerable advantages, those with the ability to limit family size will do so, and the influence of the larger families of fertile individuals of low intelligence would be greater than in a society in which the penalties for large families were less severe.

For these reasons it seems possible that the spread of contraceptive knowledge has had some influence on the trend of the intelligence which is measured by tests, and a smaller and perhaps trivial influence on the genetic component in intelligence. This conclusion is based, not on the negative correlation between measured intelligence and sibship size, which could be due to biological variation, but on consideration of the extent to which contraception may have been practised by individuals of varying intelligence.

Finally let us consider whether if such a trend exists it is of any practical importance. It seems to be widely believed that a general increase in intelligence would be highly desirable, and that even a small decline, particularly of the genetic component in intelligence, would be a serious matter which would require urgent action. This opinion overlooks the fact that there exists an immense reserve of unused ability which is more accurately assessed in Gray's *Elegy in a Country Churchyard*, a poetic expression of the relationship between nature and nurture, than some discussions of the trend of intelligence. Unless we are prepared to believe that there have been some remarkable mutations at different times in history, we must conclude that it is only in certain places and for very short periods that any considerable part of the capacity available has been exploited.

Further Reading

Cartwright F. F. (1977) *A Social History of Medicine*. Longman Group Ltd., London.

Hogben L. (1945) *Nature and Nurture*. George Allen and Unwin Ltd., London.

Penrose L. S. (1963) *The Biology of Mental Defect*, 3rd edition. Sedgwick & Jackson, London.

5

The Measurement of Ill Health

Resources are limited in all societies, so that as health care has become more effective it has become more costly, and health services need to compete more for funds with other services. Thus if we are to provide the best care possible, we must know what care achieves, especially in terms of the commonest diseases, as well as what it costs. We must monitor not only the resources we deploy, but also health itself.

If health priorities are to be determined it is necessary to know what the major disease problems are, and as health resources are deployed their impact must be judged by monitoring. Until recently deaths were the only source of information about the pattern of ill health in Britain.

Measurement of Mortality

Number of deaths and age at death have been reliably recorded for more than a century; reporting of cause of death has been less reliable. The tabulations of deaths by cause published each year by the Registrar General are an analysis of what different generations of doctors with varied medical backgrounds have written on death certificates. They represent an analysis of opinions rather than facts, for fashions in diagnosis change and as knowledge advances nomenclature of disease also changes. For example, when death registration was introduced in 1838, fewer than 100 causes of death were distinguished and these included as major categories 'want of breast milk', 'convulsions', 'privation', 'diarrhoea' and 'old age'; today the current International Statistical Classification of Diseases, Injuries and Causes of Death (ICD) lists more than 1,000 diagnostic entities.

In Chapter 3 the principal causes of death in England and Wales were discussed in some detail. Table 5.1 reminds us that over one quarter of all deaths in this country are now attributed to ischaemic heart disease and

Table 5.1 Leading causes of death in England and Wales 1970 and 1980 (males and females of all ages)

ICD No.	Cause of death	1970 No. of deaths	1970 Crude death rate per 1,000 population	1970 Percentage distribution	1980 No. of deaths	1980 Crude death rate per 1,000 population	1980 Percentage distribution
410-414	Ischaemic heart disease	139,317	2.8	24.2	154,373	3.1	26.5
140-209	Malignant neoplasm	115,729	2.4	20.1	130,566	2.7	22.5
430-438	Cerebrovascular disease	79,291	1.6	13.8	71,443	1.6	12.3
393-404, 420-429	Other heart conditions	46,733	1.2	8.1	39,375	0.8	6.8
490-493	Bronchitis, emphysema and asthma	30,181	0.6	5.3	25,391	0.5	4.4
800-999	Accidents, poisonings and violence	22,701	0.5	3.9	20,296	0.4	3.5
	All other causes	141,242	2.6	24.6	139,941	2.8	24.0
	All causes	575,194	11.7	100.0	581,385	11.9	100.0

over one-fifth to cancer. Next in order of magnitude come cerebrovascular disease, other heart conditions with bronchitis, emphysema and accidents some way behind. As the table shows, ischaemic heart disease and cancer have become relatively more important, and the others less important over the past decade. But the *crude death rate* (the number of deaths per 1,000 total population) provides a very incomplete and, indeed, a misleading picture of the amount of serious disease in the population. For, other things being equal, the more old people there are in a population, the higher the crude death rate will be: the crude death rate is lower in Birmingham than Bournemouth and in Ebbw Vale than Llandudno, not because Birmingham and Ebbw Vale are healthier but because Bournemouth and Llandudno are places to which many elderly people move after retirement. Deaths in infancy, childhood and young adult life represent a much more serious loss to the community than deaths in old age. There are many ways of making allowance for age at death in comparing different populations. One is to consider only *age specific death rates*, for example the *stillbirth rate* (number of stillbirths per 1,000 total live and stillbirths registered in a year), the *infant mortality rate* (deaths of infants under 1 year per 1,000 live births registered) or death rates for 5 yearly age groups (i.e. 0-4, 5-9, 10-14, etc.). Death rates in broader age specific groups are shown in table 3.4. There are also various ways of standardizing death rates for age and of calculating standardized mortality ratios (the SMR gives an age adjusted death rate converted to a percentage of the death rate in a standard population).

However, even when age is taken into account and the cause of death given on the death certificate is reasonably reliable as it now is in Britain, it is only when there is a high *case fatality rate* (number of deaths per hundred cases of the disease) that the death rate provides any measure of the frequency with which a disease occurs. For example, in 1980 cancer of the respiratory system (ICD 160-163) was responsible for 27,720 male and 8,747 female deaths, in the same year the deaths of 1 male and 2 females were attributed to neuroses (ICD 300). The first number provides a good measure of how common cancer of the lung is because more than 90 per cent of all cases die within 5 years of diagnosis; the second gives no indication of the size of the problem presented by the neuroses.

If deaths are a poor indication of the amount of disease in a community, they are an even more inadequate measure of the suffering, disablement, inefficiency and loss of working time caused by ill-health. In national mortality data a death from an immediately fatal road accident is given the same weight as a death at the same age from mitral stenosis preceded by many years of impaired health, a major and costly operation and a period of extreme disablement. In short, therefore, although in the nineteenth century death rates forcibly demonstrated that at that time the over-riding disease problem was one of epidemic and endemic infectious disease, today, when infection is a much less common cause of death and mortality in infancy and young adult life is very much lower, more refined measures of the amount and distribution of ill-health are required. We need to know how often, for how long and from what causes people are ill as well as the rate at which they die.

Measurement of Morbidity

In addition to innumerable *ad hoc* surveys, there are now many routine sources of information about the amount of ill-health in the community. Some of the more important sources are given in table 5.2. The importance of the census is that it provides denominators, classified by age, sex, place of residence, occupation etc., for the calculation of rates.

For many reasons measurement of ill-health is more complex than measurement of mortality. There is no clear line between health and sickness as there is between life and death; death is a unique event which, with rare exceptions consequent to modern medical technology, takes place at a point in time, whereas illnesses have a duration, can recur and have different degrees of severity.

It has been pointed out that the decision whether a person is sick depends on definitions of health and the individual making the judgement. A man may believe he is ill, even if his doctor is unable to find a physical explanation. In contrast, on examination for life insurance, or as a result of a screening procedure, a man who believes he is healthy may be found to have a disease which soon will cause disability or death (e.g. chronic nephritis, or carcinoma of the lung). Clearly, although he is not conscious of ill-health, in a very real sense he is ill. The science of bacteriology drew attention to this type of difficulty by uncovering the carrier state, and the development of biochemical, haematological and other laboratory tests have underlined it by presenting the clinician and epidemiologist with comparable problems in the field of non-infectious disease for example diabetes, anaemia, cancer of the cervix, hypertension.

Difficulties also arise because illnesses have a duration and because over a given period the same person may suffer from more than one illness. Many different indices of morbidity are therefore possible. For example, in a defined population we can count all the illnesses present at a point in time (*point prevalence*), all the illnesses present at any time during a defined period (*period prevalence*), or illnesses that begin during a defined period (*incidence*). In the same way instead of illnesses we can count persons who are ill. The same person may have more than one cause of ill-health at a given time, or may suffer from more than one illness, or may develop the same illness more than once, over a defined period. These complications have given rise to a great deal of terminological confusion, so that in any statement about morbidity it is essential to define the index used.

Finally, measurement of the severity of illness presents its own problems. Indices such as time off work, confined to house or bed, out-patient attendance, admission to hospital and duration of stay in hospital all have their uses and limitations, and prevalence of various forms of impairment or disability can be as useful as prevalence of the underlying conditions (see also Chapter 28).

It should now be clear that there can be no precise answer to the question: how much ill-health is there in the population. Indeed if we accept the definition of health provided by the World Health Organization—'a state of complete physical, mental and social well being and not merely the absence of disease or infirmity'—nearly all of us are sick. But if definitions of ill-health are used which are less all embracing and more precise, answers of considerable medical interest can be provided. It is useful to look at the problem at four different but not altogether mutually exclusive levels: ill-health most frequently complained of; ill-health leading to general practitioner consultation; ill-health causing absence from work; and ill-health leading to hospital admission.

Illnesses most frequently complained of

A continuous survey of sickness in the population of England and Wales was carried out by the Central Office of Information from 1943 until 1952. The data were collected by direct interview, not from records of patients using the medical services, with the intention of assessing, among other things, the amount of ill-health which did not come to medical attention. Each month men and women in representative samples of the adult population were interviewed by non-medical field workers about the illnesses they had experienced during the previous 3 months.

Table 5.2. Sources of usual information for assessing morbidity in Britain

1. Census and Census Related Studies

(a) decennial census (OPCS)
(b) *occupational mortality* (Registrars General and OPCS based on census and death registration—also decennial)

2. Notification

(a) *Births* (to each District Medical Officer (DMO) leading to a computerized file for childhood development surveillance; vaccination schedules. Basis for school health records)
(b) *Deaths* (to each DMO) leading to some regionally organized computer analysis schemes
(c) Infectious diseases (to Medical Officer of Environmental Health)
(d) Congenital malformations (to DMO)
OPCS Monitors publish some of this information relating to (a), (b), (c) and (d)
(e) *Certain prescribed industrial diseases.* Fourteen industrial diseases are also notifiable (Department of the Environment—DOE)

3. Registration and Registers

(a) *Mortality publications* (derived from death registration). Responsibility of Registrars General, compiled by OPCS for England and Wales. Series deal separately each year with tabulations by all causes, area, time trends etc. as well as for cancer, childhood conditions, infectious diseases etc.
(b) *OPCS monitors* (publish more frequently information under 3 (a))
(c) *Master age-sex registers* (lists by age, sex and address of all patients under the care of a general practitioner held by Family Practitioner Committee—FPC)
(d) Age-sex register and with increasing frequency disease register (held in accessible form by increasing numbers of general practitioners)
(e) Cancer register (data collected in several centres and co-ordinated by OPCS in England and Wales; nationally in Scotland and Northern Ireland)
(f) Blind and partially sighted register } maintained by Local Authority Social Service Departments
(g) Disabled persons register

4. National Health Service Records

(a) Annual hospital statistical returns (SH3) in England and Wales (inpatient data overlap with 4 (b) but are the only routine source of outpatient information)
(b) i) *Hospital Acitivity Analysis* (from Regional Health Authorities) and *Hospital Inpatient Enquiry* (published jointly by DHSS and OPCS) both concerned with England and Wales
ii) *Scotish Hospital Inpatient Survey* (published by the Information Division of the Common Service Agency—ISD)
(c) *Mental Health Enquiry*, inpatient statistics (published separately for England, Scotland and Wales by DHSS, ISD and the Welsh Office)
(d) Systems for *linking records*
i) Scottish National Data (ISD)
ii) Oxford Record Linkage Study (health, including primary care records and demographic data) for populations resident in Oxford RHA and neighbouring locations
(e) Prescription costs in General Practice (FPCs to Prescription Pricing Authority)

---

5. Surveys and Enquiries

(a) *National Food Survey* (entire United Kingdom; Ministry of Agriculture, Food and Fisheries)
(b) *General Household Survey* (entire United Kingdom; OPCS)
(c) *Confidential Enquiry into Maternal Mortality* (DHSS, England and Wales)
(d) *Confidential Enquiry into Perinatal Mortality* (RHAs and Health Boards)
(e) *General Practice Morbidity Survey* (Royal College of General Practitioners; OPCS and DHSS)

---

6. Other Sources

(a) *Social Security Statistics*
(b) *Industrial Health Service Records*
(c) *Prescribed Industrial Diseases*—diseases, including the notifiable industrial diseases, which entitle workers to compensation (see table 18.1) (DoE and DHSS)

The definition of illness was broad and included anything the individual considered to be a disturbance of his health during the period.

There are obvious weaknesses in morbidity statistics based on what a person remembers and is prepared to tell a non-medical interviewer about recent ill-health; nevertheless they provide useful information that cannot be obtained in any other way. Two out of three persons reported an awareness of some ill-health during the month before the interview, and, as expected, awareness of ill-health increased steeply with age. Less expected was the finding that at all ages females complained of more ill-health than males. These findings have subsequently been supported by several analyses of attendance at general practices and by similar surveys in the USA and elsewhere. In spite of the very high proportion of the population reporting awareness of ill-health, only 1 in 4 of those complaining had seen a doctor and only 1 in 8 had lost time from work or been confined to the house during the month. Rheumatism, digestive disorders and colds, influenza and other respiratory conditions were the illnesses most frequently reported (table 5.3). This type of survey draws attention to the fact that there is a great deal of minor and ill-defined illness in the population which causes little incapacity and rarely leads to consultation with a doctor.

Illnesses for which people consult general practitioners

The General Household Survey obtains information every year about some 15,000 households selected from the population of England,

Table 5.3 Illnesses most frequently complained of (Survey of Sickness, 1949)

Nature of Illness	Number of Illnesses	Percentage of Total
Rheumatism	16,133	12.1
Digestive disorders	14,642	10.9
Colds, Influenza	14,115	10.6
Other Respiratory Illnesses	9,642	7.2
Eye Affections	6,370	4.8
Dental disorders	5,289	4.0
All other illnesses	67,129	50.4
Total	133,320	100.0%

Scotland and Wales by random procedures. Procedures for collecting information are broadly similar to those which were used in the Survey of Sickness, although the information itself is of a much more general nature. Questions are directed towards economic and social matters, as well as health and health behaviour including the use of health services. Table 5.4 shows the reasons given by respondents who consulted their General Practitioners over a 2 week period in 1971.

Although there is much minor ill-health for which medical advice is not sought, about two-thirds of all patients on a doctor's list consult him either in their own homes or in his surgery at least once during a year; and over the same period he gives an average of 4 consultations per patient on his list. Much the commonest reasons for consultation in both sexes are upper and lower respiratory diseases, followed in men by trauma and cardiovascular disease, and in women by cardiovascular disease and ill-defined symptoms (table 5.4). This pattern of ill-health is not unlike that reported by people in morbidity surveys but is very different from that displayed by mortality statistics (table 5.1). Indeed, cancer, responsible for 20 per cent of the deaths in the country, does not appear among the first 10 reasons for general practitioner consultation.

Illnesses which cause absence from work

Medical certificates of incapacity for work are required by the Department of Health and Social Security to support claims to sickness or injury benefit. Analysis of the claims provides information of great administrative importance, and on the face of it should also be a valuable source of data about morbidity in the population. From this point of view, however, the data have to be interpreted with caution. In the first place, the whole population is not covered, for even in times of plenty many women and some men are not gainfully employed. Second, much minor illness is excluded, for short spells of incapacity are not normally subject to benefit. Third, duration of absence is not a very reliable measure of the severity of an illness. A man's attitude to his work, his employer's and fellow workers' attitude to him, the security of his job, the loss of income involved (whether he is also entitled to benefit from private insurance, works sick club, etc.) and many other factors may affect the period of absence. Finally, the reason given on the medical certificate for sickness absence is imprecise and sometimes unreliable or even misleading, for the general practitioner knows that his certificate will be

Table 5.4 Consultations with National Health Service General Practitioners by group of diseases causing consultation over 2-weeks in 1971

Males Disease Group	%	Rank	**Females**	%	Rank
Diseases of the respiratory system	26.9	1	Diseases of the respiratory system	19.3	1
Fractures, dislocations, sprains and other injuries	10.4	2	Heart disease, hypertension and other diseases of the circulatory system	9.5	2
Heart disease, hypertension and other diseases of the circulatory system	10.0	3	Symptoms and ill-defined diseases	7.7	3
Diseases of the digestive system	8.7	4	Arthritis and rheumatism and other diseases of the musculoskeletal system	6.6	4
Symptoms and ill-defined diseases	7.6	5	Diseases of the nervous system and sense organs	6.6	4
Diseases of the nervous system and sense organs	6.9	6	Mental disorders	6.4	6
Intestinal and other infectious diseases	6.4	7	Intestinal and other infectious diseases	6.1	7
Arthritis and rheumatis and other diseases of the musculoskeletal system	6.3	8	Diseases of the genitourinary system and breast	6.1	7
Diseases of the skin and subcutaneous tissue	4.0	9	Fractures, dislocations, sprains and other injuries	6.1	7
Mental disorders	3.9	10	Diseases of the digestive system	6.0	10
Diseases of the genito urinary system and breast)	1.7	11	Diseases of the skin and subcutaneous tissue	4.0	11
Other	7.2		Other	15.6	
	100			100	
Total consultations reported by sample	1,960		Total consultations reported by sample	2,946	

seen by the patient and by a number of lay persons, including possibly the patient's employer. Hence the diagnosis he enters is often intentionally indeterminate. The stated causes must therefore be interpreted with caution, although it is consistent with information from other sources that hypertension and ischaemic heart disease should have increased in absolute and relative importance, while bronchitis and emphysema have decreased. Details for males in 1975 are given in table 5.5 which shows that also of great importance are mental illness, accidents, digestive disorders, other diseases of the respiratory system and arthritis and rheumatism—a very different pattern from that displayed by mortality, but recognizably related to general practitioner consultations. Recently there have been changes in government regulations concerning notification of absence from work the full impact of which has yet to be determined.

Table 5.5 Leading causes of absence from work, Great Britain (males only) 1975

Diagnostic Group	Millions of days lost	Percentage distribution
Bronchitis and emphysema	27.13	11.1
Hypertension and ischaemic heart disease	25.26	10.4
Accidents, poisoning and violence	24.58	10.1
Mental disorders	20.18	8.3
Arthritis and Rheumatism	17.11	7.0
Other disease of circulatory system	15.27	6.3
Disorders of digestive system	15.12	6.2
All other conditions	98.92	40.6
Total	243.57	100.0

Illnesses treated in hospital

Since hospitals are the most costly segment of the medical services, a regular flow of information about use, staffing and cost of hospital beds is important administratively. Case records also provide a useful index of the amount of serious illness in the population. Hospital discharge data for non-psychiatric hospitals analysed by each regional health authority are known as Hospital Activity Analysis (HAA). In addition a 10 per cent sample of such hospitals have over some decades participated in the

Hospital Inpatient Enquiry (HIPE) and sent data to the Office of Population Censuses and Surveys which jointly with the Department of Health and Social Security publishes tables which permit inter-regional comparisons and the study of time trends. The Mental Health Enquiry provides analogous statistical information about the use made of mental illness and mental handicap hospitals. No other source of morbidity satistics provides data about diagnosis with so much detail and reliability, but the sample of illness is highly selected by the referral system in the health service. Nearly every case of some conditions (such as perforated peptic ulcer or acute schizophrenia) is admitted to hospital. But for many others the decision whether to admit or to treat at home is influenced by social class, domestic circumstances, availability of beds, interests of general practitioners and other factors which vary from area to area and time to time and are only loosely related to severity of illness. The analysis of reasons for hospital treatment (table 5.6) reveals a pattern of disease greatly influenced by the need for surgery. This is the pattern medical students see during their clinical years and it bears little resemblance to

Table 5.6 Estimates of leading diagnoses for discharges and deaths from non-psychiatric hospitals, England and Wales 1980

	1980	
Diagnosis	Number of discharges and deaths	Percentage distribution
Fractures, dislocations and other injuries	544,560	11.5
Cardiovascular disease	534,340	11.3
Diseases of the digestive system	514,370	10.9
Malignant and benign neoplasms	473,440	9.9
Diseases of respiratory system	397,050	8.4
Female genital system including disorders of the breast	272,610	5.7
All other conditions	1,999,080	42.2
All conditions	4,735,450*	100.0

*Excludes discharges from maternity beds

the pattern of ill-health reported by the general population or seen by general practitioners.

Further Reading

Cartwright F. F. (1977) *A Social History of Medicine*. Longman Group Ltd., London.

Wadsworth M. E. J., Butterfield W. J. H. and Blaney R. (1971) *Health and Sickness: The Choice of Treatment*. Tavistock Publications Ltd., London.

6

Mortality and Morbidity in Britain Today

The decline of mortality in Britain which began at least 2 centuries ago has continued until recent years. Death rates from nearly all causes have been falling, but a few major diseases have shown increases that warrant the description of epidemics. Moreover it is not surprising that it is possible to identify subgroups of the population which differ widely in experience of disease, since there are large differences in living standards and medical services are by no means uniformly adequate.

Modern Epidemics

During the past 60 years, for both males and females, there have been increases in the frequency of ischaemic heart disease and cancer of the lung of epidemic proportion. Because of changes in the International Classification of Diseases, the ageing of the population and advances in diagnostic precision, it is not possible to judge precisely the magnitude of the increase over the whole period. However we can be much more confident about the last 2 decades than the preceding period. Table 6.1 shows how in both sexes mortality has been increasing from ischaemic heart disease and cancer of the lung, although the rate of increase has in each case fallen. Cancers of certain reproductive organs in the two sexes have also become commoner causes of death, and the rate of increase for cancer of the prostate and testis in males, and cancer of the breast in females is accelerating. It should be mentioned that, when corrected for the change in the age structure of the population over the 2 decades some of these percentage increases are a little reduced. Although 2 of these epidemics (ischaemic heart disease and cancer of the lung) are known to be due largely to personal habits (cigarette smoking, unsatisfactory diet and lack of physical exercise: see Chapter 10), it has not yet been possible to control such influences. At every age death rates for most causes are

Table 6.1 Modern epidemics in England and Wales (certain causes of death for which death rates are increasing)

		Males				
ICD		Death rates per million			Percentage increase	
No.	Cause of death	1960	1970	1980	1960-1970	1970-1980
410-414	Ischaemic heart disease	2,927	3,392	3,738	16	10
162	Malignant neoplasm of bronchus, lung and trachea	852	1,045	1,117	23	7
185	Malignant neoplasm of the prostate	165	164	210	−1	28
		Females				
ICD		Death rates per million			Percentage increase	
No.	Cause of death	1960	1970	1980	1960-1970	1970-1980
410-414	Ischaemic heart disease	2,032	2,324	2,562	14	10
162	Malignant neoplasm of bronchus	131	214	332	63	55
174	Malignant neoplasm of breast	382	424	482	11	14
183	Malignant neoplasm of ovary	124	144	146	16	1

lower for females than for males, but death rates for cancer of the lung are increasing more steeply for females than for males as is the amount of cigarettes they smoke. The reasons why cancers of some sex glands have been on the increase in recent years are unclear. Moreover, a fall in mortality from cancer of the testis from 10 to 7 per cent million between 1960 and 1980 has masked a steady rise in incidence over the same period because treatment has become very much more effective.

Regional Differences in Disease Incidence

When death registration was made compulsory in 1838 it was immediately obvious that there were striking regional differences in death rates. Broadly speaking the death rates increased with latitude and this is still true today—death rates tend to be lowest in the south and the east and highest in the north and the west.

This pattern is well illustrated by the stillbirth and infant mortality rates for 1980 (table 6.2). The trend is due in part to recognizable differences in living conditions; the young infant is very sensitive to adverse

Table 6.2 Stillbirth and infant mortality rates by region (England and Wales 1980)

	Rates per 1,000 total births		Rates per 1,000 live births	
English regional health authorities and Wales	Stillbirths plus infant deaths	Stillbirths	Postneonatal deaths	Infant deaths
East Anglian	16.4	5.9	3.9	10.4
South West Thames	16.5	5.5	4.6	11.0
North West Thames	17.0	5.9	4.5	10.9
Oxford	17.6	6.0	3.9	11.4
Trent	17.8	6.9	3.5	11.9
Wales	17.8	6.0	3.4	11.4
South Western	18.1	6.5	4.1	11.5
Wessex	18.1	6.0	4.9	12.0
South East Thames	19.4	6.7	4.7	12.3
North East Thames	19.8	7.5	4.5	12.0
Mersey	20.0	7.0	4.9	12.8
Northern	20.6	8.4	3.9	12.4
North Western	21.0	7.9	4.5	12.9
Yorkshire	21.1	8.4	4.6	12.9
West Midlands	21.3	8.2	4.4	13.1

environmental influences. Death from infectious disease or accident may result from a low standard of maternal care, overcrowding, malnutrition, and bad housing which is often associated with inadequate facilities for washing, cooking and food storage; defective sanitation; and unsatisfactory arrangements for room heating and refuse disposal. There is less overcrowding in the south than in the Midlands and north of England, which still have a legacy of congested and insanitary working class housing from the nineteenth century.

Regional rates for the postneonatal period (from the beginning of the second to the end of the twelfth month of life) follow a different pattern from that for stillbirths. However, although the denominators are different rough comparisons can be made. Pneumonia, gastroenteritis and bronchitis still make a substantial contribution to the death rate during that period, and mortality from these diseases is greatly influenced by adverse living conditions. That *perinatal mortality* (stillbirths and deaths during the first week of life per thousand total births) should also show a regional pattern is less expected, for the leading causes of death are of natal and prenatal origin (congenital malformation, immaturity, birth injury). Many influences are involved: for example, standards and availability of health service vary from area to area, as does diet, fresh vegetables are more widely consumed in the south and east and starchy foods in the north; even within the limited range of latitude of England and Wales climate may play a part in determining regional differences. Climate is certainly associated with the regional pattern of mortaility from respiratory infections and chronic bronchitis, which is much the same as that for infant mortality.

Among the striking regional differences in disease incidence, for which as yet there are no convincing explanations, are cancer of the stomach for which death rates are more than 30 per cent higher in Wales than in England, and the neural tube defects (anencephalus and spina bifida) for which the incidence in South Wales is among the highest in the world. The malformations of the central nervous system are particularly common in the mining communities of Glamorgan and Monmouthshire.

Urbanization and Disease

When related to the size of the urban community in which they occur, death rates tend to be highest in the so-called conurbations and decrease through large and medium sized towns to their lowest level in small towns and rural areas. Urban-rural gradients for mortality, expressed as SMRs, in 1973 the last year in which this analysis was published, are shown in table 6.3. The conditions are ranked according to the gross number of deaths each caused during the year.

The association of death with city dwelling is almost all due to an increase of death rates from respiratory diseases with increasing size of town (table 6.3). People living in and near large cities have been subject to very much higher death rates from bronchitis, cancer of the lung, respiratory tuberculosis and pneumonia than those living in the country. Death rates from most other conditions, including ischaemic heart disease and cerebrovascular disease (together now responsible for nearly half all deaths), bear little or no relation to size of town. Exposure to the irritants which in the past poured into the atmosphere of cities from coal consumed in domestic grates and in the ovens and furnaces of industry is the likely explanation for much of the urban excess (see Chapter 13). It may also be due to the increased risk for city and town dwellers of contracting airborne infection when travelling to work or at work, or in places of entertainment. In the past this played an important part in the spread of respiratory tuberculosis.

For many medical and most surgical conditions hospital admission rates are also higher for town than for country dwellers and are highest for those living in the conurbations. The reason is not clear. Utilization of health services is determined as much by the facilities available as by the need for them, and whether admission rates for such conditions as uterine fibromyoma, haemorrhoids, tonsillar hypertrophy and hernia are much higher in conurbations than in rural districts because these conditions are commoner among city dwellers or because there is a greater demand for treatment and a much readier access to hospital services in the cities is a matter for investigation. The only group of diseases which shows a clear-cut trend in the opposite direction is motor vehicle accidents. Although there are fewer cars and in gross numbers fewer accidents in the rural areas, the speed at which they occur is much greater. Compared with the 4,690 fatal motor vehicle traffic accidents in 1973 there were 4,045 in 1981 and this number has been further reduced since the legislation compelling those in the front seat to wear restraining belts.

Occupation and Disease

An industrial society presents a wide range of occupational environments and patterns of work which may affect health. In Chapter 15 the impli-

Table 6.3 Standardized Mortality Ratios for males (England and Wales = 100) for certain causes of death related to population aggregation for 1973

ICD No.	Cause of death	Conurbations	Large towns	Medium towns	Small towns	Rural areas	Total deaths
410-414	Ischaemic heart disease	102	103	100	103	96	87,158
140-209	Malignant cancer (all sites)	111	105	99	95	86	64,804
430-438	Cerebrovascular disease	97	101	103	105	97	31,082
162	Cancer of trachea, lung and bronchus	117	97	101	88	80	26,032
480-486	Pneumonia	113	111	100	91	87	20,411
490-492	Bronchitis and emphysema	118	107	105	97	75	19,851
E810-819	Motor vehicle accidents	84	90	96	104	121	4,690
400-404	Hypertension	109	98	95	95	96	3,805
011	Tuberculosis of respiratory system	123	136	48	86	70	637

cations of this fact are discussed in relation to control of disease. Here we shall consider briefly occupational mortality at national level.

Information about occupation is obtained from relatives at death registration and occupation is recorded for the whole population at each census. At or near the census years, therefore, deaths can be related to the working populations in which they have occurred to give occupational mortality rates. William Farr was influential in developing census natality and mortality information and made the first official study of this type. Using data from the census of 1851, he calculated mortality rates for males in several hundred different occupations. For the age group 45-54 he found that farmers had the lowest and innkeepers the highest mortality (table 6.4).

Table 6.4 Occupational mortality for males aged 45-54 at the census of 1851 (after William Farr)

Occupation	Mortality per 1,000 living
Farmer	11.1
Shoemaker	15.0
Weaver	15.4
Grocer	16.5
Blacksmith	16.5
Carpenter	16.7
Tailor	16.7
Labourer	17.3
Miner	20.1
Baker	21.2
Butcher	23.1
Innkeeper	28.3
All males	17.9

For various reasons data such as these are difficult to interpret. First, mortality in many occupations is influenced by the type of men recruited into them. For example, jobs making heavy physical demands tend to attract the fitter and more active members of the working population, while men with respiratory tuberculosis, cardiovascular disease and chronic bronchitis often seek jobs which make light physical demands. Thus apparently safe jobs such as repairing shoes and watches can be associated with high mortality (see table 6.5). Second, mortality in hazardous occupations, such as coalmining and foundry work, is understated because workers whose health has been seriously undermined by such employment may transfer later in life to less exacting occupations and these are recorded at death registration. Third, information about occupation given by relatives is not always reliable; the relative may not know the job of the deceased, or may upgrade it. Finally, a difficulty arises from the different age structures of persons in different occupations. To take an extreme example, there would be little point in comparing mortality of medical students with that of senior physicians; some allowance is made for the last difficulty in the standardized mortality ratio. The SMR has many uses. For example, different occupations can be compared in respect of all causes of death taken together. Table 6.5 shows that at the time of the 1971 census bricklayers and deck and engine room ratings were subject to death rates more than twice the national average and five times the death rates of university teachers. Mortality among registered medical practitioners was 81 per cent of the national average.

Occupations can also be compared in relation to a specific cause of death. Table 6.6 shows, not unexpectedly, that publicans and inn-

Table 6.5 Some occupations with high and low SMRs for all causes. Males aged 15-64 (England and Wales 1970-72)

High ratios	SMR
Bricklayers, etc.	273
Deck and engine-room ratings, barge and boatmen	233
Steel erectors, riggers	164
Shoemakers and shoe repairers	156
Publicans, innkeepers	155
Watch and chronometer repairers	154
Low ratios	
University teachers	49
Paper product makers	50
Managers in building and contracting	54
Ministers of the crown; MPs senior government officers	61
Electrical and electronic fitters	67
Medical practitioners	81

Table 6.6 Some occupations with high and low SMRs for cirrhosis of the liver. Males aged 15-64 (England and Wales 1970-72)

High ratios	SMR	Rank in top 20
Publicans, innkeepers	1,576	1
Deck, engineering officers and pilots of ships	781	2
Fishermen	595	5
Electrical engineers	319	13
Medical practitioners (qualified)	311	14
Low ratios		
Draughtsmen	27	
Company secretaries and registrars	25	
Sawyers and woodcutters	25	
Turners	19	

keepers have a mortality from cirrhosis of the liver 15 times the national average and 63 times that of sawyers and woodcutters. The hazards of the publican's life have evidently changed little since Farr's day.

Mortality from specific causes of death in a particular occupation can also be compared with the national average. In addition to cirrhosis of the liver (see table 6.6) doctors have a much higher than average mortality from accidental poisoning and suicide with SMRs of 618 and 335 respectively and a much lower than average mortality from cancer (particularly lung cancer), bronchitis and tuberculosis. Their death rates from coronary disease and cerebrovascular disease are a little higher than the national average.

Standard of Living and Disease

For more than a century it has been clear that standard of living has an important influence upon the pattern of mortality and morbidity, but the magnitude of the influence is difficult to measure. The concept of standard of living is complex and imprecise, including as it does housing, nutrition, education, recreation and many other inter-related influences. Family income would provide a good index of material prosperity but many difficulties stand in the way of collecting reliable information about it. A rough and ready measure of standard of living is provided by the occupation of the head of a family, as used by the Registrar General since the census of 1921. All occupations are divided into 6 'social classes' on the basis of their standing in the community, the skill they demand and the income they command.

Class I	Higher professional and administrative occupations,
Class II	Employers in industry and retail trades and the lesser professions,
Class IIIN	Non-manual skilled occupations,
Class IIIM	Manual skilled occupations,
Class IV	Partly skilled occupations,
Class V	Unskilled occupations.

The classification is arbitrary and takes no account of personal circumstances (housing, family size, private income, etc.) other than those indicated by the stated occupation. Nevertheless it has provided much valuable information about the association between disease and social circumstances and is still a useful research tool.

Infant mortality particularly after the neonatal period increases regularly and sharply with social class, so that a child born into the family of an unskilled worker in 1971 who survived the first 4 weeks of life was 5 times as likely to die in the next 11 months as a child born into a professional family. A similar difference existed in 1921, but infant mortality has declined so much in all classes that by 1971 the infant in social class V had a better expectation of reaching its first birthday than the infant in social class I of 40 years earlier. Such differences exist between countries too, for example in 1980 infant mortality in the Scandinavian countries was between 7 and 8 per thousand live births (compared with 12 in Britain) but in many other countries it was over 100 and in parts of Africa, South America and Asia, for which statistics are not available, was probably over 300.

That the percentage difference between mortality in class I and V in England and Wales should have remained about the same throughout a period when infant mortality as a whole declined dramatically was unexpected. In the first place welfare legislation (child benefits, social security, health services, local authority housing assistance etc.) was thought to have been of more benefit to the poorer sections of the community than to the better off and this might have been expected to reduce the social gradient of infant mortality. And secondly, there was more scope for reduction of mortality from infection and other 'preventable' causes in class V than in class I. Yet because the percentage decline of total infant mortality has been about the same for both classes I and V, the proportionate decline from 'preventable' causes has evidently been greater for class I. Two possible influences may be mentioned in explanation of this apparent paradox; the better educated and well-to-do parents have earlier access to and make better use of social and medical advances; and because of improvements in the educational system among other things, there is more social mobility now than formerly, so that those in class V today are more likely to be there because of ill-health or lack of ability than those in class V 60 years ago.

Some causes of first year death show much greater social class differentiation than infant mortality as a whole. The death rate from both acute bronchitis and pneumonia is five times greater in class V than in class I, a striking illustration of the importance of social circumstances in determining whether or not infants die from what are now treatable diseases.

It is commonly believed by the general public that dying of high blood pressure and of coronary disease or stroke, its sequelae, or of duodenal ulcer is the lot of the business executive working under stress. Table 6.7 shows that this is not the case and that for all these conditions there is a trend rising from class I to V which, with the exception of ischaemic heart disease, is consistent from class to class. No individual disease shows a consistent trend in the opposite direction, although this is found when all neoplasms in women are combined. This is shown in table 6.7 which also includes some diseases in which the pattern is irregular, but the SMR is higher in class I than in class V. For some conditions such as bronchitis social class gradients have been constant throughout the years since 1921, when mortality data were first published by occupation and social class, but for others this has not been the case. Table 6.8 shows three examples of diseases for which the reported mortality has changed in this way. The differences may not be real, however, and changes in the International Classification of Disease and in diagnostic fashion have both been offered as explanations for the differences between the social distribution of acute coronary disease in 1931 and 1971. Explanations for the shifts in diabetes and cancer of the rectum (table 6.8) are conjectural although it is unlikely that either is a statistical aretefact.

Table 6.7 Standardized mortality ratios for certain causes by social class (aged 15-64 England and Wales 1970-72)

ICD No.	Cause of death	Social class I	II	IIIN	IIIM	IV	V
Some SMRs which increase with declining social class (men only)							
010-012	Tuberculosis of respiratory system	26	41	84	89	124	254
151	Malignant neoplasms of stomach	50	66	79	118	125	147
161	Malignant neoplasm of larynx	65	65	81	102	132	194
162	Malignant neoplasm of bronchus, trachea and lung	53	68	84	118	123	143
400-404	Hypertensive disease	71	85	104	104	112	141
410-414	Ischaemic heart disease	88	91	114	107	108	111
430-438	Cerebrovascular disease	80	86	98	106	111	136
532	Ulcer of the duodenum	45	67	81	103	115	201
Some SMRs which do not increase with declining social class							
186	Malignant neoplasm of testis	157	106	125	89	105	86
173	Malignant neoplasm of skin	118	117	107	96	90	113
446	Polyarteritis nodosa and allied conditions	126	117	109	94	111	81
574, 575	Cholelithiasis and cholecystitis	114	102	99	88	127	80
	All malignant neoplasms in women	122	115	108	101	96	87
174	Malignant neoplasm of female breast—married	117	112	116	109	108	92
	unmarried	131	117	117	111	107	120

Sex Differences in Disease Incidence

All countries with reasonably complete registration report an excess of males at birth (about 105 male for every 100 female infants). Throughout postnatal life, however, most cause specific death rates are higher for males than for females, with the result that in elderly populations there are normally more females than males. A measure of the sex difference in mortality is provided by expectation of life at birth, which in 1979 was 5 years less for males than for females (70 and 75 years respectively). It may be good fiscal policy, but it is otherwise anomalous that women should become pensionable at 60, when they have an expectation of a further 21 years of life; while men must wait until 65, when their expectation of life has dwindled to 13 years.

Table 6.8 Some examples of changes through time of patterns of mortality by social class (SMRs for males aged 15-64, England and Wales 1970-1972)

ICD No.	Condition	Social class I	II	IIIN	IIIM	IV	V
19	Angina pectoris						
	1930-32	237	147	96 (IIIN and IIIM combined)		67	67
	Acute myocardial infarction						
	1970-2	88	92	115	107	108	108
250	Diabetes mellitus						
	1921-23	129	149	93 (IIIN and IIIM combined)		75	66
	1970-72	84	93	111	98	111	128
154	Malignant neoplasm of the rectum						
	1959-63	79	89	106 (IIIN and IIIM combined)		98	120
	1970-72	84	90	103	114	106	108

The reasons for the excess male mortality in postnatal life are complex. Table 6.9 shows that in England and Wales at the present time the heaviest contributions to the excess are made by ischaemic heart disease, cancer of the lung and bronchitis. For these major causes of death much of the difference between the sexes is attributable to the different environments in which men and women live and work and to differences in their social habits (occupation, diet, tobacco, alcohol etc.). On the other hand some of the variation in mortality experience is clearly biological in origin. Although as we have seen cancer of the reproductive organs is causing more deaths in both sexes, cancer of the breast and genital organs is much commoner in females, as are endocrinological, and particularly thyroid disorders. For many sex differences there is so far no obvious explanation.

Although as we have seen there are more liveborn males than females, more males than females are stillborn (about 105 to 100) and there is some evidence of an excess of male abortions. This suggests that more males than females are conceived. This possibility can be reconciled with the chromosome mechanism of sex determination, which supposes the production of equal numbers of X and Y bearing spermatozoa, by assuming the presence of sex-linked, gamete-lethal genes or of environmental influences affecting unequally the mobility or fertilizing ability of the two types of spermatozoa. It is not certain, however, that there is an excess of males at conception. Although more males are stillborn, among

Table 6.9 Sex differences in mortality rates (England and Wales 1980)

ICD No.		Crude death rate per million		
Some conditions with relatively high male mortality		Males	Females	M/F
	Malignant neoplasm of:			
162	Trachea, bonchus, lung	1,117	332	3.4
188	Bladder	123	51	2.4
140-149	Buccal cavity and pharynx	40	25	1.6
151	Stomach	267	178	1.5
154	Rectum and rectosigmoid junction	138	115	1.2
490-493	Bronchitis, emphysema, asthma	882	299	2.9
E810-819	Motorvehicle traffic accidents	168	68	2.5
010-019	Tuberculosis	16	8	2.0
E950-959	Suicide	110	67	1.6
410-414	Ischaemic heart disease	3,738	2,561	1.5
Some conditions with relatively high female mortality				F/M
	Malignant neoplasm of:			
174	Breast	3	482	160.7
193	Thyroid	4	10	2.5
156	Gall bladder and bile ducts	5	13	2.6
180-186	Genital organs	224	280	1.2
240-246	Thyroid disease other than neoplasm	4	17	4.2
393-398	Chronic rheumatic heart disease	38	92	2.4
E880-887	Accidental falls	63	108	1.7
250	Diabetes mellitus	83	110	1.3
430-438	Cerebrovascular disease	1,140	1,746	1.5
574-576	Diseases of the gall bladder and biliary tract	16	22	1.4

stillbirths there are 3 times more females than males with gross malformations of the central nervous system (namely anencephaly and spina bifida). Information about the sex-ratio of abortions, although suggesting an excess of males, is not very reliable, for collections of early embryos are almost always unrepresentative. In view of the high abortion rates in early pregnancy, no great excess of females among early abortions would be required to make the observed preponderance of males at birth consistent with equal numbers of males and females at conception.

Although mortality is higher for males than females throughout life, the reverse appears to be true of morbidity. As table 5.4 shows, females consult general practitioners more than males at a ratio of 3 to 2; in addition they are admitted to hospital more frequently, and sickness surveys all show a considerable excess of morbidity among females. The reasons are even more complex than the reasons for the mortality differences. It does not follow that women are more often sick or disabled although some studies suggest that they are. The explanation may lie in part in a sex difference in awareness of minor departures from health, and in readiness to seek medical advice. And since fewer women are in full-time employment, they have more opportunity to consult their general practitioners.

Further Reading

Morris J. N. (1975) *The Uses of Epidemiology*, 3rd edition. E. & S. Livingstone, Edinburgh.

Townsend P. and Davidson N. (1982) *Inequalities in Health*. Penguin Books Ltd., Harmondsworth, Middlesex.

7

The Role of Clinical Medicine

This chapter examines medical advances in the care of some important non-infective conditions, the postponement of death in other fatal disease, and the treatment of non-fatal disease. As we have shown the chief requirement for an understanding of health in the past is an explanation of the rise and fall of infectious diseases. In relation to the future, however, assessment of achievements with non-communicable diseases is, arguably, more significant. In developed countries, they are now the predominant causes of sickness and death, and what has been achieved in the understanding and control of such conditions is therefore a valuable, if incomplete, indication of future possibilities.

The cure of non-infective disease

Unfortunately it is very difficult to assess the achievements. In the first place, because non-communicable diseases vary greatly in severity, duration and the extent of associated morbidity and disability, mortality is a far less satisfactory index than in the case of the infections, where the outcome was usually either death or complete recovery. Secondly, many clinical procedures have never been satisfactorily evaluated, and their use has been based on clinical impressions or indirect laboratory evidence. A short assessment of the medical contribution to longevity and the improvement of health can therefore be little more than a list of conditions in which clinical intervention is generally believed to be effective.

In his thoughtful examination of medical advances in the period 1950-75, after discussing the management of infectious diseases Lewis Thomas a contemporary American medical philosopher concluded that the list of decisive new accomplishments is not much longer than the contents of the following paragraph.

"There have been a few other examples of technology improvement, comparable in decisive effectiveness, since 1950, but the best of these have been for relatively uncommon illnesses. Childhood leukemia and certain solid tumours in children, for example, can now be cured by chemotherapy in a substantial proportion of cases, but there are only a few thousand of these per year in the country [the USA]. Endocrine-replacement therapy has become highly effective and relatively inexpensive ('relative' considering the cost of caring for untreated endocrine abnormalities) for a variety of disorders involving the adrenals, pituitary, parathyroid, ovary, and thyroid; in particular, the biochemical treatment of thyroid dysfunction has improved markedly. Hematology has offered new and effective replacement treatment for certain anemias. Immunological prophylaxis now prevents most cases of hemolytic disease of the newborn. Progress in anesthesia, electrolyte physiology, and cardiopulmonary physiology has greatly advanced the field of surgery, so that reparative and other procedures can now be done which formerly were technically impossible.*"

His paragraph provides a reasonable summary of decisive advances, some of which were launched before 1950. To them should be added the treatment of hypertension. Successful measures also include the treatment of accidents, defibrillation and surgical treatment of cardiac and pulmonary conditions, relief of prostatic obstruction, renal transplants and cure of a minority of cancers. Treatment of obstetric conditions may be life-saving, as the valuable investigations of maternal mortality in Britain have shown. So too is intervention in other emergencies such as abdominal obstruction, and perforated peptic ulcer. There are many therapies (referred to below) which postpone rather than prevent death from a specific cause, or provide relief of symptoms without affecting expectation of life, which in many disorders is not threatened.

The importance of these advances is that they are not restricted to preventable disorders, such as accidents, which in an ideal world would not occur. They include conditions which are relatively intractable. The prevention of rhesus haemolytic disease is a remarkable example of an advance made possible by a combination of genetic and clinical knowledge. The identification and abortion of a fetus affected by Down's disease is another solution of an apparently intractable problem made possible by application of genetic knowledge. Equally impressive in a quite different way is the immense technical accomplishment which restores a child with a patent ductus arteriosus or an atrial septal defect to a life of normal duration and quality. Such achievements suggest that further investigation may make it possible to prevent, eliminate or treat success-

* Thomas, L., 'On the science and technology of medicine' in *Daedalus* (Winter, 1977), p. 37.

fully some of the most difficult disorders with which medicine is now confronted.

Postponement of Death

The use of the decline of mortality as the main index of improvement in health is sometimes said to overlook the contribution of medical intervention which postpones death but does not change its cause. Diabetes is cited as an example of a disease in which the extension of life is not reflected in the trend of mortality, among other reasons because the same cause often appears later on a death certificate.

The interpretation of death-rates is admittedly complex. As we have seen they are based on the number of dying (the numerator) over the total population (the denominator). If deaths from a disease are reduced, the death-rate from that disease and the death-rate from all causes, assuming no other changes have occurred, both fall, because the numerator is smaller and because a larger proportion of the population is still alive the denominator is larger. This is true whether the cause of death is eliminated, as in typhoid, or postponed, as in diabetes and ischaemic heart disease. Moreover, in both cases the rates are permanently lowered, because the number dying in a year remains smaller in relation to the population at risk. Hence the postponement and prevention of death from a specific cause are both reflected in the index.

We have also seen that when examining the trend of mortality over a considerable period it is important to standardize for age changes in the population. The need for this procedure is evident from a comparison of death-rates from diabetes before and after insulin. In England and Wales the crude rates were 107 per million in 1911-20 and 125 in 1973, which would seem to imply that mortality increased over this period. When standardized to the 1973 population, the death-rate in 1911-20 was 188.

However, standardization does not remove all the difficulties of interpretation. Diabetes appears to be more common than in the past, but it is not possible to dissociate the effects of improved survival, better diagnosis and possibly other influences. Survival of diabetics has been gravely prejudiced by the increased frequency of smoking during the period when effective treatment by insulin and oral diabetic drugs has been available. And finally for diabetes in particular, mortality statistics are very unreliable, because many diabetics die from arterial degeneration and these deaths are by international convention attributed to disease of the kidneys, heart and brain.

With due regard for these difficulties, useful evidence of the effect of treatment can be obtained from examination of age of death of diabetics. Figure 7.1 shows (for England and Wales) the number of survivors of cohorts of 1,000 females exposed to the mortality rates of 1911-20 and 1973. The difference in mean age at death at the 2 periods was approximately 10 years.

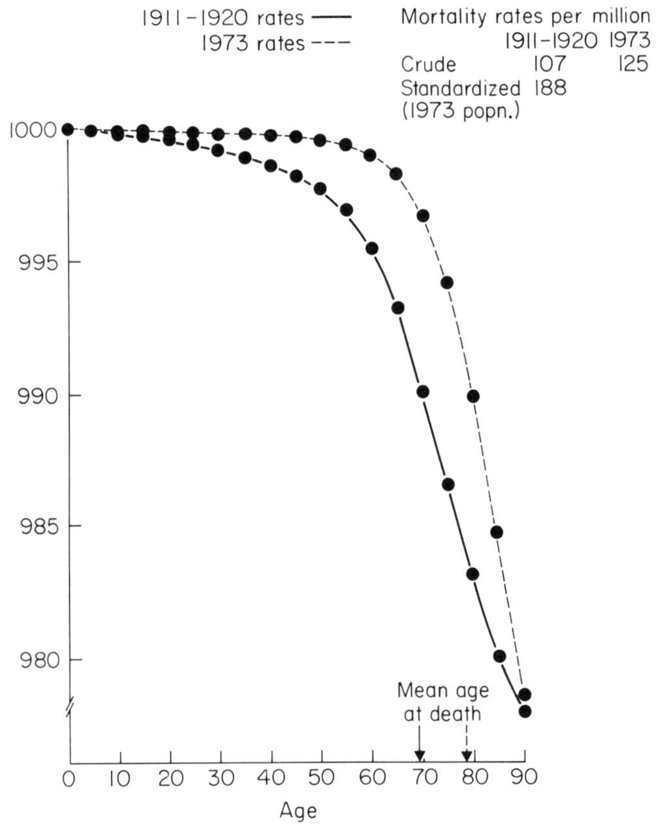

Figure 7. 1. Survivors from a cohort of 1000 females exposed only to mortality from diabetes at rates of 1911-20 and 1973.

It may seem surprising that mean age at death could be so late—nearly 70 in 1911-20 and nearly 80 in 1973. This is explained partly by the fact that even before insulin most diabetics died relatively late in life. The age at death in 1911-20, and the extension of life which has resulted from treatment, would of course be vastly different if the analysis were restricted to juvenile diabetics. But the late age of death is also determined by the fact that deaths of diabetics from all causes other than diabetes could not be included in the cohort, and those dying from a single cause, diabetes or any other, are highly and favourably selected in respect of length of life.

Treatment of Non-Fatal Diseases

When presenting the results of his experiments on himself, a distinguished biologist seemed to say: Take one average human being, for example, J. B. S. Haldane. Adopting the same unconventional statistical approach, we can illustrate the relation between morbidity and mortality by considering the experience of one lakeland poet. William Wordsworth followed most of the rules for health now advocated by life stylists. He did not smoke or drink; unlike some of his best friends he avoided opium; he lived and worked in the open air, added little weight and took an amount of exercise which would have daunted most joggers. De Quincey (who did take opium) estimated that Wordsworth walked between 175,000 and 180,000 miles during his life, and if so he must have averaged nearly 10 miles a day for 60 years.

Predictably, according to the health rules, he had a long life. However, he and his sister both suffered a good deal from minor morbidity—headaches, toothaches, bowel upsets and numerous other unspecified complaints—recorded meticulously by Dorothy in her *Journals* during their years in Dove Cottage. As for his mental health, it has been suggested that he had an abnormal relationship with his sister, but although many of her references to him are highly suggestive, there is no evidence that it was ever consummated. What Wordsworth's history illustrates is that there is no necessary close relation between morbidity and mortality. The diseases that diminish the quality of daily living are rarely those that shorten our lives.

In the present context, however, we are concerned with medical achievement through treatment of diseases and disabilities that do not kill. In this assessment account must be taken of both the frequency and the seriousness of a condition: the common cold affects most people fairly frequently; rheumatoid arthritis and schizophrenia are much less common but far more disabling for those who are afflicted.

With one notable exception, there is no wholly effective treatment for the non-fatal illnesses which trouble most people from day to day. These are the acute respiratory infections, digestive disorders, the skeletal and muscular disabilities referred to as rheumatism, and a variety of mental illnesses, particularly the neuroses and psychoneuroses. The exception is dental disease. As the history of many famous people illustrates, dental diseases were formerly among the most common causes of serious discomfort; today they can be prevented and treated, and in the 1949 Survey of Sickness in Britain they accounted for only 4 per cent of the illnesses of which people complained most frequently. It would be interesting to have an estimate of their frequency in the past, say in the age of Pericles or the court of Louis XIV. Louis himself suffered grievously from his teeth, and no doubt would gladly have exchanged his painters, dramatists, one or two mistresses and several peers of France for a modern dentist.

Of course a good deal can be done to relieve discomfort from the common complaints; it might also be said that many, although by no means all of them, are transient and present no permanent threat to the quality or duration of life.

There have been advances in treatment of many uncomfortable and, in some cases, disabling conditions, including hernias, piles, varicose veins, Parkinson's disease, pemphigus and ulcerative colitis. Although neither rheumatoid arthritis nor osteoarthrosis can be cured, symptomatic relief can be provided and surgical treatment is sometimes remarkably successful, particularly by replacement of the diseased hip, one of the outstanding achievements of contemporary medicine. The major psychoses, schizophrenia and manic-depression, are still unexplained, but drug therapy has been beneficial and, by making patients more manageable, has reduced the difficulties involved in their care. There has been little advance in the treatment of mentally subnormal patients, although they can be assisted by educational and occupational opportunities as well as personal care.

Because the non-fatal diseases vary greatly in frequency, duration and severity, achievements in their treatment are difficult to summarize. It is a recognition of the difficulties they present rather than a criticism of medical research and practice to say that while symptomatic relief can be provided for some, perhaps all patients, with some notable exceptions the underlying pathological conditions cannot at present be cured. This is true both of the relatively benign diseases which trouble most people from day to day, and of the less common causes of serious disease and disability.

Further Reading

Hampton J. R. (1983) The end of clinical freedom. *British Medical Journal* **2**, 1237.

Illich I. (1976) *Limits to Medicine. Dream Mirage or Nemesis?* Penguin Books Ltd., Harmondsworth, Middlesex.

McKeown T. (1979) *The Role of Medicine.* Basil Blackwell, Oxford.

Thomas L. (1984) *The Youngest Science: Notes of a Medicine Watcher.* Oxford University Press, Oxford.

2

Methods of Promoting Health

8

Society and Protection from Disease

A classification of prevention which is widely used is that of the late H. R. Leavell*, formerly Professor of Public Health at Harvard, who described three levels based as follows:

1. *Primary prevention*
Health education, genetic counselling, etc.
Specific protection against disease which includes immunization, protection from carcinogens, etc.
2. *Secondary prevention*
Early diagnosis and prompt treatment; this includes screening.
Limitation of disability.
3. *Tertiary prevention*
Rehabilitation, prevention of relapse.

These are based on the natural history of disease and their widespread application is a measure of their value not only in a public health but in a clinical setting because most activities at the second level and all of those at the tertiary level comprise routine care of the sick rather than prevention of sickness.

In this book our central concern is the origins and control of disease in society at large, rather than in its individual members. Just as the scheme in figure 1.2 serves as a basis for understanding the causes of disease, so it can serve as a basis for bringing about its prevention and promoting health. We have already seen that the severity of most infectious disease has been greatly reduced by indirect means, principally the improvement of diet. This and other purely social and economic factors still have an important role to play in the promotion of health. As we indicated in Chapter 1 we have defined the ways in which the health of

* Leavell H. R. (1953) *Preventive medicine for the doctor and his community*. McGraw-Hill Book Co., New York.

society can be protected and they can be grouped under two headings:

1. primary protection which controls factors that cause disease without the direct participation of individual members of society;
2. secondary protection which can only be brought about by deliberate individual action or change in behaviour.

Primary protection

Reference to the concept of primary protection has already been made in Chapter 1. It is an approach which has led to control of the inanimate environment by providing clean water safe sewerage and clean air, and aspects of the animate environment have been made safe by the control of arthropod vectors of disease such as the anopheline mosquito which carries malaria and *Aedes aegypti* which transmits yellow fever and dengue to man.

There are generally four steps in the provision of primary protection, namely:

1. epidemiological and laboratory research which establish the existence of a causal relationship between a clearly identifiable component of the environment and a disease or a group of diseases, which are very likely to follow exposure to the factor and have a high case fatality rate. For instance, water or food contaminated with *Salmonella typhi* or *Vibrio cholerae* or air laden with gaseous or particulate matters which cause a wide range of lung diseases;
2. development of procedures capable of controlling the noxious environmental agent(s). This usually involves sciences other than medicine such as chemistry, biology or engineering;
3. drafting and passage of laws to make the control procedures enforceable. This is often a slow process because social change and expenditure of tax revenue will be involved which experience has shown sections of the public and many politicians may oppose. Evidence indicating that children can safely be protected from dental caries by adding small quantities of fluoride to the drinking water is overwhelming, yet a small, highly organized group of people with conscientious objections has for years successfully blocked the introduction of the necessary regulations in many British local authorities. Indeed in one borough which was practising fluoridation the group had this regulation repealed (see Chapter 9);
4. introduction of the programme which will probably not be in the

hands of doctors, but of scientists, engineers and administrators. Primary protection is also well established in industry where a complex code of regulations and procedures has been established through the years to reduce to a minimum the risk of accidents and of diseases caused by substances and equipment to which the workers are exposed.

Thus, there are many highly efficient and effective ways in which society can promote the health of its members without them necessarily being aware that anything is being done for them let alone doing anything themselves. In countries where they are available people take clean water and clean air for granted.

Secondary protection

Deliberate action from individuals some of which may be inconvenient or even unpleasant can in a wide variety of ways further enhance health. We have seen how the availability of good food has probably done more to improve health than any other single factor. This in terms of the scheme in figure 1.2 can be described as modifying the phenotype; phenotypic modification can also be brought about by means of artificially stimulating antibody formation. In the first instance co-operation is immediately gratifying but in the second it is not, partly because injections are painful, but also because successful immunization programmes of young children depend upon parents travelling to attend a clinic, and even in a school attended by a doctor parental consent must be obtained before a vaccine can be administered. Similarly programmes which set out to screen an adult population, for example for hypertension or carcinoma of the cervix depend on the willingness and ability to co-operate of each individual in the group which is to be protected. Unwillingness or even inability to act in the interests of health is evident in exaggerated from when the noxious environmental agent is the basis of a pleasurable or addictive habit as is the case with tobacco smoke or alcohol.

The law can influence individual health behaviour, however, and it can do this in a variety of ways. Direct penalization of people who are considered to be putting themselves at unnecessary risk, such as those who do not wear seat belts in cars, is one which has been adopted by many societies. Others include control of the sale of alcoholic beverages by limiting the hours during which they can be sold; and with them and tobacco by raising the cost by high taxation and setting out special regulations as to how and where commercial advertisements for their sale can be displayed.

Secondary protection is also promoted by health education which has been classified as taking three forms:

1. learning about the body and how to look after it;
2. providing information and advice about access to health care resources and their most appropriate use;
3. learning about the structures and processes in the environment at large which damage health.

Clearly a proper understanding of the second and third will depend upon some understanding of the first, and understanding alone is not sufficient to provide motivation. Nevertheless health education is one of the most important ways of changing health behaviour and if enough individuals give up smoking, reduce their weight or take more exercise for such behaviour to become fashionable, then social pressure is added to understanding, and helps to motivate those who find a change in behaviour difficult.

Integration and co-ordination of primary and secondary protection

Situations commonly arise when health promotion and disease prevention require the integration and co-ordination of both methods of protection. For instance improvement of the living or the working environment can offer primary protection by the provision of, for example, clean water, good lighting, effective exhaust systems, or structures free from damp, but their influence can be greatly enhanced by appropriate behaviour such as the wearing of eyeshields and other forms of protective clothing, cleanliness of the hands (important in the home, but because of the numbers at risk even more important in the food industry) and so on. Neither these secondary nor the primary procedures are sufficient if implemented singly. Finally an improved environment can have an important direct effect. Well designed structures in a harmonious urban or rural setting can go a long way towards promoting a sense of well being and contentment even though not clearly associated with the absence of any particular disease.

Further Reading

Smith A. (1982) *Recent Advances in Community Medicine, Volume 2*. Edinburgh: Churchill Livingstone. Chapters 2 and 3.

9

Control of the Genetic Constitution of Human Populations

Control of Genetic Stock

When they wish to improve their stocks, plant and animal breeders do not hesitate to manipulate the environment, or to control reproduction by selection of one or both parents. Choice of one or both these methods is determined by effectiveness and cost. The marked improvement in the quality of livestock which followed the introduction of root crops in the eighteenth century is an example of the first method; the modern through-bred racehorse and improvements in the protein content of maize are examples of the second.

It should be noted that the use of selection as a means of improving crops and livestock preceded the establishment of the science of genetics. To farmers who knew nothing of genes and chromosomes it was clearly worthwhile to select parents on the basis of their characteristics or those of their offspring. In practice this procedure has not been greatly altered by genetical knowledge. Breeders of racehorses still assess the value of a sire according to both his own record in competition and the performance of his offspring.

The characteristics of human beings have also been determined by selection. Infectious disease, for example, must have had a profound influence on human evolution, since it killed large numbers of people—until recently the majority of those born—before they could reproduce. There is, however, an important difference between this kind of selection and the purposeful selection practised by farmers. With rare exceptions, such as the Inca royal family, there has been no conscious control of human breeding, and to a visitor from Mars it would no doubt seem remarkable that humans have not applied to their own kind the methods which have had such conspicuous success with plants and other animals.

We shall consider the reasons for this restraint in relation to three themes: ethics; effectiveness; and desirability.

Ethics

The first question is an ethical one: Would it be right to control human breeding? It is not surprising that there are wide differences of opinion about the answer. On religious grounds some people believe that in no circumstances would it be right to interfere with the 'natural' pattern of reproduction. Others consider that the evolution of the human race is too important to be determined by the sexual attraction between two individuals, and that human beings should eventually transfer their reproductive functions to the laboratory.

These are extreme views and most people take an intermediate position. While they do not object in principle to some control of breeding, they are concerned about the methods of achieving it and the purposes for which it is to be employed. They are particularly doubtful about the use of compulsory powers.

Effectiveness

The second question to be considered is whether control of breeding would be effective. This question must be made more precise. Would it be possible either to eliminate or reduce the frequency of undesirable genotypes, or to increase the frequency of desirable genotypes? In relation to the first question we shall refer separately to the few conditions which appear to be attributable to a single gene, and to the much larger number including most important diseases which are not.

With due regard for a reservation referred to below (mutation), in the case of conditions due to a single gene the effectiveness of suppressing reproduction depends upon the extent to which it is possible to identify those who carry the gene. By preventing reproduction of affected persons it would be possible to eliminate dominant genotypes which are completely manifested before reproductive age. This requirement is more or less met in only a few rare abnormalities, for example in achondroplasia, and in a certain type of juvenile cataract. In most dominant genotypes the requirement is not met, either because the abnormality is not completely manifested in all environments, or because it does not appear until after reproduction. Huntington's chorea is an example of a condition due to a dominant gene which cannot be eliminated in this manner because it becomes evident in middle life when those affected may have reproduced.

As a rule single genes which cause abnormalities are recessive, and manifested only in the homozygous state. The number of individuals who carry the gene but are not themselves affected (the heterozygotes) is much larger than the number of affected (the homozygotes). For example only about 1 in 20,000 individuals exhibit albinism (i.e. are homozygous), whereas about 1 in 70 carry the gene but are not affected (are heterozygous). Hence only a small proportion of those affected have affected parents, the suppression of whose reproduction would have relatively little effect on the frequency of the gene. Reduction of the incidence of a sex-linked recessive condition, such as haemophilia, would be more feasible, but would require restriction of breeding of daughters and sisters of affected males, as well as of the affected males themselves.

We have so far ignored the fact that genetically-determined abnormalities also result from mutation, the reservation referred to above. The mutation rates so far estimated in man are relatively low, but they are by no means insignificant. In haemophilia, for example, the frequency of mutation is apparently high enough to maintain the incidence of the disease at a fairly constant level, in spite of the fact that until recently most affected males died before reproductive age. Control of reproduction would not reduce the incidence of a genetic condition below the level which results from mutation.

In most human diseases the genetic mechanisms are not understood. But it is clear that they are not attributable to a single gene, and that they are influenced to a considerable degree by the environment. There is therefore no basis for exact prediction of the effects of control of reproduction although in most cases they would undoubtedly be small. For example, most mentally handicapped persons have normal parents, and prevention of reproduction of those affected would have little influence on the incidence of mental handicap in the general population.

It is even less certain that control of breeding would make it possible to increase the frequency of desirable genotypes. There are some qualities—honesty, intelligence, vitality, etc.—which most people would regard as desirable. But little is known about the respective contributions of inheritance and environment in determining these qualities, and nothing is known about the related genes. It seems probable that if parents were selected with no other object than an increase in stature it could soon be achieved. It is far from certain that the same is true of intelligence, or of the other unmeasured, and perhaps unmeasurable, qualities regarded as desirable. Moreover although cattle are bred with a single object such as increased milk yield or improved quality of beef, no single object would be acceptable in man. It is also conceivable that improvement of one feature might be accompanied by deterioration of another.

We may summarize our conclusions about the possibility of control of human inheritance by quoting a statement by a group of well-known geneticists. 'At the present level of genetic knowledge we cannot improve the genes with which we are born, and there is little we can do to determine which genes we pass on to our children.'

Desirability

Finally, if it were permissible and effective, would it be desirable to control human inheritance? Again the question must be put more precisely. No one is likely to quarrel with the statement that the elimination of many genetically-determined diseases and abnormalities would be desirable if brought about by acceptable methods. But some people also suggest that it would be useful to increase the proportion of genetically well-endowed people. This claim requires closer scrutiny.

The belief that it would be desirable to increase the proportion of gifted people presupposes that improvement in human affairs is at present restricted by lack of them. It is difficult to accept this view. The fact that achievement has been outstanding only in certain places and for short periods—in Italy during the Renaissance, for example—suggests that at most times the environment is unfavourable. The alternative explanation—that there have been some remarkable mutations at different times in history—is not credible. Hence it seems probable that there is a large reserve of ability which is not exploited.

Moreover it might not be possible to provide suitable employment and rewards for a larger number of gifted people. There are perhaps few jobs which could not be done better by intelligent than by less intelligent people; but many occupations already demand abilities which they do not fully reward and others give little satisfaction because they do not use fully the capacities of those employed in them. Modification of the proportion of individuals with different levels of ability might therefore create more problems than it would solve.

Controlling the Individual Genotype

Francis Galton (1822-1911) developed 'the study of agencies under social control, that may improve or impair the racial (i.e. inherited) qualities of future generations, either physically or mentally'; this he called eugenics. Galton's views about how this was to be done changed considerably during his own lifetime, as he became more aware of difficulties. In general his emphasis passed from the negative to the positive aspect of the subject; from concern about those who should not breed, to interest in those who should. This trend characterized the "eugenics movement", which has latterly been interested in social policies which might encourage "desirable" parents to have larger families.

The discussion which follows is concerned with the limitation of genetic disease. We shall consider three approaches, prevention of conception, termination of pregnancy, and withholding treatment of affected individuals after birth. It should be noted that in the progression from conception to pregnancy to birth, the ethical acceptability of intervention diminishes; contraception is more acceptable than induced abortion and abortion than withholding treatment. But in the same progression the effectiveness of the procedures increases, for whereas withholding treatment can be restricted to abnormal births, this is less true of abortion and clearly does not apply to contraception. Since the relative specificities of the three procedures are known, the choice between them is more an ethical than a technical matter.

Prevention of conception

(*a*) *Compulsory*. The most severe measure is sterilization of persons believed to be unfit to reproduce. It is not practised in Britain, but has been used in Germany, and in the United States where many States have laws which permit or require sterilization of individuals affected by certain conditions. About twenty-four conditions are included, but as each American State makes it own decision, only a few are common to most States—idiocy, imbecility, feeblemindedness, insanity, and epilepsy. We should note three points about these classes. In the first place, none of them is a genetic entity; for example, the mentally subnormal include a few types which have a simple genetic basis, and a very much larger number which do not. Secondly, with perhaps the exception of epilepsy, little or nothing is known about the genetic background of the majority of cases included in each class. And thirdly, it is very doubtful whether suppression of reproduction of affected persons would have much effect on the incidence of the defects. It should of course be said that sterilization is sometimes advocated not only on genetic grounds, but also on the social grounds that individuals suffering from these conditions are incapable of providing a reasonable home environment for their children.

An alternative method used to suppress reproduction is to segregate affected individuals, at least during their reproductive years. This procedure makes it possible to provide supervision and care; but since it requires separation of the sexes, and restriction of leave, it can hardly be considered more humane than sterilization. If a choice were to be made between segregation and sterilization, it would seem most reasonable to base it upon the affected individual's need for institutional care rather than upon the relative effectiveness of the two methods in suppressing reproduction.

(*b*) *Voluntary*. Another approach is the provision of advice to parents or prospective parents about the risk of occurrence of undesirable traits in their children. This is known as genetic counselling and there are now consultants in the National Health Service who specialize in it. The question may be raised by persons about to be married, by married couples contemplating pregnancy, or by a woman who is pregnant. The common reasons for concern are that parents or prospective parents are closely related (usually cousins); that one or both have an undesirable trait; or that previous children or other relatives have had such a trait.

The expectation of a reduction of incidence of disease by discouraging parents likely to have affected offspring seemed realistic when genes were believed to be numbered in thousands rather than millions, and when distinction between normal and abnormal genes was thought always to be possible. Recent knowledge of the nature of genetic disease has made it difficult to see how a population can benefit substantially from attempts to influence fertility on medical grounds. This approach is feasible in the rare disorders due to dominant genes; it may also have a limited use after the birth of a child with an abnormality such as anencephalus, the genetical background of which is obscure, but for which increased risk of recurrence in later children of the same sibship has been estimated empirically to be high. But even if applied consistently such restrictions on reproduction could only make a trivial contribution to the reduction of incidence of disease; moreover, they would lead to the prevention of a large number of normal pregnancies.

Screening and termination of pregnancies

Although fetal diagnosis has long been practised by obstetricians concerned with the management of pregnancy and labour, it has only recently been extended to identification of genetic disorders by amniocentesis. But from the time (1956) when it became possible to define the sex of the fetus from the presence or absence of sex chromatin in fetal cells in the amniotic fluid, it was recognized that methods might be developed which would permit the identification and abortion of some abnormal embryos. Since then fetal cells have been shown to be capable of multiplication *in vitro*, allowing the study of any characteristics revealed by tissue culture, either in the cytoplasm or the nuclei, in addition to the analysis of the amniotic fluid. These methods can now be used in chromosomal disorders, such as Down's syndrome and in certain genic disorders, such as Tay-Sachs disease and gargoylism. At present, they are impractical in the commoner conditions such as fibrocystic disease, phenylketonuria and haemoglobinopathies.

Unfortunately there are considerable difficulties in making full use of this knowledge. In the first place, the procedure has been generally practicable only from the 14th week of pregnancy, when amniocentesis becomes reasonably safe, until about the 21st week, when termination becomes decreasingly acceptable. However a new technique involving chorionic biopsy in the early weeks of pregnancy is extending the scope of antenatal diagnosis. Secondly, screening of all pregnancies is not at present feasible, and when investigation is restricted to pregnancies of mothers who have had an abnormal birth, the reduction in the frequency of chromosomal and genic disorders is relatively small. Its value is undoubtedly greatest in relation to a condition such as haemophilia, where a substantial reduction in incidence could be achieved by preventing haemophiliacs from having daughters.

Withholding treatment after birth

The procedures referred to above have four major limitations: (*a*) even if fully applied they would not prevent the conception and birth of a large number of abnormal children; (*b*) their full application would require either avoidance of conception or abortion of many normal individuals; (*c*) amniocentesis followed by abortion involves risks for the mother which, if not great, are not negligible; and (*d*) the technique of amniocentesis itself exposes the fetus to some risk.

These objections are absent or much less serious in the case of withholding treatment. This procedure does not carry with it a risk of destruction of normal births nor does it present a physical risk to the mother. It is true that not all major abnormalities can be recognized soon after birth, but the proportion missed is much smaller than before or during pregnancy. The objections to it as a means of eliminating serious malformations are essentially of a personal and ethical kind. The loss of a child after birth is much more stressful for parents than contraception or abortion. Death of a live born child is unacceptable on ethical and legal grounds, particularly when it is caused by active measures. To many people it is also ethically unacceptable when it results from withholding treatment. These issues were touched upon in Chapters 3 and 4.

Further Reading

Bresler J. B. (ed.) (1973) *Genetics and Society*. Addison Wesley Publishing Co., Reading, Mass.

Burnet M. (1971) *Genes, Dreams and Realities*. Medical and Technical Publishing Co. Ltd., Aylesbury, Bucks.

Dobzhansky T. (1946) *Heredity and the Nature of Man*. Harcourt, Brace and World, New York.

Primary Protection

10

Water

Without water there can be no life. The need for it directs the wanderings of nomadic tribes and determines the site and size of agricultural communities. Navigable rivers have been the cradles of civilization and population growth has often been influenced by the extent to which arid but potentially fertile land bordering rivers can be irrigated. The Tigris and the Euphrates watered Babylonian civilization and Egypt is still dependent upon the Nile.

For the maintenance of health, particularly in congested urban communities, a good supply of clean water is essential. If the supply is inadequate for personal and public hygiene (bathing, washing clothes and domestic utensils, cleaning streets and removing sewage and trade effluents) the spread of diseases associated with domestic and communal squalor is encouraged; and if it is not protected against contamination with pathogenic organisms and toxic substances, outbreaks of water-borne disease are likely to occur.

An Adequate Water Supply

The rate at which water is used in modern towns varies considerably from town to town and from country to country. Most big cities in Great Britian use about 250 litres per head per day; in the cities of the United States the consumption is twice that amount. Although it is conventional to define the amount of water used in terms of consumption per head, in large industrial towns less than half the total quantity consumed is used for domestic purposes; the rest is needed for municipal purposes (removal of sewage, cleansing of streets, fire-fighting and supplying public baths and ornamental waters) and for industry (about 750,000 litres are used in the manufacture of one motor car).

In many parts of the world the direct storage of rain in cisterns and tanks is still a common method of ensuring a minimum supply of water, but in Great Britain, except in a few isolated communities, this source is no longer relied upon. Urban needs are met by water from natural and artificial lakes in upland districts and from rivers and underground sources. Upland water is usually soft, that is to say free from calcium and magnesium salts in solution, underground water is commonly hard, and river water before it is purified is often grossly polluted.

A Safe Water Supply

A safe water supply is more important to the health of a population than any drug in the Pharmacopoeia, yet in many parts of the world it remains a pressing health need.

Contamination with pathogenic organisms

With few exceptions (guinea worm infestation is one), the major water-borne diseases are transmitted by contamination of water supplies with infected human faeces or urine, so for practical purposes a safe water supply is one protected from contact with human and other excreta and treated to destroy any pathogenic organisms inadvertently introduced.

Cholera is the outstanding example of a major epidemic disease spread through the contamination of drinking water by human faeces, although it can also be transmitted by infected food and by direct contact. It is a disease of great historical interest. For centuries it has been endemic in Bengal. In the nineteenth century it became pandemic and on 6 occasions reached Europe, where it gave rise to devastating epidemics and hundreds of thousands of deaths. In 1831, 1848, 1853, and 1865 explosive outbreaks of the disease in the overcrowded, unsanitary and rapidly expanding industrial towns of England and Wales caused great public alarm and helped the Public Health Movement to gather momentum. During the epidemic of 1848 alone 53,000 deaths were attributed to cholera and a further 19,000 to diarrhoea. John Snow traced the spread of infection to the contamination of drinking water by the excreta of cholera patients and suggested that the disease might be due to invisible living organisms. In 1883, 34 years later, Koch discovered the cholera *Vibrio*.

Typhoid fever is the only other major water-borne infectious disease of which we in England and Wales have had any great experience; like cholera it can contaminate food. In 1875 the death rate from typhoid was 370 per million; in 1905 it was 115, and now years can pass without any deaths from it. When the disease was common, as it still is in many parts of the world, it was due to wholesale pollution of drinking water with the faeces and urine of cases and of carriers. From 2 to 5 per cent of patients continue to excrete the organism for months and sometimes for years after they have recovered from the disease; and the organism can remain alive in water for long periods although it does not multiply there. In countries with high standards of sanitation and water purification localized outbreaks still occur. They may be due to accidental pollution of the water supply, as in Croydon in 1937, when there was a carrier in the gang of men employed to clean out a deep well who urinated into the water. More commonly they are due to contamination of food, in particular of milk and its products and canned meats. Shellfish feed by filtering very large quantities of water, and can concentrate numbers of bacteria and viruses in their bodies. If they are caught in sewage-contaminated water and eaten raw they can cause outbreaks of typhoid, hepatitis A, and dysentery.

Other water-borne diseases of international importance include amoebic dysentery which is common in Africa, India, South America and the Far East, and schistosomiasis which takes various forms and is widespread in Egypt, the rest of Africa and the far East. Between them these two diseases are responsible for an enormous amount of ill-health.

Even in countries with stringent regulations to protect and purify drinking water, accidental gross contamination can still occur. In 1926 because of a faulty mains connection Poplar was for a short time supplied with unpurified river water, and in 1936 a chalk well in Surrey became polluted by seepage from an unsuspected fracture in a nearby sewer. Characteristic localized explosive outbreaks of non-specific diarrhoea and vomiting resulted.

The virus of poliomyelitis is excreted in the faeces of patients and carriers and can be isolated in sewage effluents during and for some time after an epidemic; but modern methods of water purification kill the virus and drinking water has not been implicated in the epidemic spread of the disease.

Contamination with toxic substances

Deep well water can cause diarrhoea when it is heavily impregnated with soluble sulphates; a suspension of microscopic particles of sand or mica, can also cause diarrhoea; and very occasionally minute quantities of arsenic find their way into upland water from sheep dip and weed killer applied in the catchment area.

Lead pipes were commonly used for domestic cold water systems. Some alkaline waters contain salts which react with the lead in such a way that the inside of the pipes becomes lined with insoluble compounds rendering the system safe. Acid waters, however, are plumbo-solvent and concentrations of lead as low as one part per million have been known to cause symptoms of lead poisoning. Upland waters from peaty districts are particularly dangerous. An outbreak of chronic lead poisoning from this cause was reported in Sheffield as long ago as 1885. To reduce plumbo-solvency, lime or sodium silicate is added to water supplies of this type. Better still, lead pipes are removed and replaced by copper.

Protection of supplies

The problem of preventing epidemic water-borne disease resolves itself largely into a matter, first of purifying the domestic water supply, and second, of providing an efficient sewage disposal system.

With appropriate treatment even grossly polluted water can be made safe. Many large towns use as their main sources of water rivers heavily contaminated with sewage effluents from upstream towns, and with untreated waste from isolated factories, farms and houses on their banks. Londoners may drink the sewage effluents of Maidenhead, Reading and Oxford.

In the towns of this country water carriage systems are almost universally employed to remove domestic discharges and trade effluents from the neighbourhood of purified water supplies. Gross solids are screened from the sewage and most of the remaining solid matter is allowed to separate out as sludge in special tanks. Finally the organic matter in the tank liquor is biologically oxidized into simpler and less offensive compounds and the resulting effluent is discharged into neighbouring streams or rivers. However, the final effluent may still be contaminated with coliform organisms, and pathogens may sometimes be isolated from it.

Appraisal of Services

The introduction into Great Britain of efficient water purification and sewage disposal schemes in the second half of the nineteenth century undoubtedly made an important contribution to the decline in mortality at that time. It is impossible now to assess the extent of that contribution, but while water-borne disease is still a leading cause of death and disability over much of the world, in this country cholera has disappeared from the epidemiological scene, typhoid fever is a rarity and the incidence of dysentery and non-specific gastroenteritis have declined dramatically. Today the safety of the water supply is so much taken for granted that we remember the importance of the services only on the rare occasions when they break down. Three important problems remain; the pollution of coasts and rivers with sewage effluents and trade wastes; the question of fluoridation of water supplies; and the question of the relation between softness of water supplies and mortality from cardiovascular disease.

As towns have become cleaner, coasts, lakes and rivers have become progressively more filthy. Many of our coastal and lakeside holiday towns persist in the nasty habit of pouring their largely untreated sewage directly into the open water. A Medical Research Council Memorandum reported in 1959 that many samples of sea water contained thousands of coliform organisms per 100 ml, and counts of over 100,000 were recorded. The importance of this is that when the coliform count in water from a public supply rises much above 10 per 100 ml an outbreak of water-borne disease is likely. However, there is little or no evidence that bathing in polluted sea-water gives rise to bowel infection or to poliomyelitis and objections to that practice rest on aesthetic grounds and the temperature of the water surrounding the British Isles.

River pollution is more serious. Rivers have a strong propensity to purify themselves by oxidizing organic contaminants, but their ability to do this is limited. As the amount of sewage effluent and industrial waste (acids, alkalis, phenols, cyanides) poured into them mounts, a point is reached beyond which purification no longer takes place. Fish die, putrefactive bacteria multiply and the water cannot be made safe for domestic use even after extensive treatment. Ninety years of exhortation, special reports, Royal Commissions and legislation have slowed down this unsavoury trend and in some instances even reversed it—the Thames, for instance, is now so much cleaner than it was in the 1960s that it has proved possible successfully to restock it with fish.

For a long time it has been known that drinking water containing 4 or more parts per million of fluoride produces a permanent mottling of dental enamel in children. More recently it has been observed that children who have been drinking water containing fluorides at concentrations below that which causes mottling show a relative immunity to dental caries. In 1944 it was reported that the incidence of dental carries among 12 year-old children in South Shields (1.4 parts of fluoride per million) was 45 per cent less than among children of the same age and comparable social status in North Shields (0.25 parts per million). All available evidence indicated that fluorides at this concentration are harmless to health, so controlled experiments were carried out in the United States, in Canada and more recently in Britain in Anglesey, Watford and Kilmarnock to assess the effect of artificial fluoridation to the level of 1 part per million. In each experimental area there was a striking improvement in the teeth of young children. In the British studies there was a 66 per cent reduction in caries among 3 year-old children born after the introduction of fluoridation. We have already referred (Chapter 8) to the small minority which opposes this; it was so effective in Kilmarnock that in 1962, 6 years after the introduction of fluoridation, fluoridation was discontinued. The amount of decay in the children's teeth in that Scottish burgh subsequently rose again to prefluoridation levels.

Finally, the association between mortality from cardiovascular disease and the softness of local water supplies merits mention. In Britain, Japan, the United States, Sweden and some other countries, areas with a hard water supply appear to have lower death rates from cardiovascular disease, in particular from ischaemic heart disease, than areas with soft water. If the cardiovascular disease death rate for men aged 45-64 in England and Wales as a whole were as low as in towns with very hard water supplies, there would be 8,000 fewer deaths each year. But rainfall, latitude and social factors as well as water calcium which have been shown to be associated with cardiovascular mortality, are associated with one another. This is an example of the need for caution in interpreting correlation as evidence of causation. The relationship may perhaps be causal in the sense that metal or other contaminants in soft waters in some way increase the risk of death from coronary disease or the mineral content of hard waters may in some way protect against it. But much more research is needed including research on the technical problems of increasing water hardness before a controlled trial of hardening soft water supplies, analogous with the fluoridation trials, would be justified.

Further Reading

Snow John (1855) *On Mode of Communication of Cholera*. John Churchill, London, [republished (1965) as *Snow on Cholera*. Hafner, New York].

Department of Health and Social Security, etc. (1969) *Reports on Public Health and Medical Subjects No. 122*; *The Fluoridation Studies in the United Kingdom and the Results Achieved after Eleven Years*. HMSO, London.

11

Food

We shall consider in Chapter 14 the favourable effect of an adequate and well-balanced diet on general health, but the adulteration and contamination of food is also the source of much ill-health. The gastrointestinal tract is the usual portal of entry for many infectious and parasitic organisms, and food-stuffs readily become contaminated through human, insect and other intermediaries. In addition, a number of organisms pathogenic to man are natural pathogens of domestic animals and of rats and mice; and toxic chemicals may be introduced into food accidentally or deliberately at any stage between production and consumption.

Control of the cleanliness and composition of food is clearly important, but it is more complex and difficult than ensuring a safe water supply. We have seen how when the danger to the community of faecal or urinary contamination of drinking water had been recognized control was left to engineers and bacteriologists, for it demands little or no co-operation from the consumer. The effectiveness of legislation concerned with the conditions under which food is prepared, stored, distributed and eaten must always depend to some extent upon the individual.

Detailed study of the many ways in which food may become contaminated with pathogenic microorganisms lies in the domain of bacteriology; and the problems associated with the introduction of chemicals into food are primarily a matter for pharmacologists and toxicologists. The discussion in this chapter will be limited to brief accounts of some of the major sources of contamination with microorganisms and toxic chemicals and to a summary of the evolution and present status of control of those hazards.

Contamination with Microorganisms

Food contaminated with microorganisms may lead either to food poisoning or to transmission of infectious disease. Epidemiologically and bacteriologically these two hazards overlap; but in clinical and public health practice it is useful to treat them as separate entities.

Food poisoning

Clinically, food poisoning is characterized by an acute gastroenteritis of abrupt onset and short ingestion-to-onset period affecting several and sometimes many people simultaneously. The majority of outbreaks are due to the presence of the salmonella group of organisms, usually in processed and made up meat (shepherd's pie, cold ham and bacon, pork pies, etc.) and in milk and eggs (particularly duck eggs) and their products, but occasionally in fish, fruit and vegetables. The organisms multiply readily in cooked and uncooked food kept at room temperature, and from 12 to 18 hours after they are ingested give rise to a short-lived but prostrating gastroenteritis. Apart from the salmonellae, the only common causes of bacterial food poisoning are certain strains of *Staphylococcus aureus* and *Clostridium welchii.* These organisms also proliferate in cooked and uncooked food stored at ordinary temperatures, but growth is inhibited at refrigerator temperatures and food poisoning is due, not directly to the bacteria but to their toxins. These toxins are heat-stable, so that infected food may give rise to poisoning even after it has been cooked or reheated. Another well-known but fortunately rare cause of bacterial food poisoning is *Clostridium botulinum* a soil anaerobe which sometimes finds its way into processed meats, fish products and canned and bottled foods. This organism produces a powerful neurotoxin which has caused death from respiratory paralysis in about half the reported cases.

The spread of communal feeding in factory canteen, school dining room and restaurant has led to a considerable increase in the number of reported outbreaks of food poisoning in recent years.

Transmission of infectious disease

Many bacterial and some viral and parasitic diseases are transmitted by contaminated food. Sometimes the food is infected at source (bovine tuberculosis and brucellosis). More often the pathogen is introduced into the food because it has been handled by someone carrying the infection (dysentery, typhoid and paratyphoid) or it has come into contact with contaminated water. The typhoid epidemic in Aberdeen, 1964, was traced to corned beef, tins of which had been cooled in contaminated water after sterilization, and the bacteria had entered through minor defects in the seams and possibly through pin holes in the tin plate itself.

In the past, milk was probably the most important cause of food-borne disease. It forms an excellent culture medium for many pathogens and has frequently been responsible for outbreaks of dysentery, typhoid and paratyphoid fever, streptococcal sore throat and infantile gastro-enteritis, as well as for bone, joint and glandular tuberculosis and brucellosis. Occasionally it causes outbreaks of scarlet fever, diphtheria and staphylococcal infection. The struggle to free Britain from bovine tuberculosis was protracted and in this matter we lagged behind the United States, Canada and Scandinavia. Abdominal tuberculosis in children under 15 has nearly always been due to infected milk, so mortality from that condition provides a good index of the amount of bovine tuberculosis. In 1921 the death rate in England and Wales was 94 per million children under 15; today, children in Britain very rarely die from abdominal tuberculosis, for nearly all our milk is pasteurized and dairy herds are tuberculin negative. Nevertheless tuberculosis remains a problem among immigrants from Asia.

Mortality from intestinal infectious diseases is today less than one-fiftieth of its level at the beginning of the century. Not all this improvement is due to cleaner food: as we have seen typhoid fever is commonly water-borne; a great deal of dysentery is spread by direct contract; and in recent years more effective therapy has made a contribution. However, much of the improvement is undoubtedly due to statutory control of cleanliness of food, and an increased awareness in society of the hazards of unhygienic food preparation.

Young children are particularly susceptible to bowel infection from contaminated milk. In 1908 the Medical Officer of Health for Croydon reported that the infant mortality rate from diarrhoea was 8 per 1,000 for breast fed children, 65 for children fed on fresh cows' milk and 129 for children fed on condensed milk. In 1911 infant mortality per thousand from diarrhoea in England and Wales was 36; in 1970 infant mortality from all causes was only 18 and mortality from enteritis was 0.3.

Chemical Contamination

A steady rise in real wages has brought an increasing demand for a varied and attractive diet. At the same time, more than half of our food is imported and three-quarters of the population live in large towns. These factors have led to an unprecedented increase in the quantity and variety of chemicals used in the production, preparation, preservation and presentation of food. During these processes, toxic chemicals may get into food by accident or they may be introduced deliberately.

Accidental contamination

Until recently, accidental chemical contamination of food on a large scale was uncommon. An often quoted example (also referred to in another context) is the epidemic of lead poisoning in the eighteenth century due to the use of lead pipes, containers and presses in the preparation of Devonshire cider. Today the hazard of accidental contamination is less obvious and more widespread. In the first place harmful chemicals find their way into foodstuffs during production; many are used in agriculture to protect plants against animal, insect and fungal pests. The Working Party on Toxic Chemicals in Agriculture and Residues in Foods set up by the Ministry of Agriculture, Fisheries and Food in 1963 listed more than a hundred preparations, some of them powerful poisons, that present a serious hazard to agricultural workers handling them. In addition, the antibiotics and hormones used in animal husbandry are not without danger. For example, penicillin in the milk of cows treated for mastitis may give rise to unpleasant reactions in sensitized persons and may lead to sensitization in others. Harmful chemicals may also be introduced accidentally into food during processing and storage. Disinfectants, catalysts and bleaching and clarifying agents are all widely used in the food industry and the possibility of contamination of canned food with metals, particularly zinc and lead, is a matter of concern.

Since an alarming epidemic of irreversible and gross damage to the nervous system of people living around the estuaries of Minamata and Niiagatu in Japan where fish was the staple diet, there has been much concern about the pollution of fishing waters with industrial effluents containing mercury. The rising levels of methyl mercury found in the fish in certain lakes in Sweden and North America has increased that concern.

Chemical manipulation

In the eighteenth and nineteenth centuries alum, chalk and even bone ash ('the charnel bones of the dead are raked to add filthiness to the food of the living') were added to flour to give it bulk; lead preparations were used to sweeten and clear cheap wines of sediment; infusions of oak chips were added to diluted sulphuric acid and sold as vinegar; and poisonous mixtures of sulphuric acid, turpentine and alum were sold as gin. Fraudulent adulteration of food is no longer common, but chemical manipulation of food to preserve and 'improve' it is widespread and difficult to control. Recognized practices include the addition of antioxidants, moisture retaining agents and surface protections to preserve food; sweeteners, acidifiers and spices to heighten flavour; dyes, bleaching agents, clarifiers and glazes to improve appearance; and emulsifiers, thickeners and tenderisers to improve consistency. During the course of a year each of us is now consuming with our food about 6 pounds of chemical substances which are not natural constituents of that food and the amount is increasing. It must be remembered, however, that the nutrition of the malnourished and rapidly expanding world population has become more and more dependent on pesticides, antibiotics, hormones and chemical methods of food preservation.

Services for the control of food-borne disease

As far back as records go there have been prosecutions for selling adulterated foods. But the casual prosecution of a few of the worst offenders made little mark upon the problem and the evil remained practically unabated until the middle of the nineteenth century. Social control was impossible so long as there were no local authorities to operate the machinery of the law and no way of defining purity except in terms of taste, smell and appearance.

By the eighteenth century a modification of Robert Boyle's hydrometer was in fairly general use for the praiseworthy purpose of keeping the water out of the wine, and a few simple tests had been devised to detect and measure some of the commoner inorganic poisons that found their way into food. The turning point was the campaign launched by the *Lancet* in the middle of the nineteenth century, when it set up its own 'Analytical and Sanitary Commission'. Nearly 3,000 wholesale and retail purveyors of food were found guilty of selling grossly adulterated products and their names were published in the columns of the Journal. The first Food and Drugs Act (1860) was the direct result of the public outcry.

Today the control of the purity and cleanliness of food is largely a responsibility of local government. Most of the measures are to be found in the Food and Drugs Act, 1955, and in regulations made under that Act. They include food sampling for chemical analysis, and the routine inspection of meat, milk and other foods for the presence of pathogens. An authorized officer of the local authority may at all reasonable times examine food intended for human consumption, and if it appears unfit he may seize it and a magistrate will decide what further action should be taken. Minimum standards are laid down for the construction, equipment and cleanliness of premises on which food is handled, prepared or processed and particular attention is paid to the inspection of dairies and the control of persons with access to milk.

Medical practitioners have an important role to play in the control of food-borne disease. Food poisoning, enteric fever and dysentery are compulsorily notifiable and the doctor in charge of a suspected case of food poisoning should retain for bacteriological examination a specimen of faeces or vomit and if possible the remains of the suspected meal.

The problem of controlling chemical additives is a formidable one. Tests for general toxicity are expensive and time consuming. Tests for long-term toxic effects, and in particular for carcinogenicity, are even more expensive, take much longer and can never be entirely conclusive. Nevertheless there is clear need for such tests. For example nitrosamines, which are highly carcinogenic, have been found in foodstuffs intended for human consumption, and it is known that the nitrates traditionally used in the smoking of fish can react with certain amines produced in fish to form nitrosamines. With the increasing volume of international food traffic, the problem has become worldwide and a joint committee of the Food and Agriculture Organization (FAO) and the World Health Organization is actively concerned with international standards.

Further Reading

World Health Organization (1983) *Mass Catering*, Regional Publications European Series, No. 15, Copenhagen WHO.

12

Air

Disease Borne by Droplets and Dust

In Britain, respiratory tract infections are the leading cause of absence from work, and a common reason for practitioner consultations. The common cold is a universal and, so far, an uncontrollable nuisance. Pneumonia, despite effective therapy, remains an important cause of infant mortality and a major cause of death in old age. And in epidemic years morbidity and mortality from influenza are a matter for national concern. When we remember that the specific infections of childhood namely chickenpox, whooping cough, measles, mumps, scarlet fever and diphtheria are also air-borne, it is evident that the control of this method of dissemination of infection is at least as important as the control of water-borne and food-borne disease. It is much more difficult to achieve.

Air had been suspected of playing an important part in the spread of epidemic disease since at least Galen's time. In the second century he wrote 'When many sicken and die at once, we must look to a simple common cause, the air we breathe'. But until Pasteur discredited the notion of spontaneous generation of pathogenic poisons by demonstrating that living organisms can be conveyed through the air (and water), there was no rational basis for the control of airborne infection. The control of water-borne disease preceded the science of bacteriology. Lister's attempt to control airborne surgical sepsis by the use of carbolic acid sprays in operating theatres was derived from it.

Despite the remarkable advances in bacteriological knowledge since Lister's time, control of airborne infection is still far from satisfactory. Technically air is much more difficult to sterilize than water or food. Elimination of organisms from all the air we breathe is quite impossible and is difficult even in the limited environments where there is special need for it such as hospital wards and operating theatres. Control of the sources of airborne infection is further complicated by the ubiquity of the common respiratory diseases, by the fact that many of them are infectious before they are clinically apparent or indeed without ever becoming apparent, as in a subclinical attack or the carrier state, and by the facilities for their spread unavoidably provided by society such as schools, places of work, public transport and public buildings.

Modes of Transmission

There are two main methods, droplet transmission and dust transmission, by which infection is spread through the air. The first of these, droplet transmission, can be further divided into two systems: large droplet transmission; and droplet nuclei transmission.

Droplet transmission acts directly from person to person via droplets bearing microorganisms or, more important, by the much smaller droplet nuclei which remain airborne for longer. Dust transmission acts indirectly by dust from bedding, clothes, carpets and floors. The methods are not necessarily disease specific. Thus though smallpox, pulmonary tuberculosis and streptococcal infections are predominantly transmitted by means of droplet nuclei, they may also be spread by dust. Some of the infections that are normally airborne may be spread by contamination of food, usually milk, for example streptococcal sore throat and diphtheria. Not all contaminated droplets are expired by living creatures. For instance in applying his technological discoveries to make his environment more comfortable, man has created at least one new disease, Legionnaires' disease, which is a pneumonia caused by a gram negative rod *Legionella pneumophila* which is normally a soil organism. The bacteria now grow in the water of air conditioning systems, and have caused outbreaks in hotels. Although the disease is not common it can be lethal.

Droplet transmission

During quiet breathing very few droplets are expelled. They are produced by talking, and in much greater numbers by coughing and sneezing; a sneeze may expel as many as 1 million droplets. The largest droplets fall rapidly to the ground or onto the clothes or bedding of the person producing them. Droplets of less than 100 μm in diameter fall more slowly, evaporating as they fall. Depending upon their size, the atmospheric humidity, air movement and other factors, a proportion of these smaller droplets lose all their moisture before they reach the ground and remain suspended as droplet nuclei until removed by ventilation. It follows that for infection to be transmitted by large droplet spray the susceptible host needs to very near the source of infection. A child standing close to an infected person is in a particularly vulnerable position. Diseases disseminated mainly by this method are often associated with overcrowded sleeping conditions, as in the case of cerebrospinal meningitis among service personnel, or with close family contact, as in the case of whooping cough. Droplet nuclei, on the other hand, can be as small as 1 μm and carry infection over much greater distances. Tubercle bacilli and the viruses of measles, chickenpox and smallpox are commonly disseminated in this way. Because of their small size and low settling velocity the nuclei are readily carried into the alveoli, and it is therefore possible for a susceptible person to become infected from the inhalation of a very small number of them.

Dust transmission

Large droplets, when they fall to the ground, dry out and any particulate matter they contain becomes part of the dust of the room. If they contain pathogens resistant to drying, the dust may then act as a reservoir of infection for a long time; tubercle bacilli have been known to survive in dust for 3 months and haemolytic streptococci for 6 months. Organisms from soiled surgical dressings, skin scales, dried sputum and other secretions can also become part of the dust of a room and these sources have often been shown to cause cross-infection in surgical wards. However, apart from special places such as hospitals, dust is not now a common vehicle for the transmission of air-borne infection. For although huge numbers of particles containing living organisms become air-borne when the dust in a room is disturbed by domestic activities such as sweeping, bed-making and brushing clothes, such organisms are no longer likely to be pathogenic.

Control of Disease due to Organisms

There are three ways in which control of air-borne infection may be attempted: by removing the source of infection; by interrupting its lines of communication; and by protecting susceptible persons.

Removing the source of infection

In the past the only method which offered any hope of limiting the spread of infection was to isolate from the community those suffering from infectious disease as well as those who might be incubating an infection because they had been in contact with it. This was the main reason for building fever hospitals in the nineteenth century, although it is doubtful whether they limited the spread of any of the air-borne infections, with the possible exceptions of smallpox and diphtheria, because there was no satisfactory way of ensuring that those in the prodromal phase of disease were isolated let alone their contacts. Sanatoria, on the other hand, by isolating for long periods patients with open pulmonary tuberculosis probably contributed to the decline of mortality from the disease during the first half of the present century. The unexpected case of smallpox arising from the laboratory is still routinely admitted to isolation in hospital. Mortality from the other air-borne infectious diseases namely measles, whooping cough, scarlet fever, diphtheria, meningococcal meningitis, influenzal pneumonia, and pulmonary tuberculosis, is now so low, and the risk of acquiring a complicating cross-infection in hospital is relatively so much higher, that the crucial reason for hospital admission has become the need for diagnostic and therapeutic facilities rather than for isolation. Indeed, cross-infection is so dangerous to debilitated and susceptible young children that for this reason alone it is preferable that sick children should not be admitted to general or paediatric hospitals, and there are also compelling psychological reasons for home treatment.

The classroom, with its crowding together of susceptibles, provides a particularly favourable environment for the transmission of air-borne infection, so children with infectious disease should be kept away from school. The exclusion of contacts, however, although advisable in certain circumstances, is no longer enforced.

The number of streptococci and staphylococci expelled during ordinary conversation, even from the mouths of known carriers, is small. Nevertheless, the wearing of face masks in operating theatres and delivery rooms remains a sensible precaution. The type of mask is not as important as it was once thought to be, for the organisms are first expelled in droplets, not in droplet nuclei, and almost anything placed in front of the mouth will catch them. It is more important that any member of theatre or ward staffs found to be carrying pathogenic organisms in the nasopharynx, for example *Streptococcus pyogenes* or strains of *Staphylococcus aureus* of certain phage types, should be removed from duty until free from infection.

Interrupting lines of communication

The dissemination of infection by droplets and droplet-nuclei is favoured by confined and crowded working and living conditions. In the open air, infective nuclei are dispersed so rapidly after expulsion that their chance of being inhaled by a susceptible person is negligible. Good ventilation and avoidance of overcrowding are probably still the most effective, as they are certainly the cheapest, methods of reducing the risk of air-borne infection indoors. Florence Nightingale observed that 'if nothing is done for ventilation, the hospital atmosphere becomes more and more fatal'. In northern latitudes the common respiratory infections and most of the specific fevers of childhood reach their peak incidence during the winter months, when people are crowded indoors, and windows in homes, schools and factories are closed against the weather.

In recognition of the dangers of overcrowding, standards of spacing, usually in terms of floor space per person, are laid down for private houses, and for most public buildings, and building byelaws require provision of certain facilities for ventilation of domestic and public buildings. Although the risk of spread of air-borne infection is reduced by ventilation, experimental work suggests that to eliminate this risk 60 air changes an hour are needed. Ventilation of this kind can be obtained by air-conditioning plants which are costly but it cannot be achieved by ordinary methods without intolerable draughts and insoluble heating problems. An alternative, therefore, is to support normal ventilation by some method of destroying pathogens in the air.

When used as atomized sprays, sodium hypochlorite, propylene and triethylene glycol, resorcinol, hexylresorcinol and lactic acid have all been shown to sterilize air-borne particles effectively in the laboratory. Field trials, however, have been disappointing.

Control of dust-borne infection is as we have seen of great importance in hospitals. Floor-sweeping and bed-making disturb myriads of dust particles, and staphylococci and haemolytic streptococci can readily be recovered from the floors and bedding of surgical wards. During the Second World War, cross-infection in military hospitals was not uncommonly traced to this source, and the emergence of antibiotic-resistant pathogens has heightened the need for control. Oil treatment of floors and bedding reduces very substantially the amount of dust in wards and the use of vacuum cleaners with appropriate filters is even more effective. At points of high risk, such as operating theatres, burns units and labour wards, dust can be removed from the incoming air by filtration or electro-static precipitation, the air sterilized by ultraviolet irradiation, and the dispersal of infective particles checked by introducing clean air from above and removing it at floor level. It must be remembered, however, that these protective measures do not eliminate the risk of cross-infection from droplet spray or direct contact, methods of spread favoured by resistant strains of *Staphylococcus aureus*. Human reservoirs of infection must therefore also be identified and treated.

Protecting susceptible populations

It is so difficult to block all the channels by which air-borne infection can be transmitted that for the common respiratory infections prophylactic immunization discussed in some detail in Chapter 15 appears to offer the only hope of full control. By this means diphtheria has already been virtually banished from Britain, and an effective vaccine has practically eliminated mortality from whooping cough. Procedures for controlling tuberculosis among indigenous children and young adults in Britain have proved so successful that the need for BCG as a routine procedure among them is being seriously questioned. It still has an important role to play however, both among immigrants, especially from Asia, and among medical and health workers. Measles vaccine is also proving effective, and gamma-globulin can be used to prevent or modify the disease in very young or sick and debilitated older children. Progress towards the control of influenza is slow. Virus-specific vaccines provide reasonable protection, but vaccines are of limited value when the epidemic virus has a different antigenic pattern from the viruses in the vaccine. Whisky remains one of the pleasantest of the many ineffective prophylactics against the common cold.

Disease Caused by Pollution

Pollution of the air from domestic and industrial sources is also an important cause of disease. The relation between tobacco smoke and ill-health is discussed in Chapter 17 and the effects and control of air pollution at place of work in Chapter 19.

In towns, clean air like safe water, depends on the control of domestic and industrial effluents; but whereas the problem of controlling the pollution of water supplies was well on the way to being solved by the end of the nineteenth century and was the first and most notable success of the public health movement, the problem of controlling urban atmospheric pollution is still with us. This is partly because pollution of the air is more difficult and costly to control, and partly because its connection with ill-health is more complex and took longer to demonstrate. In Britain the cholera epidemics of the middle of the nineteenth century provided alarming and unmistakable evidence of the need to separate sewage from drinking water. It was not for another hundred years that the London smog disaster of 1952, the last of a long series, gave an equally dramatic demonstration of the need to control atmospheric pollution.

Causes and Composition of Pollution

The main sources of atmospheric pollution are the domestic and industrial combustion of solid fuel, coal and coke, and of petroleum products such as kerosene, diesel oil and petrol by motor cars. In Britain over recent decades the sources of energy and heat for domestic and industrial purposes and rail transport have been changing rapidly. The use of natural gas and petroleum oils has increased, but that of solid fuels has fallen. In 1983 about half the solid fuel and 5 per cent of all oil consumed were used in private homes.

The solid components of pollution may be classified as grit, dust and smoke. Grit consists of gross particles upwards of 76 μm in diameter, dust of smaller particles down to 1 μm, and smoke of particles of less than 1 μm. Nearly all the grit and dust discharged into the air comes from industrial sources. In domestic fireplaces the large particles remain behind in the grate as ash, but in industrial furnaces they are driven up the chimneys by the much higher temperatures. Because of its weight, grit tends to settle in the immediate neighbourhood of industrial chimneys, but dust particles are dispersed more widely. On the other hand nearly all the smoke pollution comes from incomplete combustion of coal. Oil and coke fuels make a very small contribution. Although before the Clean Air Acts of 1956 and 1968 only about one-sixth of the national consumption of coal was used for domestic purposes, half of the low-level smoke in industrial districts came from domestic grates which burn raw coal very inefficiently. In industry, coal is used more efficiently, and the combustion products are usually discharged into the upper air from tall chimney stacks. There is an appreciable quantity of benzpyrene in coal smoke and minute but measurable amounts of that known carcinogen are present in the atmospheres of our towns and cities.

The combustion of coal and oil produces a wide range of gaseous pollutants. From British coal several million tonnes of sulphur dioxide have been discharged into the air every year. In large industrial towns the mean atmospheric concentration of sulphur dioxide during the winter months may be 0.2 parts per million, and in smog episodes it has risen to over 1 part per million. Nevertheless its emission has fallen from 6 million tonnes in the 1970s to 4.7 million tonnes in 1980, mainly because of the reduction in the use of coal by low and medium emitters. Concentrations in the atmosphere of urban areas have fallen on average by 60 per cent since 1960.

The nitrogen oxides emitted from the chimneys of industrial furnaces and exhausts of internal combustion engines may also be of pathological significance. They are present as a regular pollutant in the air of the cities of Britain at concentrations of about 0.1 parts per million. There is very little carbon monoxide in flue gas, but it constitutes 10 per cent of the exhaust gas from internal combustion engines. Concentrations of 2 parts per million are common in traffic congested city streets, and may reach 30 or more times that level in traffic tunnels or in traffic jams. Fuel burning produces huge quantities of carbon dioxide (it is poured into the atmosphere at a rate of over 200 million tons a year) but it is diluted so rapidly that it does not constitute a toxic hazard. Another consequence is causing serious concern, however; solar heat is being retained in the lower atmosphere, with the result that the polar ice caps are receding. This is sometimes called the greenhouse effect. Another general deleterious effect of burning fossil fuels in industrial plants and power stations is that carbon dioxide is dissolved in the moisture in the atmosphere to form carbonic acid. This subsequently falls down wind as acid rain, and among other things is harmful to forests. It is believed that damage due to British effluent is being caused in Norway.

The concentration of pollutants in the atmosphere of a town is determined in the first place by the quantities discharged into the air from local industrial and domestic sources. An important secondary influence is the rate at which pollutants are subsequently removed from the air. Particles of grit and dust settle by gravitation. The rate at which smoke and gases are dispersed depends upon rainfall, the direction and force of prevailing winds, and upon air turbulence created by geographical contours and thermal gradients. The sun warms the earth and this sets up convection currents by warming the air at its surface. The warm air rises, carrying with it and dispersing the pollutants. When local weather is controlled by a high pressure system and there is a local topography which restricts air flow, a temperature inversion may occur with the warm air above and the cold air below. When this happens there is no upward movement of air, and in a heavily polluted area pollutants can accumulate to produce a 'smog episode', with immediate effects on the health of the local population (see below).

Effects Upon Health

For a number of reasons the effect of atmospheric pollution on health is difficult to measure. In the first place the acute effects are nonspecific; smog episodes produce an increase in morbidity and mortality among those already suffering from cardiac or pulmonary disability rather than a new, specific and clearly recognizable illness. In this respect they differ from the disastrous epidemics of infectious disease. Second, the long-term effects can be estimated only by their contribution to the complex, multifactorial aetiology of chronic bronchitis and cancer of the lung. Third, atmospheric pollution has as we have seen many different components, particulate and gaseous, and their effects are unusually difficult to separate. Even in the controlled environment of the animal laboratory the effects of pollution are difficult to separate and to measure. It has been shown, however, that when mice are exposed to quite low concentrations of sulphur dioxide their growth is stunted and they develop recognizable pathological changes in the lungs. It is also known that skin and lung cancers can be produced by exposing them to the polycyclic hydrocarbons found in the atmosphere of cities.

Immediate effects

Charles Dickens in the opening lines of *Bleak House* vividly described how the skipper of a Thames barge coughed and wheezed in a London smog. In recent decades the immediately harmful effect of gross atmospheric pollution has been impressively demonstrated by three major smog episodes: in December 1930, in the Meuse Valley, Belgium; in October 1948, in the city of Donora, United States; and in December

1952, in London. All three episodes were characterized by anticyclonic weather conditions, high atmospheric humidity producing suspended particles of water (fog) which acted as a solvent, and an unusually persistent thermal inversion which allowed pollutants to accumulate and dissolve in the still air for several days. In London all the pollutants were products of coal combustion, but in the Meuse Valley and in Donora some of them came from heavy industry (coke ovens, blast furnaces, zinc reduction plant, etc.).

In the London episode the pollutants began to accumulate on December 5th and reached their maximum concentration within 3 days. The amount of sulphur dioxide in the air increased 7 times and the concentration of suspended matter (smoke) 10 times; but it was only after retrospective analysis of mortality and morbidity data that the gravity of the episode was appreciated. In the smog area there was an excess of 1,600 deaths during the first 3 weeks of December, mainly among infants and the elderly. Table 12.1 shows that much of the excess was due to a very large rise in mortality from all the major respiratory diseases; but the number of deaths attributed to coronary disease and myocardial degeneration also increased substantially. From hospital admissions, sickness claims and general practitioners' records there is evidence that although the amount of respiratory illness in the population increased steeply, the increase was less than might have been expected from the number of deaths. The general conclusion drawn from the evidence was

Table 12.1 Deaths registered in London Administrative County for the smog episode of 1952

Cause of death	Number of deaths: (a) Week of Smog	Number of deaths: (b) Week before Smog	Ratio a/b
Bronchitis	704	74	9.3
Respiratory tuberculosis	77	14	5.5
Influenza and pneumonia	192	47	4.1
Other respiratory diseases	52	9	4.8
Coronary disease and myocardial degeneration	525	206	2.6
All other conditions	934	595	1.6
Total	2,484	945	2.6

that the main effect of the smog was to exacerbate illness and precipitate death among people with pre-existing respiratory or cardiac conditions.

The eye and lung irritating photochemical smogs of Los Angeles are produced by an interaction of ozone and the hydrocarbons and oxides of nitrogen from the exhausts of motor vehicles in the still air and bright sunlight of that city. In Britain the necessary concentration of motor vehicles exists in some of the large cities, but there is not enough still air in bright sunlight to cause this unpleasant phenomenon.

Long-term effects

There is much evidence to suggest that in industrialized communities atmospheric pollution plays some part in the aetiology of chronic bronchitis and carcinoma of the lung. It is difficult to assess the precise part, however, for the evidence is indirect, most of it derived from epidemiological studies in Britain and difficult to interpret.

The high, though falling death rate from chronic bronchitis in the United Kingdom is often attributed to enthusiasm for coal fires. But bronchitis is a notoriously imprecise diagnosis, and some of the excess may have been due to the national tendency to give bronchitis as the cause of death. There are also considerable differences between countries in smoking habits, and tobacco is a very important aetiological influence (Chapter 17). Then there is the relation between size of town and mortality from bronchitis and cancer of the lung, referred to in Chapter 6, which may be due in part to the higher concentration of pollutants in larger towns; but other features of urban life may also be important, for example overcrowding, which increases the risk of recurrent respiratory infection, and the gross pollution of the air immediately around them to which some men are exposed at their place of work.

The case that atmospheric pollution is in part a cause of the increase of bronchitis and lung cancer mortality with increasing population density is strengthened by the observation that mortality from bronchitis in the county boroughs was directly related to intensity of air pollution. Even more convincing are the results of a survey of sickness absence, premature retirement and death among postmen, in which indices of population density, household crowding and atmospheric pollution were defined and morbidity and mortality rates calculated by cause for different areas. Disablement and death from bronchitis were found to be closely related to urban pollution but not to area or domestic crowding. In contrast, mortality from carcinoma of the lung was much more closely related to population density; and morbidity from influenza was related to household overcrowding.

The rapidly increasing density of the traffic on the roads raises questions about the possible effects on health of the carbon monoxide and lead expelled at street level from motor exhausts into the air of our towns. The levels of carboxyhaemoglobin registered in the blood of people exposed to atmospheric pollution from heavy traffic are regularly exceeded by the levels found in the blood of cigarette smokers not exposed to traffic pollution, but it must be remembered that the two effects can be additive. So far the blood lead levels recorded in people exposed to motor exhaust fumes in cities, although some cause for concern, have been well below the levels at which overt lead intoxication occurs.

In conclusion, there is little doubt that long-term exposure to atmospheric pollution has contributed to the high prevalence of bronchitis and lung cancer in Britain, although the effect is difficult to quantify. It is also likely that by increasing the general gloom and squalor of industrialized cities it makes a contribution to mental ill-health, and by screening the sunlight it may still stunt the growth of city children.

Control

In Britain awareness of the smoke nuisance and the need for its control has a long history. In 1273 the burning of coal in London was prohibited by statute and in 1306 an artificer was executed for the offence. Queen Elizabeth I was 'greatly grieved and annoyed with the taste and smoke of the sea-coals'. In 'Fumifugium: or the smoke of London Dissipated', John Evelyn in 1661 submitted to Charles II a plan to control the 'hellish and dismal cloud' which enveloped London. And since the middle of the nineteenth century there has been an accumulation of statutory attempts to control pollution from industrial sources. Yet, after 7 centuries of endeavour, atmospheric pollution remains a major problem in the field of environmental control. The reasons are not far to seek. For centuries coal has been the cheapest and most accessible source of power for industry and of heat for the home. Growth of population and industrial expansion have continued to outpace unpopular attempts to control pollution, unpopular because they tend to increase the cost of industrial processes, and because the open-hearth fire is a long established feature of domestic architecture and winters are not quite cold enough to make a break with tradition easy. Before reviewing the present position, we will mention briefly some of the problems of control.

Cleaning the air of cities requires control of emission of pollutants from the burning of fuel for domestic and industrial purposes. There is little prospect of developing domestic apparatus for burning raw coal without smoke, and the solution to the domestic problem is the use of gas, electricity and oil or of solid smokeless fuels such as coke, anthracite, coalite and phurnacite in properly designed appliances, supplemented possibly by district heating schemes. Control of emission of pollutants from conventional power stations and from industrial processes is more complex. If appropriate methods are used, almost any fuel can be burnt without the emission of dust or smoke. But control of harmful waste gases, particularly sulphur dioxide, is more difficult. The long-term solution to the sulphur dioxide problem lies in increasing use of sulphur-free fuels and of nuclear and hydroelectric sources of power. In the meantime aesthetic considerations are put aside and we rely upon rapid dilution of irritant flue gases to safe levels by discharging them into the upper air through tall, unsightly chimneys.

For the first half of the twentieth century, legislation to control atmospheric pollution was fragmentary, permissive and never very effective. The London smog of 1952 disclosed the urgency and magnitude of the problem. The following year the Government appointed a Committee 'to examine the nature, causes and effects of air pollution and the efficiency of present preventive measures; to consider what further preventive measures are practicable; and to make recommendations'. The Committee reported in 1954 and the Clean Air Acts of 1956 and 1968 embodied most of the recommendations. Emission of black smoke from chimneys is prohibited; new industrial furnaces may not be installed unless they are provided with grit arresting equipment and are capable, so far as practicable, of being operated without emitting smoke; and local authorities are empowered to declare 'smoke control areas' in which the emission of smoke from chimneys is an offence. In 1974 further legislation gave the government authority to control the composition and content of fuel used in motor vehicles, and the sulphur content of oil used in furnaces or engines. Since the Acts the amount of smoke discharged into the atmosphere from industrial sources has been uniformly reduced. The effect upon domestic sources of pollution has been slow but steady. London and a few large cities led the way by substantially lowering the levels of atmospheric pollution with a noticeable effect upon age standardized death rates from bronchitis. Other cities and towns followed with the result that the more easily maintained oil and gas fired central heating systems are replacing the open grate as the norm in Britain.

Further Reading

Editorial (1984) Acid rain: toxic metals. *Lancet* **i**, 659-660.

Report of the Royal College of Physicians (1970) *Air Pollution and Health*. Pitman Medical and Scientific Publishing Co. Ltd., London.

Reports on Public Health and Medical Reports (1954) *Mortality and Morbidity during the London Fog of December 1952.* HMSO, London.

13

Animal

Even if man himself is set aside, it is difficult to exaggerate the importance of the animal kingdom in the transmission of disease. Mammals, arthropods, molluscs and lower organisms can amongst others all play a part. The way this is done is varied and may be complex. Some diseases, known as the zoonoses are diseases of animals, and only infect man by accident; examples are rabies and yellow fever. In others, such as malaria and schistosomiasis, man provides an environment for an essential phase in a complicated life cycle. In the former, a vector, the anopheline mosquito carries the pathogenic organisms to man; in the latter he exposes himself to them by immersing his unprotected skin in water in which swim the larvae of a blood fluke whose intermediate host is a water snail. Probably the simplest form of vector borne transmission is coincidental. For instance the housefly can contaminate its feet by walking on faeces containing organisms which cause diarrhoea or dysentery and the fly can then carry them to food which will not be cooked before consumption.

The rat with its fleas has carried bubonic plague from area to area in devastating epidemics since the beginning of history. The body louse, by transmitting typhus, has been responsible for the deaths of more soldiers than all the pre-atomic weapons of mankind. Malaria and yellow fever, and trypanosomiasis, have depopulated and kept under-populated millions of square miles of fertile land. Even today animal-borne diseases are so widespread and so debilitating, that they profoundly depress agricultural productivity in a world chronically short of food.

The subject is so large that only its more important aspects can be referred to here. We shall be particularly concerned with the control of some vectors, reservoirs and carriers.

Modes of Transmission

More than a hundred of the communicable diseases to which man is subject are known to have animal links in their chains of transmission. All known infective agents are implicated (viruses, rickettsiae, bacteria, fungi, protozoa, and helminths) and the animal vectors include all the common domestic mammals and birds, and many wild vertebrates (mammals, birds and fish), insects and molluscs. In relation to control the way in which the diseases are transmitted is of great importance.

Direct transmission

(*a*) *Physical contact with infected animals.*

A number of important infections are acquired by physical contact with infected animals or their carcasses. For example rabies is directly transmitted to man by the bite of an infected animal, particularly dog or cat but others such as foxes, rats, and vampire bats, can also spread it. The main source of human anthrax is contact with the carcasses, wool, hair or hides of infected animals or with the feeding stuffs and fertilizers made from the bones and other parts of such animals. Cowpox, rat-bite fever and certain of the dermatomycoses (for example, cat, dog, cattle and horse ringworm) are further examples of diseases directly transmitted by infected animals.

(*b*) *Ingestion of the tissues of infected animals.*

Salmonella food poisoning can be transmitted by the ingestion of meat from infected pigs and cows, and eggs from infected ducks. In many parts of the world including western Europe milk from infected animals is responsible for much brucellosis and bovine tuberculosis.

(*c*) *Contact with the excreta of infected animals.*

A good example of this type of transmission is provided by Weil's disease. The causal organism, *Leptospira icterohaemorrhagica* is excreted in the urine of infected rats and it can survive for several weeks in water, from which it enters the human host through the skin. As a result of this mode of transmission Weil's disease tends to be associated with occupations such as coal mining, sewer work and fish-handling, which bring workers into contact with rat infested waters. Throughout the world salmonellosis is endemic in a wide variety of animals such as poultry, swine, cattle and rodents, and food contaminated with the faeces of infected animals can give rise to food poisoning.

Indirect transmission

Much more important are the many infections transmitted indirectly through intermediaries or vectors which maybe vertebrate or invertebrate.

The modes of transmission are varied and often complex. The vector may as we have seen act only as a mechanical vehicle for carrying the infecting parasite from one host to another. In this way the house fly can transfer the organisms of bacillary dysentery from infected faeces to food and cooking utensils—although the usual method of transmission is handling food with contaminated fingers or by direct, person to person contact. More commonly the vector is involved biologically in the process. For example, the rickettsiae of typhus multiply in the cells of the louse midgut and because the louse defaecates as it bites, the human host inoculates himself with the infected faeces when he scratches. Sometimes the animal vector plays an essential part in the life cycle of the parasite; (the sexual cycle of the malaria protozoa takes place only in anopheline mosquitos).

The nature of the animal vector, arthropod, mollusc or vertebrate has an important bearing on the control of indirectly transmitted infections.

(*a*) *Arthropod vectors*

Malaria, yellow fever, typhus and trypanosomiasis, all with arthropod vectors, are of the greatest international importance.

- Malaria is conveyed only by anopheline mosquitoes. The sporozoites find their way into the insect's salivary glands from which they are injected into the human blood stream when the female mosquito is feeding. The clinical features of the disease are determined by the species of plasmodium involved, and its epidemiological pattern by the habits of 50 or more species of anopheline vectors. All depend upon water for their larval stage, but the choice of water (clean, brackish, tidal, sunlit, shady), flight range, feeding habits and choice of resting place vary from species to species. Climatic conditions are also important; a temperature of not less than 20°C is required before the sexual cycle of *Plasmodium falciparum* (the cause of malignant subtertian malaria) can be completed in the mosquito and a temperature of 15°C is needed for the other species. For this reason it is believed that in historical times malaria was never common in Britain, although indigenous cases still occasionally occur. For example in the years immediately following the First World War 359 cases were notified in Kent, the disease having been transmitted by infected anophelines in the Thames marshes.
- Yellow fever, a virus disease, in its epidemic form is transmitted between humans only by *Aedes aegypti*, a domestic mosquito which will breed in any small collection of rain water (such as in a discarded tin or

motor tyre or the bottom of a boat). The mosquito demands for its life cycle a mean temperature of at least 24°C, so it is confined to the tropics. Although the vector is common in Asia and the Pacific, yellow fever is found only in Africa and South America. In endemic form (jungle yellow fever) the disease occurs sporadically in the scattered rural communities of the tropical rain forests of Africa and South America. This form of the disease has its reservoir in certain species of monkey which live high in the tropical rain forests and is transmitted from them to man by forest mosquitoes.

• Rickettsial diseases of which typhus is the most important are transmitted by many different arthropods—lice, fleas, ticks and mites. There appears to be no animal reservoir of epidemic typhus, which has been the destroyer of armies and the scourge of hospitals and prisons. As has been stated it is transmitted from man to man by the body louse, which almost always dies of the infection. The many other typhus fever are primarily animal infections, transferred from animal to animal by arthropod vectors and occasionally transmitted to man when he is walking or living in wild country by the bite of those arthropods. Murine typhus is a world-wide infection of rats, sporadically transmitted to man by infected rat fleas. Dogs and rodents throughout the world are also subject to tick-borne typhus infections, and these are occasionally transmitted to man as in the examples of Rocky Mounted spotted fever and North Queensland and Kenya typhus.

• Trypanosomiasis, in Africa, is transmitted by the bite of the tsetse fly, which is biologically involved in the developmental cycle of the protozoa. The different species of the vector are often very specific in their environmental needs, some living only near rivers and streams, others requiring for survival certain shrubs and trees in scrub and bush country. In consequence the human form of the disease, sleeping sickness, is essentially a rural disease, for the vectors cannot survive in an urban environment. Trypanosomiasis of cattle (ngana) is of social and economic importance because of its effect upon human nutrition, for it has delayed the development of vast tracts of good grazing land in Central Africa. In South America the Triatomid bug is responsible for transmitting another form of trypanosomiasis known as Chagas' disease of which the armadillo is the animal reservoir.

(*b*) *Molluscs*

Oysters and mussels are as we have seen sometimes responsible for the spread of typhoid and hepatitis A but by far the most important of the molluscs are the freshwater snails which are essential to the life cycle of *Schistosoma*, the trematode worm responsible for human bilharziasis the African name for the form of the disease which in other parts of the world is called schistosomiasis. This debilitating disease is widely distributed in Africa, South America, China, Japan and the Philippines. In these countries it is found wherever man comes into barefooted contact with water suitable for the appropriate species of snails. The adult worms live in the human portal system, but the eggs are excreted in the urine or faeces depending on the species of organism. In water the eggs hatch and the trematode continues its developmental cycle in the tissues of a vector snail, from which it again enters the water to gain access to a human host through the unbroken skin. The disease is very difficult to control and irrigation schemes are introducing it into many fresh areas so that it threatens to replace malaria as the leading vector-borne disease.

(*c*) *Vertebrates*

Some of the many worms which parasitize man are transmitted by vertebrates. Sometimes several animal intermediaries are involved before a new human host becomes infected: for example the adult fish tapeworm *Dyphyllobothrium latum* inhabits the human intestine; the eggs are excreted with the faeces, and in fresh water produce free-swimming larvae; the larvae enter the next phase of their development when they are ingested by certain small crustaceans; they undergo further development when the crustaceans are swallowed by small fish; when the small fish are swallowed by larger fish, the larvae invade and become encysted in the muscles of the new hosts; and the cycle is completed when man eats the raw, smoked or pickled flesh of the infected large fish. The human tapeworms *Taenia saginata* and *Taenia solium* have cattle and pigs as their intermediate hosts. Gravid segments of the worm are passed in the faeces of infected persons, and the eggs, if swallowed by the appropriate animal vector, liberate embryos which find their way into the skeletal muscles, where they encyst. Man acquires the worm by eating such muscles raw or incompletely cooked. Man sometimes becomes involved in the life cycle of *Echinococcus granulosus*. The common definitive host of this small tapeworm is the dog and the usual intermediate host the sheep. Man develops hydatid disease by ingesting the eggs excreted by infected dogs. The disease is an important health problem in many parts of the world and still occurs from time to time in Britain. In a survey of farm dogs in Mid Wales 1 in 5 was found to be infected.

Control

It might be expected that of all the major communicable diseases, those in which animals are involved would be most amenable to control, for their epidemiology is well understood, and it should be possible to block the channels of spread by controlling the animal vectors. Yet animal-borne disease remains a major health problem throughout the world. The reasons for this are apparent if we remember what has been achieved in Britain and then consider some of the difficult problems facing less advanced countries.

In Britain the four major animal-borne diseases of historical times have been plague, typhus, bovine tuberculosis and rabies. Plague died out after the devastating epidemic of 1665, although it remained in parts of Europe for another century. There is no satisfactory explanation for this. Typhus disappeared at the end of the nineteenth century, an unplanned consequence of a rising standard of living, in particular of improved water supply which enabled people to wash themselves, and of being wealthy enough to change their clothes. Nutrition may also have been important since the disease in its epidemic form has often accompanied famines. In contrast, bovine tuberculosis has been deliberately brought under control by law, aimed first at pasteurization of milk and later at elimination of diseased cattle. Rabies has been eradicated by a combination of chance and choice. The English Channel provides a natural barrier against the entry of infected wild animals and makes it much easier to enforce quarantine on imported animals including household pets. The spread of the disease over the past decade into France together with the huge rise in cross channel motor traffic have increased the need for rigid enforcement of this legislation.

We are left with a number of less important animal-borne diseases—salmonellosis, brucellosis, leptospirosis, tape-worm infestation and hydatid disease—incompletely controlled by complex statutory machinery concerned with port health, rodent control, refuse disposal, meat inspection and the hygiene of food establishments, slaughter houses and dairies. Control is incomplete because behaviour expressed in terms of standards of personal hygiene and the cooperation of individuals is also involved.

At a world level the control of the major animal-borne diseases presents formidable problems. The difficulties are well illustrated by the WHO campaign to eliminate malaria, one of the most ambitious health projects of recent times. The plan was to achieve global eradication by way of area and regional programmes. The strategy of area eradication was well defined and consisted of four phases: a preparatory phase usually of about 12 months, in which the malarious area was surveyed and field-workers trained; an attack phase in which all habitations in the area were sprayed 2 or 3 times a year for 4 years with residual insecticide at the end of which period almost all malarial infections could be expected to have died out spontaneously; a consolidation phase during which the whole population is kept under surveillance and blood samples are taken from all fever cases in the area, until no new case has been detected for 3 years; and a maintenance phase to guard against recrudescence or importation of the disease until it has been eradicated in the rest of the world. By these methods malaria has been eradicated in continental Europe, the Mediterranean Islands, the United States and parts of South America, and campaigns are in the consolidation phase in Ceylon and much of India. In many other parts of the world, however, progress is slow. This is partly due to resistance of anopheles to insecticides and of plasmodia to drugs, and partly the failure of those responsible for planning and supplementing the control programmes to recognize and make allowance for the importance of behaviour and attitudes of local populations. These derive from cultural and social influences, but are also dependant on health. Filipino farmers, whose health had benefited from a control scheme, cleared areas of virgin forest thereby creating new breeding grounds for anopheles.

Other causes of incomplete success have been breakdown of surveillance during the phase of consolidation through lack of financial, technical resources, and the behavioural problem of poor cooperation. Promising progress is being made in the development of a vaccine however.

None of the major animal-borne diseases is more difficult to control than bilharziasis. As we have noted, its epidemiology is well understood; yet in most of the affected areas the disease is static and in some, as water resources are developed and irrigation schemes extended, it is spreading. In poor countries with low standards of hygiene it is impossible to prevent the pollution of irrigation water with urine or faeces as the case may be and since treatment of the disease is not very effective, agricultural workers inevitably come into contact with infected water.

Secondary Protection

14

Nutrition

D.R.R. WILLIAMS

We have already seen how food, as a component of the physical environment can, coincidentally carry disease to man. In this chapter our concern is with the kind of food people eat, the ways in which social and community forces influence the choice of food and how in turn diet is related to health. Thus although nutrition can be looked upon as the process of sustaining with food, and as such falls into the purview of biochemists and physiologists, its modification and improvement can only be brought about by changes in behaviour. In earlier chapters we have indicated that the health and longevity of the British population have over the centuries been profoundly influenced for the better by improvement in nutrition (figures 2.1 and 2.2). Nevertheless during recent decades new problems have emerged because it has become clear that nutritional factors have played a role in the genesis of the chronic degenerative diseases which are characteristic of affluent societies (Chapter 5). The paradox should be borne in mind however that the effects of undernutrition are still frequently to be found in one country among communities living side by side with others suffering chronic disease from the surfeit and imbalance of what they eat.

Changes in Food Consumption

Studies of food consumption suggest that considerable changes in eating habits have occurred in many countries since the beginning of this century, that these have accelerated since the Second World War, and are still occurring. The Organization for Economic Co-operation and Development (OECD) and the Food and Agriculture Organization (FAO) regularly publish food consumption estimates for the populations of their member countries. Although calculated indirectly, these estimates can serve as indicators of changes in eating habits over time, and of differences in nutritional standards between countries. As examples, OECD consumption estimates for the populations of West Germany, Japan and Portugal are given in table 14.1, where the most recently available statistics (1977 or 1978) are contrasted with the period 1955-59, the earliest period of which comprehensive data are published. The data in this table show not only marked contrasts in food consumption between the three countries, but also dramatic changes within each of them over time.

Table 14.1 Estimated consumption (g/person/day) for selected food groups in West Germany, Japan and Portugal, 1955-59 contrasted with latest year of available data. Source: OECD Food Consumption Statistics 1955-1973 and 1964-1978

		Total Cereals	Rice	Fish	Meat	Fruit	Veget- ables*	Potato
West	1955-59	246.9	4.4	30.2	162.8	208.9	134.3	405.3
Germany	1978	192.5	4.4	18.4	266.0	313.8	209.7	251.0
Japan	1955-59	421.8	311.0	124.1	14.2	48.4	229.0	120.8
	1978	320.5	224.1	104.1	79.8	111.0	315.4	75.1
Portugal	1955-59	341.1	35.6	81.7	68.8	181.4	297.2	298.7
	1977	334.1	48.4	80.1	145.3	144.7	368.2	247.8

*excludes potatoes

The consumption of cereals and starchy vegetables such as potatoes has fallen sharply in West Germany and Japan but changes have been slight in Portugal. While fish consumption has fallen in the former countries, that of meat has risen dramatically in all three. It has more than doubled in Portugal and increased almost six-fold in Japan. Fruit intakes have more than doubled in Japan but fallen in Portugal. The intake of vegetables, other than potatoes, particularly fresh green and frozen or preserved vegetables, has risen because of improved processing and transportation.

In Britain, the National Food Survey (NFS) publishes data on food consumption as estimated from an annually conducted survey of expenditure by a national sample. The Survey does not record details for food purchased and eaten outside the home and, since there have undoubtedly been important secular changes in the extent to which food is eaten away from home, NFS data must be viewed with some circumspection. Nevertheless, they too suggest marked changes in eating habits, some of the more important of which are displayed in figure 14.1.

British households in 1980 appeared to be eating less of several important foods and food groups than they were in 1956. Less milk and bread were consumed, although the proportion of brown, wholemeal or wholewheat bread which had become unfashionable is again increasing, and was 18 per cent of all bread eaten in 1980 compared with 9.8 per cent in 1975. Poultry has become far more usual as a component of the diet. As in most other industrial countries, UK households now eat more fresh fruit and processed vegetables and fewer potatoes.

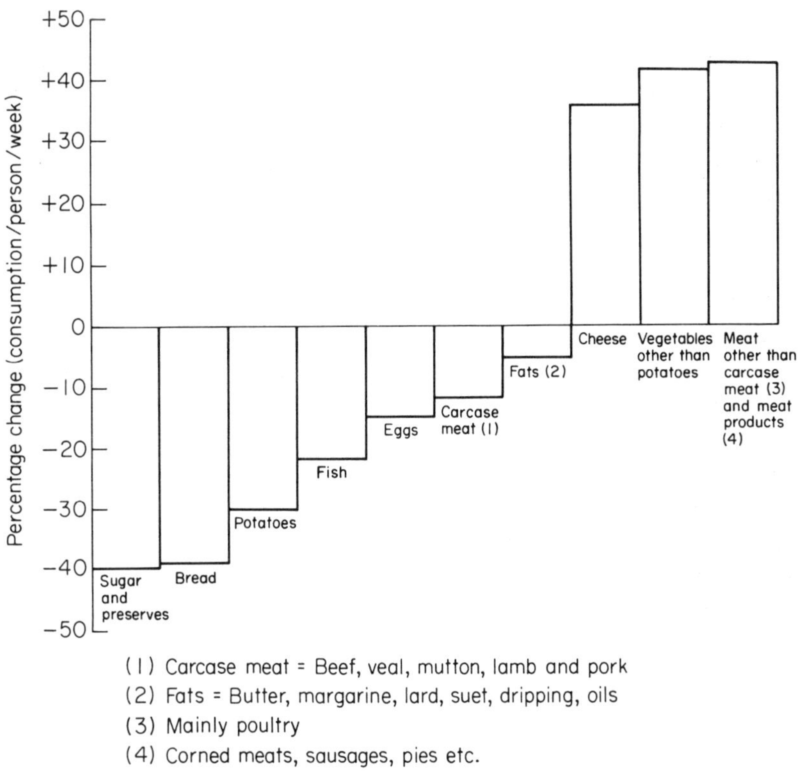

Figure 14.1 Percentage changes in domestic food consumption in the United Kingdom between 1956 and 1980.

The NFS has not yet published routine figures for the consumption of dietary fibre (non-starch polysaccharides) because these substances are of comparatively recent interest in human nutrition. Estimates of trends suggest that from the beginning of this century, with the exception of the years during and immediately following the Second World War when high extraction National Flour was in use, there has been a decline in the consumption of dietary fibre to an average intake of just over 20g per person per day by 1974. The proportional contribution of cereal fibre to this total has become less and that from vegetables has increased.

Choice of diet

In most parts of the world malnutrition is as we have seen still common; and until recently the great majority lived with the threat of famine and death from starvation close at hand. Those who are preoccupied with the problem of finding enough food to keep alive do not bother much about the relative proportions of the different components of their diet, and apart from the risk of acute poisoning are not much concerned with whether food may cause disease. They eat what they can get and this is determined by where they live: maritime communities live largely on fish: in the tropics the variety of naturally occurring roots, fruits and cereals favours vegetarianism; and people living in Polar regions depend almost entirely on the flesh and fat of seal, whale and walrus. Even in more advanced communities climate and geography have a considerable influence on diet, of which the olive oil, pasta and wine of Italy and the herrings, porridge and whisky of Scotland are examples. Moreover, in a given locality seasonal variations in availability of fruit, vegetables and animal foods are usually still reflected in seasonal changes in diet.

Brahmins, Muslims, Jews and Catholics all have strong dietetic taboos; a Frenchman will eat snails, an Australian bushman insects, a Welshman seaweed and an Englishman corned beef and cabbage. So highly conditioned is the sense of taste that each may find his own titbit delectable and his neighbour's disgusting.

Over the past century there has been unprecedented technological change in methods of producing, storing and transporting food, and climate, season and geographical position are no longer so important in determining what a community eats. In spite of these advances, food habits and standards of nutrition still vary a great deal from country to country and between different social groups. Climatic differences also account for some of the variation though because of improved transportation these influences are becoming less important. For instance, in Japan, inceases in imports have played an important part in reducing the consumption of rice (which is mostly home grown) in favour of meat and vegetables. But by far the greater part of the variation is due not to climatic influence or religious and social custom but to economics. This is true at the national as well as at the personal level. Nations, like individuals, can have as adequate and varied a diet as they can afford.

World Bank statistics attribute the lowest estimates for per caput gross domestic product (GDP) and mean personal income to developing African countries south of the Sahara, which for the period 1970-1977, was about US $100 per person per year; correspondingly the United Nations Food and Agriculture Organization estimate their energy intakes to be the lowest in the world averaging 85-90 per cent of calculated requirements. Industrialized countries, with a per caput GDP of US $3,200 in the same period, has estimated individual energy intakes of 120-130 per cent of the recommended level. Although total energy is only one aspect of food intake it is almost invariable that populations deficient in total food energy are also lacking in some if not all essentials such as vitamins, minerals and protein.

The classical studies of Boyd-Orr in Britain in the 1930s gave the first quantitative information of how expenditure on food depended on family income. Recent data on the UK population show that this relationship still holds with a clear gradient of increasing consumption of many commodities and nutritients with increasing family income. Fruit and vegetables other than potatoes show this gradient particularly clearly (the trend is in the other direction for potatoes) and, accordingly, vitamin C shows much higher levels of intake in high income groups than in the low income groups. The gap between rich and poor for intakes of this nutrient and for several others has actually widened since the post war period although the intakes of all groups have increased. Expenditure on food as a whole is relatively loosely related to price since, as food costs rise, so, almost invariably, do those of other goods and services, particularly of shelter, fuel, clothing and transport, and the individual often has less control over expenditure on these items than on food. The tendency is to reduce food expenditure relative to these items either by a general reduction or by switching to cheaper brand or commodity alternatives.

Nutrition and health

There is evidence that food choices are at least partly determined by an individual's perception of what constitutes a healthy diet. Nevertheless, as suggested, the influence of economics, social and religious customs, geography and climate are predominant. Also, the general public's nutritional information and opinions are often incomplete, out of date, misinformed or in other ways inadequate.

Breastfeeding

The influence on the health both of mother and infant, of breastfeeding, is often less important in determining the mother's practices than are social customs and commercial interests. Although the principal constituents of breast milk—protein, carbohydrate and fat—are, so far as can be ascertained, well buffered against variations in the mother's diet, volume and vitamin content are governed partly by adequacy of maternal nutrition. Hence, in populations where adult nutrition is deficient breast milk substitutes may have a place. In recent years, however, widespread commercial advertising has been able to convince many populations in the Third World to abandon breastfeeding in favour of bottle feeding even where maternal nutrition is adequate and prolonged breastfeeding a traditional practice. The reasons for concern about this consequence of commercial promotion relate to the widely accepted and important protective functions of human breast milk for human offspring, to its superiority to any substitute from the hygienic point of view, and to the emotional benefits mother and child derive from breastfeeding.

The precise way in which specific protection is achieved is not known though the transfer from mother to child of immunoglobulin (particularly IgA), complement components and the cellular elements contained in breast milk are clearly important. Whatever the exact mechanism, breast fed infants are less susceptible to all infections, (but especially those of the respiratory and gastrointestinal systems), than bottle fed infants and these differences are particularly marked where the preparation of breast milk substitutes is carried out in unhygienic conditions. Most authorities now advocate breastfeeding where possible as preferable to bottle feeding and, perhaps partly because of this, social custom in most industrialized countries is again tending to favour suckling after many decades during which it was less widely practiced.

School milk and school meals

From shortly after the Second World War until 1968, free milk at school was provided for all British children. From that year milk has only been available for successively younger age groups and since 1978 the provision of this dietary supplement has been at the discretion of Local Education Authorities. At present, children in some areas receive free milk while those in others do not. Its introduction on a national scale in 1946 was based on the observations of Corry Mann among others who, in 1926, had noted an improvement in the growth of undernourished boys when they were given a supplement of 1 pint of milk per day. The prevailing social conditions of most groups of children in Britain have changed considerably since the immediate post-war years and several studies have recently examined the possible influences of school milk provision on children's stature, growth and nutritional intake. It seems that children who drink school milk have significantly higher intakes of animal protein, calcium and riboflavin than those who do not, but these differences are not associated with clear-cut differences in height gain. It is likely however, that while socially disadvantaged children would benefit from nutritional supplements including milk, providing them free to all schools should not now be the policy of choice in Britain.

Though there has never been a time when school lunches have been available free to all British school children, their provision has in some ways followed a pattern similar to that of school milk. In 1944 all Local Authorities were required to make a midday meal available to those children who wished to take one. Standards were laid down for the composition of this meal in relation to recommended intakes of energy and essential nutrients though, in practice, these were rarely adhered to. In 1980 the obligation to provide school meals was withdrawn, and Local Authorities were allowed to determine their own standards and level of provision. Several authorities still attempt to enforce national standards especially in meals for infants and junior children.

Data on the effects of midday meal provision on the health and growth of school children are available. Like those for school milk provision, they are open to a number of interpretations but suggest that in the 1970s the growth of English school children was not related to eating school lunches, although some Scottish school children from low income families showed slower rates of growth if they took these meals than if they ate lunches prepared at home. Nevertheless, as with school milk studies, surveys of school lunch provision do not rule out the possibility that subsidized or free school lunches of an accepted minimal standard benefit socially disadvantaged children. In addition, school meals have the potential advantage not only of feeding children but teaching them what they should eat, an advantage which may be lost as free choice 'cafeteria' systems are introduced.

The proportion of British pupils arriving in school without having eaten any breakfast is surprisingly high. Even in the comparatively affluent South East, an enquiry in the mid 1970s reported this to be 7.4 per cent of children investigated. This provision of a social breakfast or mid-morning snack may be as important as the provision of a midday meal, not only for nutritional reasons, but also to ensure that pupils are able to obtain full benefit from the morning's schooling.

Nutrition and chronic degenerative diseases

Although as we have seen chronic degenerative diseases are usually afflictions of middle and old age, there is no reason to believe that the aetiological factors relevant to their development are encountered only during these periods of life. It is probable on the basis of current evidence relating to ischaemic heart disease, for example, that diet and perhaps other environmental exposures in childhood and early adult life are important determinants. Of the many issues in the general field of diet and chronic degenerative disease those currently thought to be of major public health importance are:

- the established role of sucrose in the development of dental caries;
- the role of fat (and particularly saturated fats) in the aetiologies of ischaemic heart disease, colon cancer, breast cancer and obesity;
- the issue of whether a high intake of sodium and/or low intake of potassium are important causes of essential hypertension (and hence cerebrovascular, and ischaemic heart disease);
- the role of low dietary fibre consumption in the aetiology of colon cancer and
- the issue of whether certain nutrients—such as vitamins A and C—protect from neoplasia, for instance in the lung and stomach, and perhaps from certain cardiovascular diseases.

As Doll and Peto have remarked in relation to the aetiology of cancer, 'diet is a source of both excitement and frustration to epidemiologists': excitement, since there exists a large body of evidence suggesting that dietary factors are causative or protective, but frustration because conclusive evidence is often so difficult to obtain. Their observation applies also to diseases other than cancer. The problems of investigating putative dietary causes of most of the chronic degenerative disease in free-living human populations are formidable. Nevertheless, in the opinion of many, there exists sufficient evidence to justify action in promoting sound nutrition on a population basis, action which will result in prevention of disease and the promotion of health.

Of the chronic degenerative diseases, dental caries is the most expensive in terms of treatment costs and probably also in terms of loss of work time. Fortunately the evidence incriminating an excess of dietary sucrose and deficit of fluoride in the causation of this disease in incontrovertible. Although as we have seen attempts to add fluoride to the water supply in Britain have not been successful it has over recent decades been widely used as an additive to toothpaste. Sucrose intakes have also fallen (see figure 14.1), so the state of children's teeth has improved.

Less widely accepted is the evidence relating saturated fat to ischaemic heart disease and sodium to the aetiology of hypertension though many believe that it is good enough to justify recommending reductions in dietary fat and sodium, and that the evidence also supports an increase in dietary fibre in relation to diverticular disease and colonic carcinoma. Recommendations from most authoritative bodies have suggested that these and other dietary goals be adopted on a population basis, and there are countries, for instance Norway, which have already adopted national nutrition policies along these lines. Although targets for fat, carbohydrate, fibre and sodium consumption may differ slightly between countries, the general features of most sets of recommendations are remarkably similar.

It has been argued that dietary habits are not amenable to change but this is clearly false. The observations made in the first part of this chapter demonstrate that changes are continually taking place and they are often extensive. Even though economic factors largely provide the stimulus to this change, it would be misguided to consider that food prices could not (or should not) be used to encourage dietary change for health reasons. It is also necessary to consider whether the profound changes that are already underway should be encouraged or discouraged on grounds of health. In Britain, in the period covered by figure 14.1 the proportion of food energy derived from fat rose from about 37 per cent to 43 per cent, while that derived from carbohydrate fell from around 53 per cent to 44 per cent (NFS estimates). It has been suggested that there is insufficient evidence to justify the promulgation of a healthy diet for all. No doubt there is much to be learned but we already know enough to discourage many practices and recommend others. There is no longer an excuse for inaction.

The challenges of nutritional epidemiology and social nutrition are not easy to meet. Though in most industrialized societies undernutrition is no longer evident, it still contributes significantly to the morbidity and premature mortality experienced elsewhere, and the contribution of nutritional factors to chronic degenerative diseases is evident not only in the richer nations but in the more affluent subpopulations of developing countries.

Further Reading

Doll R. and Peto R. (1981) *The Causes of Cancer—Quantitative Estimates of Avoidable Risks of Cancer in the United States Today.* Oxford University Press, Oxford.

Health Department of Great Britain and Northern Ireland (1978) *Eating for Health: A discussion booklet.* HMSO, London.

Holland W. W., Chin S. and Rona R. J. (1980) *The effect of cessation of free school milk.* In *Symposium on Nutrition* held 6-7th December in the Royal College of Physicians of Edinburgh (S. H. Davies, ed.) p. 79. Royal College of Physicians, Edinburgh.

Orr J. B. (1936) *Food, Health and Income.* Macmillan and Co., London.

Passmore R., Hollingsworth D. F. and Robertson J. (1979) Prescription for a better British diet. *British Medical Journal* **1**, 527-531.

Thomas J. (1980) The relationship between knowledge about food and nutrition and food choice. In *Nutrition and Lifestyles* (M. R. Turner, ed.). Applied Science Publishers, London.

Turner M. R. (Ed.) (1981) *Preventive Nutrition and Society.* Academic Press, London.

15

Immunization

In medical teaching there has been some uncertainty about responsibility for instruction in immunization and we must begin by clarifying our interpretation of it. Discussion of the organisms which cause infectious disease is clearly the concern of departments of microbiology. Clinical departments should deal with the clinical manifestations of the infections and, perhaps, the immunization procedures used to prevent them. Our task in community medicine is to evaluate the contribution of immunization from an organizational as well as biological point of view.

It has long been recognized that those who recover from infectious illness frequently acquire some degree of protection, and the Chinese attempted to exploit this knowledge by inoculating with material from mild cases of smallpox. This hazardous procedure was introduced to the British Isles in 1721 and appears to have been employed fairly extensively in the eighteenth century. It was replaced by cowpox vaccination from 1798, the first example of safe and effective immunization and the only one for nearly a further hundred years. The identification of bacteria led to the use of antitoxin for treatment of diphtheria from 1891. With these exceptions immunization procedures were developed in the present century, and used widely in Britain only after 1940.

For the purpose of evaluating the contribution of immunization we shall first consider diseases against which immunization is now routinely employed in Britain, and secondly diseases in which vaccines are not offered routinely but are administered in certain circumstances. As we shall see, no matter how effective a vaccine, its success as a measure for protecting society-at-large is in the event behavioural in that individuals must agree to have themselves, or as the case may be their children inoculated.

Routine Immunization

Diphtheria

Mortality from diphtheria in England and Wales has declined fairly continuously since the late nineteenth century (figure 15.1). It was then a relatively common cause of death in children. Today it is a rare disease, and many doctors who have qualified since the end of the Second World

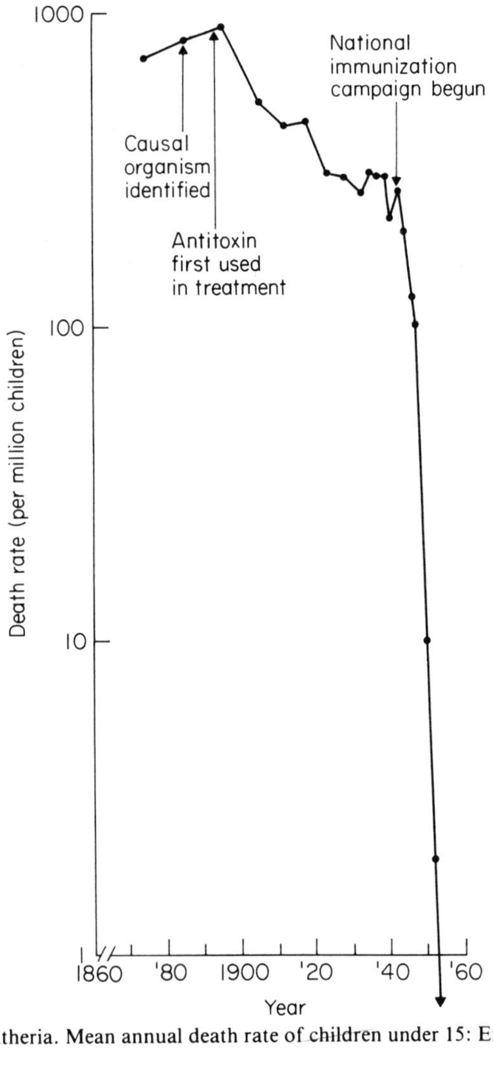

Figure 15.1 Diphtheria. Mean annual death rate of children under 15: England and Wales.

War have never seen a case of it. In the 6 years, 1965-70, there were only 9 deaths from diphtheria in England and Wales.

It is not possible to assess with any precision the relative importance of the various influences which have contributed to the decline of mortality from the disease. Antitoxin was first used in the late nineteenth century to give passive immunity and has been the accepted form of treatment since then. It is believed to have reduced the case fatality rate, which fell from 8.2 per 100 notifications in 1916-25 to 5.4 in 1933-42, while notifications remained at an average level of above 50,000 per year in England and Wales. The mortality rate increased at the beginning of the last war, but fell rapidly at about the time when national immunization was introduced (figure 15.1).

It is fair to conclude that much of the decline of diphtheria mortality between 1895 and 1922 was due to treatment with antitoxin, and the rapid fall since 1940 to immunization. But the fact that diseases such as whooping cough (figure 15.2) and measles (figure 15.4) showed a large reduction of mortality, without treatment or prophylaxis, suggests that other unspecified influences were at work. We cannot exclude the possibility that they also contributed, perhaps substantially, to the decline of diphtheria.

Tuberculosis

In Chapter 2 we discussed the trend of mortality from tuberculosis in the nineteenth century (figure 2.5) and the possible reasons for its remarkable decline. Attempts to protect by vaccination began in 1890, when Koch introduced tuberculin, an extract of dead bacteria. The method was unsuccessful, and was followed by use of living virulent tubercle bacilli. This procedure was recognized to be dangerous and was soon abandoned.

The first avirulent live vaccine, and the one in general use today was BCG (Bacille Calmette-Guérin). The bovine strain was virulent when first isolated (in 1906), but rapidly lost its virulence when cultured on potato with added ox bile. Although Calmette and Guérin first described the strain in 1908, it was not administered as a prophylactic in man until 1921, or generally released before 1924. For a few years it was used mainly in France and Scandinavia, where it was given almost exclusively to children of tuberculous parents and to tuberculin-negative adults considered to be exposed to special risks of acquiring the disease.

The policy of vaccinating tuberculin-negative individuals in the general population was accepted in Scandinavia in about 1940 and has since spread to many other countries. In Britain BCG was used from 1949 for persons exposed to special risks of tuberculosis, and in 1953 the Ministry of Health recommended vaccination of all tuberculin-negative children at age 13. By this time mortality from respiratory tuberculosis in England and Wales had declined to less than one-fifteenth of its level when first registered (figures 2.4 and 2.5).

The value of BCG vaccination has been assessed by Springett, and the following discussion is based largely on his conclusions.

If all members of a community are tuberculin positive, or if all are tuberculin negative, BCG vaccination is useless: in the first case because all are already infected; in the second because none can become infected. Between these theoretical extreme possibilities the value of BCG must be assessed in relation to the extent to which it reduces the incidence of tuberculosis in vaccinated negatives as compared with those left unvaccinated, in economic terms to the cost and benefit of the programme. In a number of trials tuberculosis morbidity or mortality was between 30 per cent and 80 per cent lower in those vaccinated than in controls. The large difference between the results was probably due to variation in the circumstances of each trial. The type of vaccine and the conditions under which it is used are therefore important.

Low levels of protection do not justify a vaccination campaign, and a 75 per cent reduction of morbidity or mortality should be the objective. Conclusions concerning the use of BCG in circumstances which are common in the world today are as follows.

- *Many tuberculin positives and high conversion rate.* Conditions still to be found in many countries of the world, especially where facilities for treatment are limited. It seems certain that BCG vaccination can effectively reduce the amount of tuberculosis under these conditions, and the main problem is to decide to which groups to offer it. In most communities of this type, very large numbers of adolescents are tuberculin positive, and the only logical use for BCG is its application to all new-born children, as at no other age is the uninfected population large enough for BCG to be fully effective.
- *Percentage positive high, but infection rate falling from previously very high levels.* The situation of many countries with well developed tuberculosis services with full utilization of adequate chemotherapy. The factor of greatest importance here is the conversion rate to be expected in

negatives; if the great majority of children are reaching adolescence tuberculin negative, then the most effective use for BCG on a community scale would be at about the age of puberty, to protect against the increase of tuberculosis experienced in adolescence and young adult life. As infection rates fall still further, the final stage may be reached of:

- *Percentage positive low.* With declining infection rates a point is reached when the disadvantages of artificial tuberculin conversion and the cost of the procedure no longer justify its use. It is argued by some that Britain and other parts of the world with well developed health services and good living conditions have already reached this stage.

The first of these three types of circumstances is to be found in developing countries, the second in technologically advanced countries (or in sub-groups of the population within them) where infection rates are not low, and the third in technologically advanced countries where infection rates are low.

The issues are complex in the first type of community, where infection is common, medical resources are limited, and social and economic conditions are poor. In such circumstances the grounds for prevention of disease are even stronger than in developed countries because treatment is likely to be more difficult, but the widespread use of vaccination raises three questions:

1. Is BCG equally effective in all kinds of society? In countries such as Britain, vaccination was not used until mortality had declined to a fraction of its initial level (figure 2.5) by which time the population had a relatively high standard of living and malnutrition was uncommon. However, experience in Algeria, Southern India and the indigenous populations of North America suggests that even in very different conditions BCG remains relatively effective.
2. Would the use of BCG prejudice the improvement of the social environment, particularly housing and diet? These measures are very effective in controlling conditions other than tuberculosis and it would be a serious loss if the use of specific protection resulted in their neglect.
3. Does vaccination make the best use of a limited number of medical and other trained workers? In a country where tuberculosis is common BCG takes precedence over treatment, particularly since it needs only a single procedure. But where the ratio of trained workers to population is very low, as it still is in many countries, benefit provided by BCG must be weighed against that of all the other tasks the doctor and his associates might perform; this is one aspect of the economic assessment alluded to above.

The value of BCG in the second and third types of community referred to above can be assessed fairly accurately, the main problem being to decide at what point vaccination is no longer justified. Certainly it should be continued so long as the cost of treating and maintaining cases which could be prevented is greater than the cost of giving BCG to the whole population (or risk group). But when the cost of vaccination exceeds the cost of case-finding, treatment and maintenance, the question becomes more difficult, not least because the answer cannot be decided on economic grounds alone.

It has been estimated that in Britain in 1969-70 the percentage of children infected at age 13 was 8 per cent, and at this level it was considered desirable to immunize routinely children aged 10-13. However the percentage infected is still falling and has now reached a level in Britain which is so low that some experts believe that the routine use of BCG in schoolchildren is indeed no longer justified. They argue that it should be reserved for those at special risk, for instance, tuberculin negative people who are likely to be exposed to active cases of the disease such as infants born to tuberculous parents; nurses; or immigrants.

Whooping cough

Figure 15.2 shows the trend of mortality from whooping cough expressed as the annual death rate of children under 15. The causal organism, *Bordetella pertussis*, was identified in 1906 but no vaccination was available for another 40 years. In the mid-nineteenth century this disease was a very frequent cause of death, particularly in young children about as frequent as measles and much more so than diphtheria; during the first part of the twentieth century it killed thousands more than poliomyelitis. Mortality has declined almost continuously from about 1870 until 1976 when there were only 2 deaths.

A vaccine consisting of whole bacterial cells became available for trials in 1952 and began to be used on a routine basis in Britain in 1956. From the outset it was recognized that it caused local pain and fretfulness in most infants and convulsions and other more serious reactions in a few. Nevertheless, the acceptance rate was in the order of 80 per cent. In 1977 an investigator reported that 1 in 50,000 inoculations were followed by permanent, brain damage, and the uptake of vaccination rapidly fell to about 30 per cent with the result that the incidence of the disease and the death rate from it both rose with 13 deaths in 1978 and 65,000 cases,

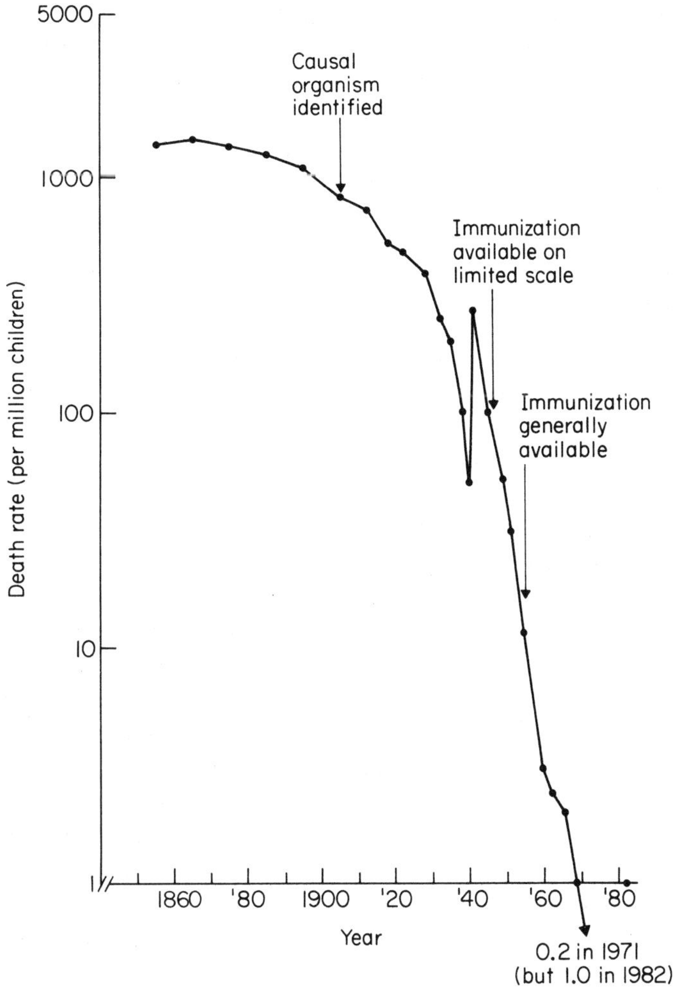

Figure 15.2 Whooping cough. Mean annual death rate of children under 15: England and Wales.

the largest annual number since the vaccination was recommended nationally. Further very careful research now puts the risk of permanent neurological sequelae at 1 in 310,000 injections; this is far lower than the case fatality rate from the disease, which in infants in their first year is nearly 1 per cent. The Department of Health and Social Security again recommended general use of the vaccine and are supporting research to make it safer. By 1982 uptake of vaccination had climbed to about 55 per cent.

No convincing explanation can be given for the great reduction of mortality from whooping cough over the hundred years between 1850 and 1950. Treatment by sulphonamides and (later) antibiotics was not available before 1939, and even now their effect on the course of the disease is questionable. Despite its importance immunization contributed only a little, for by 1952 mortality in England and Wales had declined to a small fraction of its level in 1872.

Poliomyelitis

Poliomyelitis appears to have been a rare disease before the late nineteenth century, but since that time it has occurred in epidemics in many countries. It is due to a virus which infects the alimentary tract and only occasionally causes the paralysis which is a striking feature of the disease; it is important to recognize that the number of cases infected but with few or no clinical manifestations exceeds greatly (by about 100 to 1) the number affected by paralysis. In its paralytic form poliomyelitis presents the anomaly of an intestinal infection whose incidence increases as social conditions improve, for although the polio virus is endemic in communities which lack hygiene its greatest incidence has been in countries with a high standard of living. An explanation which can be offered with reservations is that in primitive conditions children acquire immunity by early exposure to the infection whereas if hygiene is good they are protected from exposure and hence less resistant when they meet the disease in adult life. It is consistent with this interpretation that although the disease is most common in young children, its neurological manifestations are most severe in adolescents and adults.

Because of the conspicuous disabilities which are common in patients who survive, there is, understandably, some tendency to overestimate the significance of poliomyelitis in relation to other infections. In 1947, when the highest death rate was recorded in England and Wales, there were 33 deaths from the disease per million children under 15 (figure 15.3) compared with 99 from whooping cough and 69 from measles. In 1871-80, before the decline of mortality began, the last two diseases were responsible for 1,415 and 1,038 deaths (per million under 15) respectively.

Poliomyelitis was recognized as an infection in 1909. Fifty years later it was shown to be due to a filterable virus and subsequently two methods of immunization have been used widely: inactivated vaccine containing killed virus (Salk); and live attenuated virus vaccine (Sabin). The former

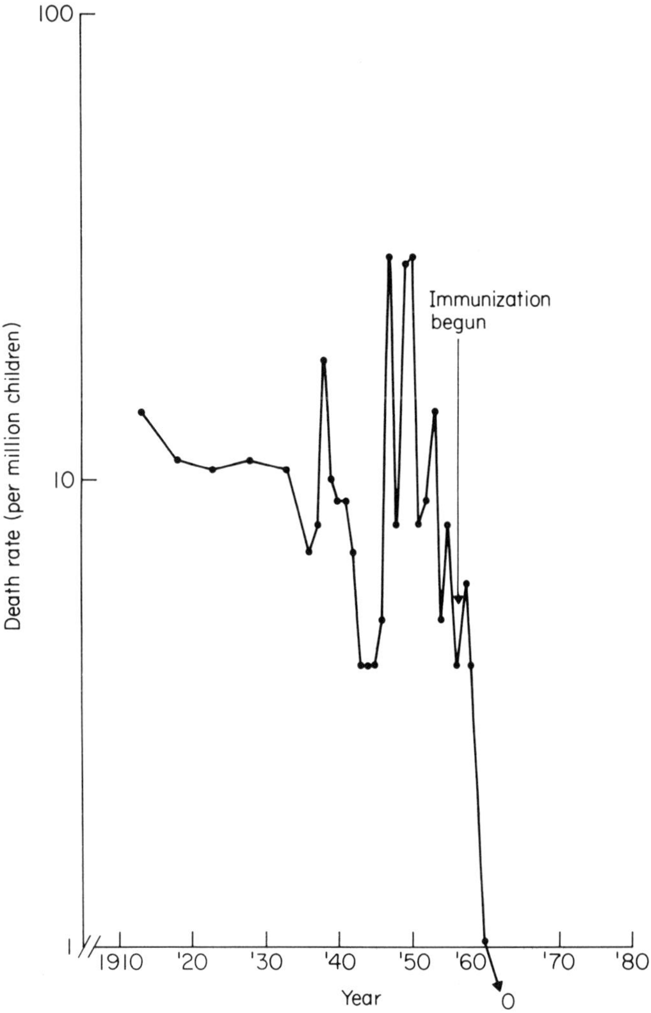

Figure 15.3 Acute poliomyelitis. Mean annual death rate of children under 15: England and Wales.

was in use in Britain from 1956, but the latter is now generally preferred since it can be given orally and the immunity conferred is greater and lasts longer. Moreover the attenuated viruses of the oral vaccine result in antibody formation in the blood and local resistance to subsequent infection with virulent poliomyelitis viruses. This reduces the number of symptomless excreters of virulent poliomyelitis virus in the community.

Figure 15.3 shows the time (1956) when immunization against poliomyelitis became common in England and Wales. Although, at about 7 per million, the death rate had been very low, it is clear that within a few years it disappeared altogether. Laboratory evidence indicates that this is because the vaccine gives a high degree of immunity, as measured by the titre of circulating antibody. Results of controlled trials have been impressive. And poliomyelitis has been almost eliminated from countries which have had effective immunization programmes, whereas it is still common in countries which have not. A surveillance scheme in existence in England and Wales shows that a slight risk of poliomyelitis induced by the oral vaccine cannot be ruled out, but the risk is considered to be so small that it does not justify restriction of the vaccination programme.

Measles

During the nineteenth and early twentieth centuries childhood mortality from measles was relatively high, but it declined rapidly from about the time of the First World War (figure 15.4). Nevertheless measles remains an important infectious disease; in 1982 nearly 140,000 cases were notified in England and there were 13 deaths, excessive figures for a disease known to be preventable.

It is now recommended that children should be immunized routinely with a vaccine containing live attenuated measles virus. In trials the living vaccine produced antibody in 95 per cent of those vaccinated and a Medical Research Council protection trial suggested that the procedure was over 90 per cent effective. On this and other evidence it was hoped that it might be possible to eradicate measles, and it was estimated that vaccination of 75 per cent or more of children at 1 year of age would result in control of the disease. The success expected has not yet been achieved, partly perhaps because the requirements for it have not been met fully. In the United States extensive vaccination programmes have totally changed the epidemic pattern of measles. Only 3,032 cases were reported in the whole country in 1981 and during that year in 15 of the 50 states there was no case caused by indigenous transmission. In Britain, on average about 100,000 cases are reported annually in a population less than a quarter of the size. An integral part of the success in the United States has been legislation which requires children to have been immunized against measles before they can be admitted to school. Efforts are being made there totally to eradicate the disease and impressive progress

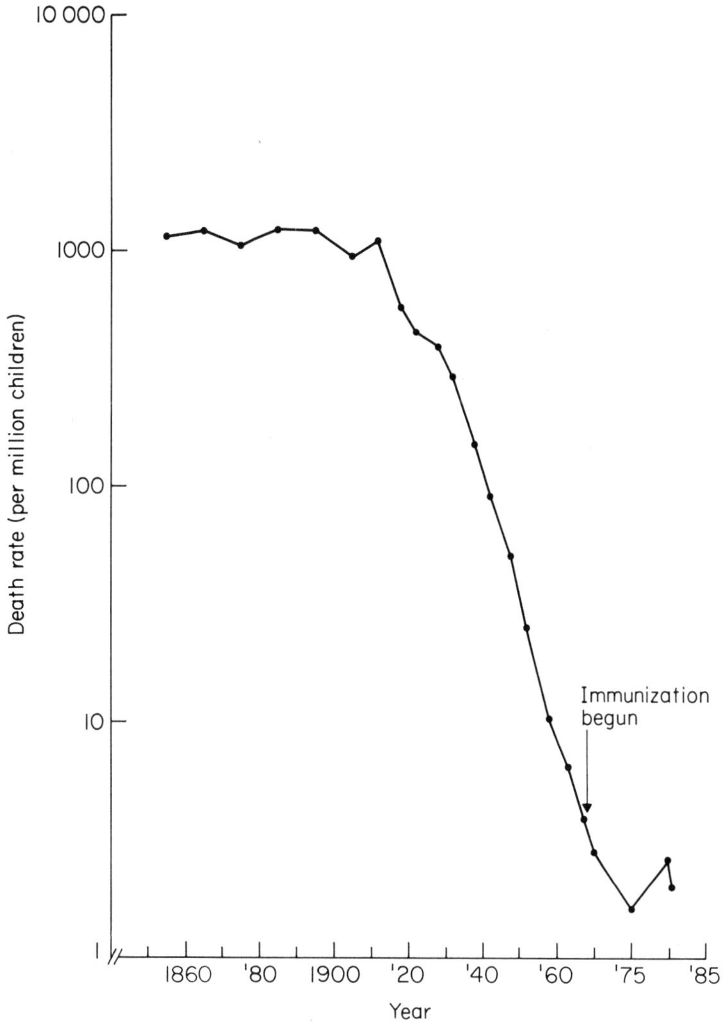

Figure 15.4 Measles. Mean annual death rate of children under 15: England and Wales.

is evident (see figure 15.5) but more stringent control will be costly and whether in the jet age this brave attempt at eradication will merit the investment is a matter for debate. Over the past century in Britain, although its incidence changed little before the introduction of immunization, the disease became steadily less serious as the fall in mortality shows (figure 15.4), but the further fall in recent years may in part be attributed to a reduction in incidence due to immunization. To judge by

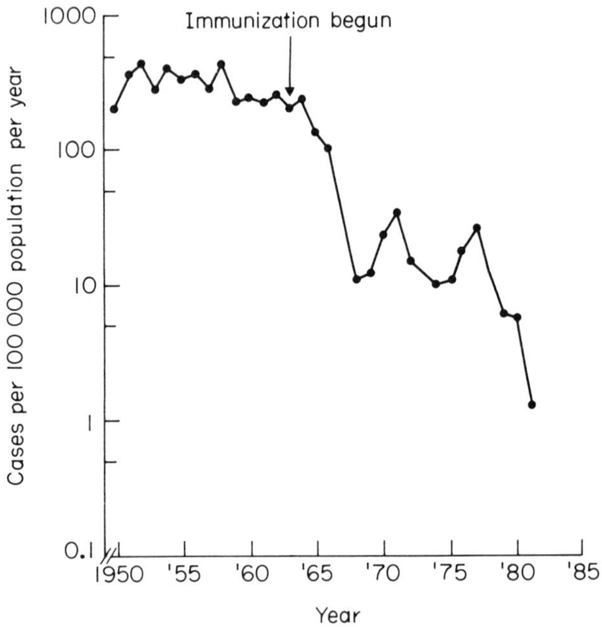

Figure 15.5 Measles. Incidence of notified cases in USA Logarithmic scale.

US experience, therefore, a marginally larger investment should prevent all deaths from this cause.

Rubella

Rubella is a very mild infectious disease which rarely gives rise to serious complications in those infected. The need for immunization was therefore unrecognized until it was observed that congenital malformations were common in children born after a pregnancy during which the mother had contracted the infection.

The virus was isolated in 1962, first from clinical cases and then from malformed infants. Subsequently vaccines were prepared which protect against the disease, and in Britain immunization is now offered routinely to all girls at ages 11 to 13. Because of the possibility of pregnancy and risk to fetus, the vaccine which is an attenuated virus is not administered routinely to women of childbearing age; but it may be used in selected groups, for example in women found to be seronegative provided they are aware of the importance of avoiding pregnancy for at least 2 months.

The only appropriate indication of the success of vaccination would be a reduction in the frequency of malformations due to rubella; or of the abortions which are usually performed once the disease is recognized during pregnancy. It is difficult, perhaps impossible, to assess this contribution, for rubella is sometimes unrecognized, and the malformations, although characteristic of the disease, may be due to other causes.

Tetanus

Before the First World War the annual death rate from tetanus in England and Wales was 7 per million of population per year. The rate has declined almost continuously since that time (figure 15.6) and is now well below 0.5 per million.

Passive immunization, in which tetanus antitoxin is given at the time of injury, has been used extensively since the First World War. However it has some serious disadvantages; it is not effective in certain cases; the protective effect is transient (about 2 weeks); it cannot be given in the large number of cases of minor injury which do not come to medical attention; and it is sometimes accompanied by the serious or minor reactions that may follow administration of horse serum. Active immunization by use of tetanus toxoid is effective and safe. In the British Army in the First World War, when antitoxin was used routinely after injury, the incidence of tetanus was at least 1 in 2,000 wounded. During the Second World War it was the policy of the US (and British) Armed Forces to immunize every man and woman with tetanus toxoid on enlistment and to give a booster dose to every casualty. Among 2,750,000 wounded Americans there were only 12 cases of tetanus. These results are not strictly comparable, but they are in accord with much other evidence that active immunization by tetanus toxoid is greatly to be preferred to passive immunization by antitoxin. A further dose of toxoid is effective after infection in a recipient who has previously received an adequate course of it, but the toxoid is useless in the non-immune. National policy is now to immunize all children, and to encourage active immunization of selected groups such as patients at accident departments of hospitals, factory workers, farm workers, students, school leavers, and amateur footballers.

It is not easy to assess the contribution of immunization to the decline of mortality from tetanus shown in figure 15.6. It cannot have contributed before the First World War, but passive immunization is believed

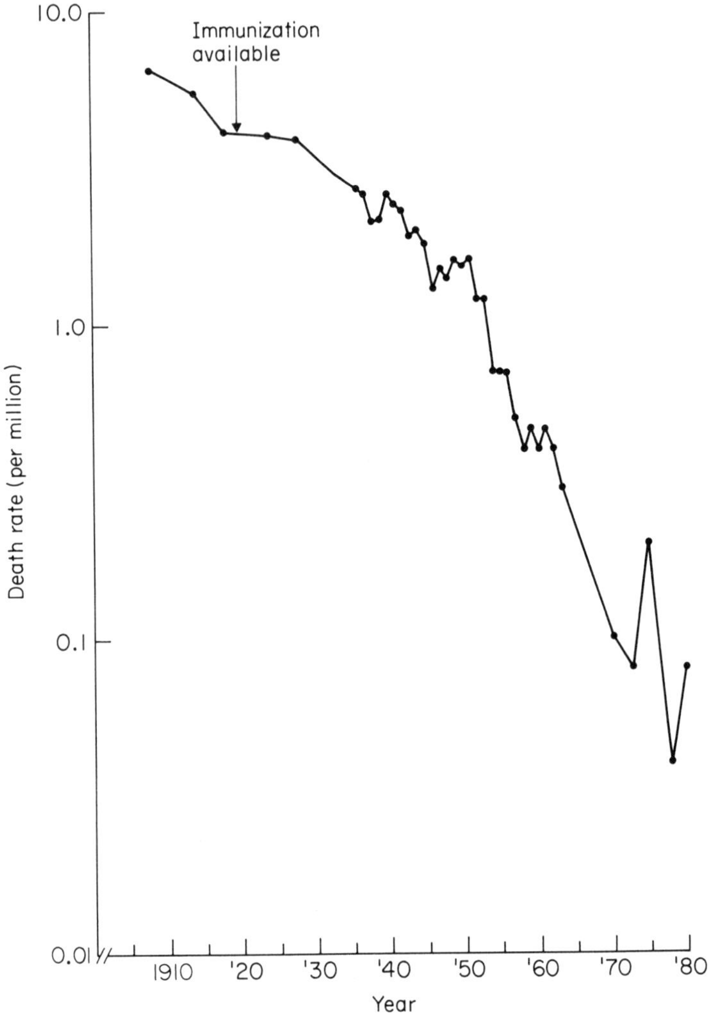

Figure 15.6 Tetanus. Mean annual death rate: England and Wales.

to have had a substantial influence since then. Although the routine active immunization of children was introduced only recently, large numbers of adults have been protected since the Second World War, including all those who have served in the armed forces. But while it is probable that both passive and active immunization have contributed to the decline of mortality, they were not the only nor, necessarily, the most important influences. Other explanations (such as the disappearance of the horse from the roads) must be found for the substantial reduction of deaths before the introduction of immunization, and in recent years there has been a considerable improvement in treatment, although the fatality rate in cases which are advanced before treatment is started remains high and the death painful.

Immunization in Particular Circumstances

Here we are concerned with diseases against which immunization may be offered only in particular circumstances; and within this class the discussion will be restricted to conditions which occur, or are likely to occur, in Britain. On these grounds we exclude yellow fever and cholera, against which people are vaccinated only when going abroad to countries where they will be at risk. Typhoid and paratyphoid fevers are also omitted, for although a few hundred cases are notified annually in the British Isles, immunization is advised only for those going to countries with low hygienic standards, and the procedure can have had little influence on the trend of the diseases in Britain. Finally we exclude rabies and anthrax. The strict quarantine regulations make it unlikely that rabies will be seen in this country except occasionally in persons who have been infected abroad, and vaccination is recommended only for those whose occupations bring them into contact with animals in quarantine. Anthrax also is very uncommon (5 cases were notified in England and Wales in 1970) and vaccination is restricted to workers exposed to risk.

The two diseases which remain are of particular interest in relation to immunization: smallpox as the infection against which vaccination was first successful, and influenza because in Britain it is probably the disease against which effective protection would now be most welcome.

Smallpox

Figure 15.7 shows the trend of mortality from smallpox in England and Wales since cause of death was first registered. Unfortunately, there are no reliable data for the eighteenth and earlier centuries, but the London Bills of Mortality suggest that epidemics of disease caused a high mortality, particularly among children. In 1796 one-fifth of all deaths in London were ascribed to smallpox. Mortality declined rapidly from the late nineteenth century and since about 1910 there have been relatively few deaths in the British Isles.

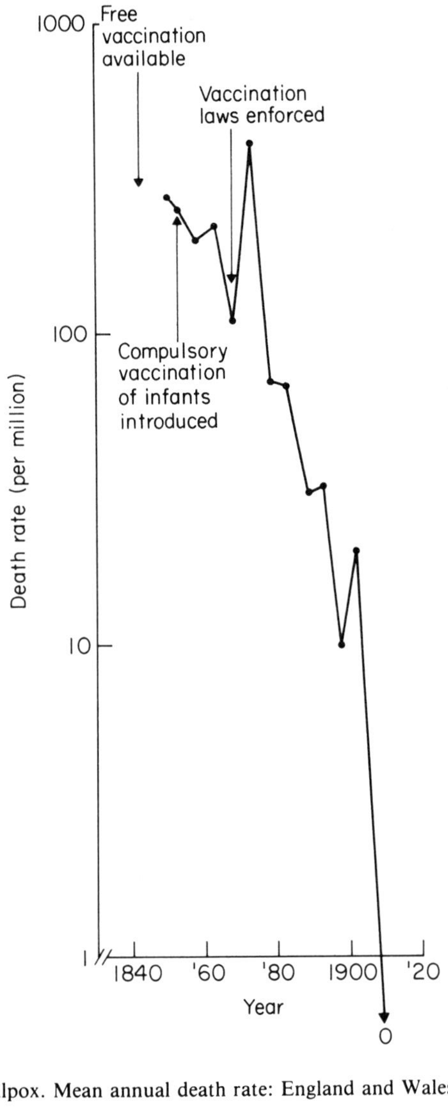

Figure 15.7 Smallpox. Mean annual death rate: England and Wales.

Vaccination was used first in 1798, made compulsory in 1852, and enforced rigorously between 1872 and 1887, when the acceptance rate for children was about 90 per cent. But parents increasingly took advantage of a clause in the law allowing objection on conscientious grounds and in 1948, when compulsion ceased, less than 40 per cent of infants were being vaccinated. In 1971 it was decided that vaccination should no longer be recommended at all as a routine procedure in early childhood.

The way in which vaccination contributes to the control of smallpox has been a subject of controversy, broadly between those who attach importance to routine immunization of the general population and those who emphasize vaccination of all persons exposed to the disease. There is no doubt that vaccination affords a high degree of protection for a limited period. But the amount of protection declines fairly rapidly and after a number of years it is greatly reduced in a population and may be absent in an individual.

On these grounds some epidemiologists with great experience of smallpox had been doubtful about how efficacious attempts at eradication would be, for they attached little importance to claims that a high proportion of a population had at some time been vaccinated unless it could be shown that the protection was maintained at a high level by repeated vaccination. Since, in a general population, this has never been achieved they argued that it would be more effective to concentrate on the vaccination of all possible contacts.

These objections notwithstanding, the World Health Organization completed some 10 years ago a global programme of smallpox vaccination by which means it claims to have eradicated the disease from all countries. Time alone will tell whether it will erupt again, but currently if there are any new cases they are in remote areas and few in number and no country any longer requires immunization as a routine. Vaccinations of course are strongly recommended for people who may be exposed to the virus in the laboratory, or should they occur, to cases of the disease.

It is not easy to assess accurately the contribution that vaccination has made to the decline of mortality from smallpox (figure 15.7); Creighton, the historian of infectious disease, considered it useless; but this view is generally regarded as perverse and inconsistent with the evidence, which is admittedly difficult to interpret. In the light of present knowledge of the high degree of protection afforded by vaccination for a limited period, however, it seems reasonable to believe that the procedure must have been very effective in the nineteenth century when a high proportion of children were immunized but endemic disease persisted.

Influenza

It is hardly necessary to emphasize the past and continuing importance of influenza as a cause of sickness and death. It is the only epidemic infectious disease which in technologically advanced countries carries with it the threat of a general epidemic with a seriously high case fatality rate. This occurred during the pandemic of 1918 when in New Britain, Connecticut, the death rate was so high and the ground so frozen that numerous coffins accumulated on the surface, and the mayor had to call in the civic engineers to bury them, a situation reminiscent of those caused by the plague and cholera in earlier times. Nowadays epidemics of influenza still kill hundreds of frail and elderly people.

Its occurrence and severity are still unpredictable, and as noted above there is no other infection from which effective protection would be more welcome, at least in developed countries.

Unfortunately this protection is not yet available. The problem is complicated by continual variation in the types of influenza virus, so that a vaccine prepared during one epidemic is more often than not ineffective against the next. This no doubt explains in part the conflicting evidence concerning the efficacy of influenza vaccines.

Influenza vaccination is not recommended for routine use nor for the attempted control of outbreaks of influenza, but it may be offered to people with certain complaints (for example, chronic bronchitis) and to persons at special risk of exposure during an epidemic. These include health service staff and children and elderly people living in residences where the disease is likely to spread rapidly.

Since vaccination against influenza was introduced quite recently, has been restricted to certain groups, has been shown to give only limited protection for a short time during inter-pandemic periods, and has not been able to counter the genetic instability of the virus, it is not likely to have reduced the incidence of the disease or mortality from it so far.

Appraisal of Immunization

There is good reason to believe that the immunization procedures now available provide substantial protection against most of the diseases referred to above. Had these measures been in general use from the late nineteenth century it would now be impossible to assess their contribution to the decline of mortality. Almost certainly we should have overestimated it. As it is, it seems probable that immunization has had a substantial effect on the reduction of deaths from smallpox (figure 15.7) and diphtheria (figure 15.1) and more recently on the smaller problems of poliomyelitis (figure 15.3) and (less certainly) tetanus (figure 15.6). The effective procedures were too late to have a maximum influence on three of the most important causes of death—tuberculosis, whooping cough and measles (figures 2.5, 15.2, and 15.4). Indeed the reduction of mortality from the last three diseases without the assistance of immunization should remind us of the other important influences which have been operating during the period of the decline of infections—a rising standard of living in general and nutrition in particular, improvements in hygiene, a reduction of family size and, latterly, better treatment. But as is the case with many other aspects of health care and preventive services, the uptake of immunization is lowest among the poorest members of society, even though it is free and all mothers are strongly encouraged to avail their children of it (table 15.1).

Table 15.1 Use of health services by children aged under 7 by social class of father (Great Britain, 1965)

	I	II	IIIN	IIIM	IV	V
Per cent not immunized against						
smallpox	6	14	16	25	29	33
polio	1	3	3	4	6	10
diphtheria	1	3	3	6	8	11

It is not possible to assess accurately the future scope of immunization in medicine but we shall refer briefly to five points which have a bearing on it.

• In what circumstances should a general immunization programme be discontinued? A short answer is: When the protection provided does not justify the cost and risks of immunization. Such a point may be reached when a disease becomes very uncommon; but the decision to stop vaccination can never be easy and cannot be taken solely on economic grounds. Some considerations which should influence the decision are: (*a*) the cost of protection which is greater if repeated doses are required, as in the case of tetanus toxoid, than if they are not, as in the case of BCG; (*b*) risks of vaccination which are not inconsiderable in the case of smallpox and whooping cough, but appear to be absent in most of the other infections discussed above; and (*c*) the possibility of effective treatment for cases which occur. This is now available for cholera.

Considerations *a* and *b* have already been responsible for the discontinuation of smallpox vaccination, and *a* and *c* are more likely to be responsible for the same decision for BCG.

• What is the scope for immunization in developing countries? This is a complex question and the answer must vary according to circumstances. In many places the frequency or severity of a disease may necessitate the use of methods, even unsafe methods, not justified elsewhere. The high mortality and serious disabilities (e.g. corneal necrosis) caused by measles in West Africa justify the use of vaccines which carry some risk for malnourished children.

But while circumstances vary, the principles of decision are the same as in developed countries. In each case it is desirable first to ascertain that the procedure is effective in the conditions in which it is used, and that its benefits outweigh its risks. If it is effective there are other questions to be considered: whether a general programme makes the best use of a limited number of medical and other trained workers; and how to ensure that it does not prejudice the application of other methods.

• Are there other important diseases against which immunization is likely to become available? To the extent that this is a technical question it must be answered by the bacteriologist and virologist; our task here is to assess where the opportunities lie. In developed countries there is little doubt that the most welcome development would be effective protection against the common respiratory infections—the common cold and influenza and perhaps bronchitis and pneumonia. In some less advanced countries, probably no specific measure would be more important than one which would prevent malaria. Immunization would of course be unnecessary in areas where the mosquito can be eliminated or controlled; but in large parts of Africa, for example, this control is impractical, and an effective vaccine might prove to be the only means of effectively preventing disease (see Chapter 13).

• The most effective vaccine is valueless unless it is administered to those in need of it, and whether or not this is done depends on a wide array of administrative, economic and behavioural factors, high among them the willingness and ability of the individual to participate. The failure of an immunization programme can very rarely be attributed solely to biological causes.

• We have repeatedly drawn attention to the interrelationship between behaviour and the origin (as well as the control), of disease. Thus, as social norms and behavioural patterns change so does the epidemiology of disease. Over the past decade the incidence of hepatitis B and genital herpes simplex have sharply increased. The former is associated with intravenous injection of addictive drugs and male homosexuality; herpes, which causes only mild discomfort in its oral form, but which is very painful in its genital form, with sexual promiscuity. There is a third disease, Acquired Immune Deficiency Syndrome (AIDS), which has a high case fatality rate, and has caused serious epidemics largely among male homosexuals. Even should immunization become available for any of them, there is no effective treatment, so control can only lie with modification of behaviour.

Further Reading

Creighton C. (1965) *A History of Epidemics in Britain*, 2nd edition. Frank Cass & Co. Ltd., London.

Department of Health and Social Security (1981) *Whooping Cough*. HMSO, London.

Dixon C. W. (1962) *Smallpox*. J. & A. Churchill Ltd., London.

Springett V. H. (1971) *Tuberculosis control in Britain 1945-1970-1995*. *Tubercle*, **52**, 136.

16

Screening

We have seen that improvement in health hitherto has been due essentially to reduction of morbidity and mortality from infectious disease. This reduction was brought about chiefly in two ways: through primary protection by preventing exposure to infection (for example from typhoid and dysentery); and through secondary protection of the individual who might become infected, either by specific measures such as immunizing him or by improvement in his general health. The contribution of all these methods is illustrated by the history of tuberculosis. Improved housing reduced the frequency of infection; BCG vaccination provided specific protection; and better nutrition increased general resistance to the disease.

However, these measures are not always successful in preventing or abating infections, and it is then necessary to provide treatment. In some diseases, such as whooping cough and measles, the acute onset of symptoms soon brings the patient to the doctor. In others, and particularly in chronic infections such as tuberculosis, symptoms may be minimal or absent, and the patient may not be seen until the disease has reached an advanced stage. It is clearly desirable to identify these patients before they complain of symptoms, so that they can be treated and measures taken to prevent the spread of infection. The purpose of cervical cytology for cancer of the uterine cervix and routine examination of blood for venereal infection is similar. This type of investigation, identification of a disease in its early, and if possible, pre-symptomatic stage, is referred to as 'screening'. It has been described aptly as 'the use of *quick* and perhaps *approximate* tests or examinations to differentiate those who probably have some disorder (*especially a latent one*) from those who probably do not'. The words in italics indicate the nature and limitations of these methods. Since tests are usually applied to large population groups, they must be quick. Being quick they can rarely be more than approximate. And since the cases identified have not usually been recognized before the screening, the disease is likely to be latent.

Screening procedures are used in infectious and non-infectious diseases. From a public viewpoint it is essential to identify a typhoid carrier; but for the patient it may be no less important to recognize a treatable non infectious disease, or a physical or mental handicap, of which the effects can be mitigated by prompt services. Treatment of phenylketonuria or infantile hypothyroidism may prevent mental retardation, and provision of a hearing aid early in life can transform the outlook for a child with impaired hearing. It is probable that in developed countries screening will have its widest application in the discovery of congenital disabilities (mental subnormality, partial sight, partial hearing, congenital malformations, etc.) and non-infectious illnesses (such as cancer and cardiovascular disease), both because they are now more prominent than the infections, and because the scope for prevention is relatively less.

Obligations in Screening

Screening is distinguished fundamentally from conventional medical practice, and the requirements that should be met before a screening procedure is accepted as suitable for general application arise from this distinction. It is due essentially to the difference in the position of the doctor in relation to the patient in the two cases: in the one when the patient seeks the assistance of the doctor; in the other when society, not necessarily through the agency of a doctor in the first place, sets out to identify those of its members who stand to benefit from medical assistance.

When the patient seeks medical advice, the doctor's ethical position is relatively simple: he attempts to do his best with the knowledge and resources available to him. He cannot fairly be criticized when the state of medical knowledge does not enable him to treat effectively or even to diagnose accurately the condition about which his advice is sought; nor can he undertake in all cases to assemble the full range of facilities for investigation and treatment from which his patient might conceivably benefit.

The position is quite different in screening, when a doctor or public authority takes the initiative in investigating the possibility of illness or disability in people who may feel quite well or not sick enough to report signs or symptoms. There is then a presumptive undertaking, not merely that an abnormality will be identified if it is present, but that those affected will derive benefit from subsequent treatment or care. This commitment is at least implicit, and except for research or the protection of public health, no-one should be expected to submit to the inconvenience of investigation or the anxieties of being screened without the prospect of medical benefit. This obligation exists even when the patient himself asks to be screened or to have a health examination, for his request is based on the belief that the procedure is valuable, and if it is not it is for medical people to make this known.

The ethical considerations are so fundamental to the concept of screening that it seems desirable to reflect them in its definition. Most definitions put the emphasis on the pre-symptomatic character of the investigations; that is to say they focus on their timing in relation to the stage of disease rather than on the circumstances in which they are initiated. A review of screening sponsored by the Nuffield Provincial Hospitals Trust led to the following definition: *medical investigation which does not arise from a patient's request for advice for specific complaints*. This was considered to comprise 'investigation of patients (*a*) who have not sought medical assistance because of signs or symptoms as with cervical cytology (*b*) who have sought medical assistance only for a screening test or health examination which they believe will be of value to them, and (*c*) who have sought assistance for a condition unrelated to a screening procedure'. This interpretation regards as the unique feature of screening to be the fact that investigation is not initiated by the patient. It is 'the medical initiative which creates the obligation which . . . makes a strict validation procedure essential'.

There is another consideration which makes it imperative to adopt for screening an approach at least as rigorous if not more than that which is followed in ordinary clinical practice: this is the scale on which a programme may be and—if it is properly validated—should be applied. The application of a new therapeutic measure is developed gradually because its use is determined by practicing physicians who assess its merits in relation to the alternative treatments available to them. But a screening programme believed to be of value invites large scale application which may involve deployment of extensive resources at local and national levels. Inevitably it is developed at the expense of other possible uses of health services, manpower and equipment. For example, a decision to introduce national screening for breast cancer would make heavy demands which could be met only by substantial new expenditure or by diverting staff and facilities from other work. This diversion may be justified, but it is clearly essential to consider how resources might otherwise have been used before accepting breast cancer screening as suitable for widespread application. The main tasks confronting those concerned with the practice of screening are therefore to decide on an appropriate validation procedure, and to apply it both to existing programmes and to new programmes before they are brought into general use.

Criteria for Screening

In the light of the obligations referred to above there are five requirements which it seems essential to consider carefully in relation to screening: reliability of identification; effectiveness and availability of treatment; assessment of risks; operational problems; and cost and benefit. These points will be illustrated by reference to screening for breast cancer.

Reliability of identification

As we have indicated, since tests used in screening are intended for large populations they will be less precise than diagnostic methods employed in ordinary clinical practice. Screening is in fact a two-stage process. The first stage consists of providing, for the largest possible proportion of the population to be screened, a test which should, in addition to being sensitive and specific (see below), also be cheap to administer, painless, and ethically and aesthetically acceptable. Most of them can be administered by non-medically trained personnel. The taking of blood pressure and electrocardiographic tracings for cardiovascular disease, the use of miniature chest X-rays and intradermal injections to identify cases of tuberculosis, and in cancers in women microscopic examination of smears from the uterine cervix and, for the breast, palpation or mammography, are all examples. Such tests allow the population to be classified into those whose results show positive and those in whom they show negative.

The second stage is to subject all those in whom the screening test was found to be positive to more definitive and elaborate diagnostic procedures which will in most circumstances involve a doctor. Because this second stage is costly in demands it makes on resources available to the health services, and in the time of the person concerned, it is essential that the test used in the first stage comes as near as possible always to identifying those, and only those, with the disease of interest. Screening procedures are judged by their *false positive rate* and *false negative rate* both of which should be kept to a minimum; in other words a test should be highly *sensitive* for and highly *specific* to the condition which it is designed to identify (table 16.1).

Table 16.1 Classification of screening procedures

		Diagnostic work-up	
		'True' Positive	'True' Negative
Screening test	Positive	a	b
	Negative	c	d
		False negative rate $c/(a+c)$ Sensitivity $a/(a+c)$	False negative rate $b/(b+d)$ Specifity $d/(b+d)$

Moreover, false negatives may lead to unjustified reassurance which delays diagnosis and treatment, or erroneous identification of disease, false positives all of whom are exposed to unnecessary anxiety and some perhaps to unnecessary treatment which may be costly, unpleasant or even harmful. False negatives can only be identified by careful follow up of those screening negative, or by re-examination of a sample of them. To do this is important when a screening procedure is being evaluated. Most screening tests have low yields and with even a small error rate the number of normals incorrectly classified may exceed the number of abnormals correctly treated. For example, in screening for breast cancer among women considered suspect after clinical examination, nearly nine-tenths were found at biopsy not to have the disease. With clinical examination and mammography combined the proportion negative was four-fifths.

Effectiveness and availability of treatment

In ordinary clinical practice it is often necessary to use treatments whose effectiveness has not been determined fully or, sometimes, at all. In screening, however, the ethical obligations and potential costs make it important to know in precise terms how effective a treatment is and whether its effectiveness can be enhanced by early diagnosis, before a test is accepted for general application. Ideally this requires a fairly complete picture of the natural history of the disease, the evidence available as a basis of screening for tuberculosis, is an example. In practice it may be necessary to accept only an evaluation of the effects of early detection and treatment on survival but even then it is important to take the natural history of the disease into account. For example, the modal expectation of life of a woman who has breast cancer treated after she has experienced symptoms is about 7 years. If the screening procedures enable cases to be identified 12 months before symptoms would normally develop, and survival is extended to 8 years, no good is achieved; she has lived for the same length of time as the 'average' unscreened woman even though she has known about her disease for a year longer. Indeed it can be looked upon as a disservice to add a year to the time that a woman knows she has cancer without adding to the length of her life. In fact no conclusive evidence available to date indicates that presymptomatic diagnosis of breast cancer through screening followed by treatment does lengthen life.

Since it is obligatory to provide the appropriate care for those discovered to require it, the operational relationship between screening and subsequent treatment services is important. It is irresponsible to leave patients to make their own arrangements, and less than satisfactory merely to inform the patient's doctor about the results of a screening exercise in which he had no part.

Assessment of risks

The obligations of screening in relation to diagnosis and treatment apply particularly to any health hazard associated with the screening procedure itself. Regrettably it must be accepted that the ordinary practice of medicine involves risks which may arise from ignorance—as seems repeatedly to be the case with drugs effective in the treatment of rheumatoid arthritis —or because the risks, like the effectiveness of treatment, cannot be fully assessed. But when the initiative in investigation of an ostensibly healthy person is taken by society, any risks must be quantified and weighed carefully in relation to the benefit from treatment. In screening for breast cancer, for example, it is not enough to believe that the risks of mammography are acceptably low; these risks must be measured accurately in relation to the frequency and type of examination and when, as with such indices, the risks are expressed as a range, it is the upper limit which should be used in coming to a decision about the advisability of screening. It is also necessary to take account of the stress and risk associated with biopsy, particularly since the majority of those investigated will be found not to have the disease.

Operational problems

In addition to the usual problems associated with the provision of all medical services, screening presents others which are unique to itself. One of these problems is that of public response to a service which is proffered rather than requested; experience of cervical cytology suggests that the response may be least from those who have most to gain from being screened. This is because the incidence of cervical cancer is highest in social class V and this class makes least use of preventive services of any kind. Another problem arises from the use of staff. Both the first and second stages of screening for breast cancer, for example, make heavy demands on the time of surgeons, radiologists and radiographers. There is some professional and public resistance to the use of less expensively trained staff, and unless this can be overcome it seems unlikely that a national service could be offered. But perhaps the largest operational issue is the relation between screening and other health services. It is not difficult to imagine the unsatisfactory position which in time would result if screening programmes were developed independently, each with its own finance, administration, staff and facilities, and all separate from the main body of medical practice. In some respects the situation would be analogous to that created by malaria eradication campaigns, before it was realized that it was essential to link them with the public health services as a whole. Hence screening should not be developed in isolation but should be linked closely in its execution and follow-up with the rest of medical, diagnostic and treatment services.

Cost and benefit

Slowly, and rather reluctantly, all health services are submitting to appraisal of their cost and benefit; but in screening, for reasons discussed above, this appraisal should precede its introduction. Clearly it is not enough to know that a programme provides some benefit; before accepting it as suitable for general use we need to know how much benefit and at what risk and cost. The final decision whether to screen turns on a value judgement, but the data on which this judgement is based should be as precise as we can make them.

Again this point may be illustrated by reference to screening for breast cancer. It would not be sufficient to show that after a number of years there are fewer deaths from breast cancer among women screened than among those not screened. As we have seen we need to know the increase in expectation of life which results from screening in a population of women and this benefit should be weighed in relation to the costs.

Appraisal of Screening Procedures

On the basis of past experience the usefulness of some types of screening can hardly be disputed. Well established procedures include tuberculin skin tests in children, examination during pregnancy of blood pressure and of the blood for anaemia, syphilis and determination of blood group, the Coombs test on the cord blood of infants of Rh negative mothers, examination of teeth, eyesight and hearing in schoolchildren, and where the prevalence of tuberculosis is high radiography of the chest. In tropical countries inspection of the blood for malaria and trypanosomiasis and of the stools for parasitic worms may be used for planning and monitoring the progress of eradication campaigns. The problems which arise in extending these methods to diseases such as breast cancer, diabetes mellitus, cervical cancer and glaucoma should not raise doubts about their usefulness in many situations.

Indeed there are grounds for thinking that a considerable extension of screening will be both possible and necessary. It will be possible because automation and electronic computers have simplified the task of analysis and interpretation of large numbers of specimens. It will be necessary because of the increasing importance of non-infectious disease, much of which can be neither prevented nor treated effectively at a late stage. Part of the answer in the case of non-infectious disease may lie in encouraging earlier reporting of symptoms by a public educated to recognize those which may be serious.

Contrary perhaps to popular belief, in technologically advanced countries screening is restricted as much by lack of knowledge as by lack of resources. Where the requirements described above are met, as was the case in the use of mass radiography for detection of tuberculosis, the method has been applied widely. The main reason for failure to employ screening for the discovery of diseases such as diabetes is that one or more of the essential requirements are not met.

Before screening can contribute significantly to the control by society of disease, there must be a considerable advance of knowledge. This requires both clinical and laboratory research, and, even more, epidemiological investigation of experience of disease in populations: the significance of signs and symptoms; observer errors; physiological variation; interpretation of departures from 'normal'; the natural history of disease; the outcome of treatment, and so on.

Finally we should refer to multiphasic or multiple screening, which has been defined as 'the application of two or more screening tests in combination to large groups of people'. The procedure may also include a medical history usually taken in the form of a symptomatic check list. Hence the system of multiphasic screening is not a screening test in the usual sense, but a mechanism for executing a number of investigations at the same time. It must therefore be judged as an operational procedure.

There is clearly no objection in principle to the coordination of a number of screening tests in time and place; indeed it is desirable that the procedures should be linked operationally to one another and to medical practice as a whole. But in multiphasic screening as currently practised most of the tests have not been validated, and this results in two major problems. First it is difficult, if not impossible, to assess the credentials of individual tests when they are incorporated in a multiphasic programme. And secondly, if multiphasic screening in its present form comes to be regarded as an established feature of medical practice, it may well displace alternative and more effective uses of the same resources. The problem is in some respects analogous to that associated with occupational and school health services, where the unvalidated practice of routine medical examinations has diverted attention and effort from other and probably more effective methods of identifying those who need medical assistance.

Further Reading

Sackett D. L. and Holland W. W. (1975) Controversy in the direction of disease. *Lancet* **ii**, 357-359.

17

Noxious Personal Behaviour and its Modification

We have already seen in foregoing chapters that there is a behavioural component in successful immunization and screening programmes, because people must take time and trouble in their own or their family's interests to do what they might not otherwise do.

Here we consider another class of behavioural influences whose effects are even more direct: we refer to aspects of an individual's personal behaviour or daily habits which may prejudice his own health. A few examples are well recognized and of long standing, as in the case of drug addiction, or sexual promiscuity leading to venereal infection. But there are other behavioural influences whose widespread ill-effects are more recent such as smoking, overeating and physical inactivity, or whose ill effects have only recently been sufficiently recognized such as steady social drinking. We shall discuss the evidence on which these habits are thought to be related to disease before considering the problems presented by their control.

Noxious Habits and their Consequences

Smoking tobacco

The tobacco leaf was introduced into Europe three and a half centuries ago. In spite of claims for its medicinal value, the practice of smoking met with opposition. James I described it as 'a branch of the sin of drunkenness, which is the root of all sins' and 'a custom loathsome to the eye, hateful to the nose, harmful to the brain, dangerous to the lungs, and in the black, stinking fume thereof, nearest resembling the horrible Stygian smoke of the pit that is bottomless'. In the Swiss Canton of Berne 'the offence ranked as only one degree less odious than adultery'. In a wide range of countries measures such as hanging, imprisonment, flogging and exile were used unsuccessfully as deterrents. But by the nineteenth century addiction to tobacco, at least by men, had become unobjectionable to most people. Its medicinal properties were discredited, but it was thought to be harmless.

This conclusion was challenged when it was reported that the proportion of smokers, and particularly of heavy smokers, was higher in male patients with cancer of the lung than in healthy men. This was the starting point for a series of inquiries into the relationship between smoking and disease. An association is now well established with cancer of the lung, oral cavity, larynx, pharynx, oesophagus and bladder; chronic bronchitis; and coronary heart disease, and the evidence is suggestive in a number of other conditions. Smoking by a pregnant woman has also been shown to cause a reduction in the birth weight of her child. Much of the evidence and almost the whole of the controversy concerning the effects of smoking have been focussed on cancer of the lung however, and we shall limit our discussion to this disease.

The earliest investigations compared the smoking habits of patients in hospital with carcinoma of the lung with those of a control group of other hospital patients. The main findings were that the proportion of smokers was much higher among patients with the disease than among controls, and that the risk of developing carcinoma of the lung appeared to increase with increasing amounts smoked. These results have since been amply confirmed and extended by prospective studies of mortality in relation to smoking habits. These prospective studies have shown conclusively that mortality from lung cancer increases sharply with increasing amounts smoked, and among those who have given up smoking, declines progressively with the length of time for which they have given up and in relation to their previous daily consumption. The association with cigarette smoking is present only for squamous-cell and oat-cell carcinoma. The less common adenocarcinoma appears to be unrelated to smoking.

These findings are consistent with the observations that deaths from lung cancer have increased with the increasing sale of cigarettes and that in general national mortality from cancer of the lung is closely related to national tobacco consumption.

Those who have challenged the evidence have done so mainly on three grounds. In the first place it is pointed out that the statistical association does not prove that smoking causes cancer. This objection is largely met by the strength and consistency of the association, by the observation that mortality from lung cancer declines in men who give up smoking and, for those who find work on experimental animals more convincing than controlled observations in man, by the production of cancer of the lung in animals which have inhaled cigarette smoke.

A second basis of objection is that smoking produces effects that are apparently non-specific, since it is associated with increased mortality from several diseases. However there is nothing surprising in the observation that smoking, like other agents as different as alcohol, the spirochaete and psychological stress, should have multiple effects. Moreover cigarette smoke is not a single chemical agent.

Thirdly, it has been suggested that certain people are genetically predisposed both to smoke and to develop lung cancer, and thus patients owe their cancer to their genes rather than to their smoking. This hypothesis was thought to be supported by certain physical and psychological differences between smokers and non-smokers; however it is inconsistent with the large increase in death rates from lung cancer during this century, and with significant decrease of mortality from the disease in first doctors and subsequently others who have stopped smoking cigarettes.

Attempts to control the habit must take into account the fact that it is not equally distributed in society. It is commoner in class V than class I, and men have had more success in stopping than women (see figures 17.1 and 17.2).

Most epidemiologists who have reviewed the evidence, taking account of the inconsistencies and the doubts which have been expressed, have no hesitation in accepting the conclusion reached in 1971 by the Royal College of Physicians 'The quantitative association between cigarette smoking and the development of lung cancer is most simply explained on a causal basis and no other explanation accounts for the facts.'

Smoking cigarettes, which is now overwhelmingly the commonest form the tobacco habit takes, was first practised in the courts of Europe and by members of the aristocracy in the latter half of the nineteenth century. Before the First World War almost all consumption of tobacco in social class V was by pipe; soldiers in the trenches changed their habits because cigarettes were available tax free, and sometimes free of any charge. Smoking amongst women only began to become socially acceptable between the wars, again starting in class I, and initially those who smoked did not smoke much. In 1980 18 million adults in Britain smoked cigarettes. As figure 17.1 shows, 42 per cent of males and 39 per cent of females had the habit. Although twice as many men as women had given up

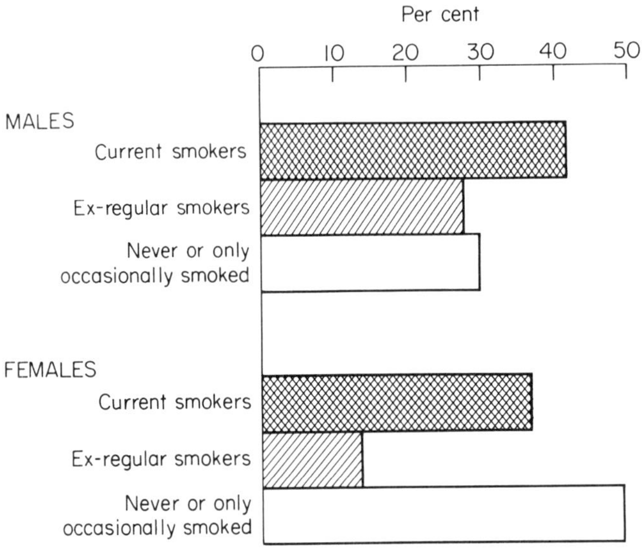

Figure 17.1. The cigarette smoking status of persons aged 16 or over: England and Wales, 1980.

smoking, more women had never smoked. Between 1972, the first year of the General Household Survey, and 1980 the average number of cigarettes consumed by each smoker increased by 4 per week in men (although there was a fall in social class I) and by 15 per week in women, a difference which is shown in every social class. Just as the patterns of smoking have changed between the sexes, so they have changed between the social classes so that by 1980, the prevalence of cigarette smoking in both sexes was lowest in social class I (figure 17.2) and in the average number they smoked weekly the women were steadily catching up the men. Social forces, or 'fashion', therefore led to a series of behavioural changes. To smoke cigarettes was considered desirable, at first amongst men of the gentry and professional class, later among manual workers and later still among women. Now it is professional men who are discarding the habit or not taking it up at all, and society at large acts against the habit (figure 17.3) so that London Transport in 1984 was able successfully to ban all smoking from its trains. Behavioural scientists, as well as epidemiologists, have contributed to our understanding of the smoking habit, and have much to offer to successful health education in this and other fields.

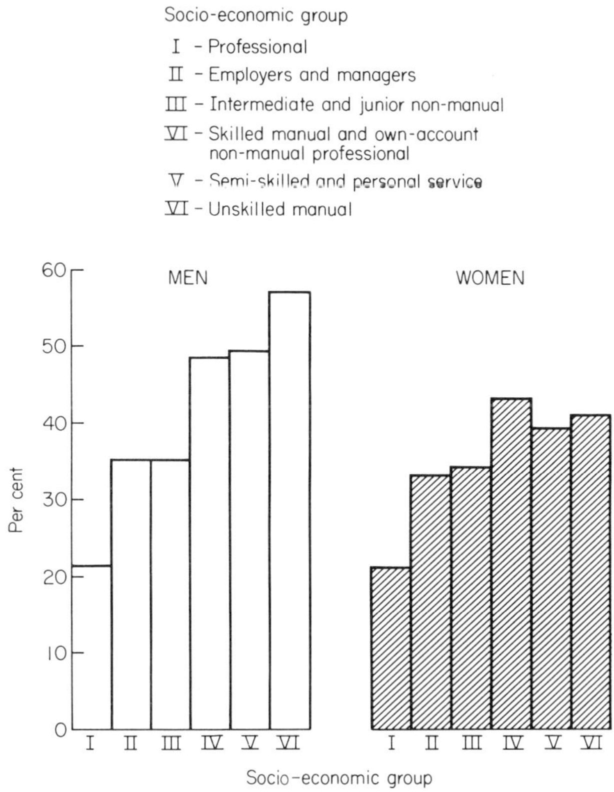

Figure 17.2. Proportion of persons in England and Wales who were smoking in 1980 by sex and socio-economic group.

Drinking alcohol

The history of the use of alcohol by man is almost as long as the history of man himself. Archaeologists have uncovered evidence of cereals having been used to brew fermented drinks from the very earliest times. Alcohol has been used and has also been abused since the beginning of history, to the harm of the individual and of society, and there have been many attempts to control the abuse. In the ninth century BC the King of Sparta decreed that all vineyards should be destroyed and the legs of drunkards cut off. In more recent times attempts have been made to enforce prohibition of alcohol with less drastic penalties, in the United States and Sweden, but with no great success. Despite heavy taxation, restrictions on the hours, places and conditions of sale, and penalties for

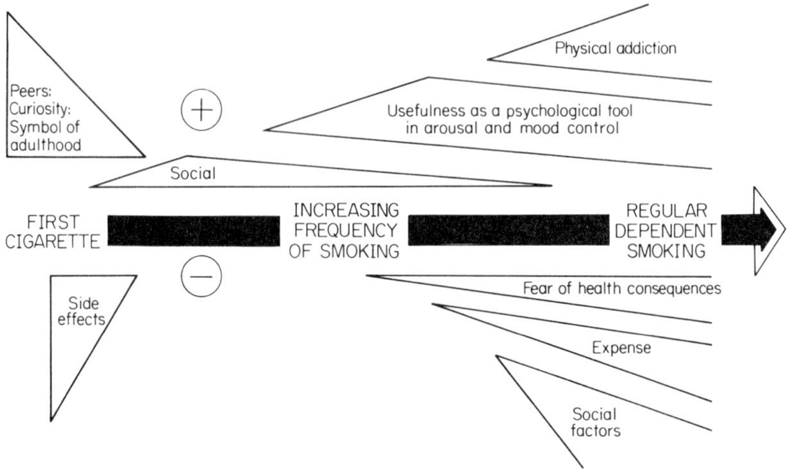

Figure 17.3. Diagrammatic representation of factors leading to the precipitation and maintenance of the smoking habit ⊕, and those preventing it or encouraging its discontinuation ⊖. (Modified from Stepney and Ashton).

driving with blood levels of over 80 mg per 100 ml, alcohol remains in this country the traditional and the most commonly used drug capable of producing dependence.

Alcohol is undoubtedly a major health and social problem, but it is difficult to assess its gravity as there is no direct measure of its effect on mortality or morbidity. An indirect and not very reliable indicator of the influence on mortality is provided by death rates attributed to cirrhosis of the liver (Table 6.6). For example, in France adults over 15 years of age drink the equivalent of more than 28 litres of pure alchohol per head per year, approximately a pint (0.47 litres) a week: in the United Kingdom the corresponding amount is about 6 litres a year or a tablespoon (15 ml) a day, to an average Frenchman less than a medicinal dose. The death rate from cirrhosis of the liver in France is 10 times the death rate in the United Kingdom. For many years mortality from cirrhosis did not increase in Britain, and between the early 1950s and the late 1960s was in the order of 30 per thousand males and 26 per thousand females. Subsequently, it has been on the increase. If the SMR for 1968 is taken to be 100, by 1978 it had risen to 130 in men and 121 for women. There are striking differences by social class and by occupation. The death rate for the professional classes (in social class I) is nearly 3 times the death rate for semi-skilled and unskilled workers (in social classes IV and V), and for hotel and inkeepers it is 15 times the average for the male population as a whole (see table 6.6).

But mortality from cirrhosis is only a small part of the death toll taken by alcohol. For example, suicides and accidental deaths are both associated with alcoholism. Though drunkness causes accidents, the relationship between these and alcohol is not necessarily one of cause and effect; both may be due to an underlying mental or personality problem. Suicide rates are nevertheless high in occupations where alcoholism is common; the suicide rate among alcoholics who have been admitted to psychiatric hospitals has been found to be 80 times higher than among men of the same ages in the general population; and in a study of men admitted for self-poisoning to hospitals in Edinburgh 39 per cent were known to be heavy drinkers. The extent to which alcohol is implicated in traffic accidents is such that in Britain and many other countries motor drivers may be stopped by the police, and if their blood alcohol, as screened by analysis of their breath, exceeds a certain level and is subsequently confirmed they may be heavily fined or imprisoned.

It is difficult to estimate the amount of ill-health in the population directly attributable to the abuse of alcohol. This is in part related to the fact that the underlying addiction is often concealed by patients. It is also related to the difficulty of defining alcoholism, when the use of alcohol ranges from occasional social drinking to regular and heavy drinking with associated morbidity which includes such varied conditions as chronic gastritis, cirrhosis of the liver, polyneuritis and mental illness, depression, reduced libido, delirium tremens and Korsakow's syndrome. The World Health Organization has defined alcoholics as 'those excessive drinkers whose dependence on alcohol has attained such a degree that they show a noticeable mental disturbance or an interference with their mental and bodily health, their interpersonal relations and their smooth social and economic functioning; or who show prodromal signs of such developments'. Within the framework of this admittedly broad definition it has been estimated that there are some 400,000 alcoholics in Britain, a quarter of whom (3 per 1,000 of the adult population) show physical and mental deterioration. On any account this represents a formidable health problem.

Indiscreet eating

During most of man's time on earth the outstanding problem connected with food has been that there is not enough of it. It is understandable that in communities where undernutrition was widespread, obesity was commonly equated with prosperity, if not with health. In the nineteenth century the wealth of the king and princes of the Wanguana in East Africa was measured by the girth of their wives. In the Journal of the Discovery of the Source of the Nile Speke reported that from early youth the women were kept with a pot of milk to their mouths, and some of them 'were fattened to such an extent that they could not stand upright and their flesh hung down like loose stuffed puddings'.

About two-thirds of the people in the world are still living in a state of chronic undernourishment, but for the first time in history there are now countries in which the opportunity to overeat or eat indiscreetly is no longer confined to a trivial minority and obesity and other consequences of dietary habits such as disturbances of sugar, lipid and urate metabolism and perhaps sodium consumption are emerging as major health hazards. For example, in England and Wales young and middle aged men are now on the average nearly 10 kg heavier than men of the same age and height in the 1930s. Life insurance statistics have provided impressive evidence of the relation between obesity and mortality. Men who are more than 25 per cent heavier than the average for their age and height have a death rate twice as high as those within 5 per cent of the average. The most striking differences are in respect of deaths from ischaemic heart disease, diabetes, some gastrointestinal cancers and accidents. Desirable standards for weight have been derived from these insurance statistics, based on the weights of men with the most favourable mortaility experience. According to these standards, middle aged men in England and Wales are now on the average about 20 lb 'overweight', and there is evidence that this overweight problem may begin in infancy—the overweight infant tends to become the overweight schoolchild and later the overweight adult. An index of inappropriate diets is the amount of food discarded uneaten.

Ischaemic heart disease is now the leading cause of death for both males and females, and the death rate for males until very recently has been steadily increasing for many decades. The increase has been most substantial for young and middle aged men, the groups that have shown the greatest increase in weight. It is reasonable to conclude in the light of all the evidence that the increase in mortality is in part attributable to increase in weight, and in part to eating a diet for which our genotypes were not selected.

Physical Inactivity

People are not only becoming more obese, but with the increasing use of the motor car, the automation of industrial processes, the availability of lifts instead of stairs etc., they are becoming less physically active and there is now evidence that those in sedentary jobs are at increased risk to death from ischaemic heart disease.

One of the first reports (1953) of the inverse relation between ischaemic heart disease and physical activity was based on sickness and mortality records of London Transport drivers and conductors aged 35-64 years. Drivers had more ischaemic heart disease than conductors; their disease also appeared at an earlier age and was more frequently fatal. The conclusion that this result was attributable to variation in physical activity was supported by similar findings in a comparison of the experience of government clerks and postmen, and from national statistics by a comparison of mortality in a wide range of occupations. The relationship of mortality to activity was remarkably consistent, even within the same social class. Since then a number of other epidemiological investigations have supported the finding that, for men, physical activity at work appears to give considerable protection against mortality from coronary disease. An enquiry related to a 16 year follow-up of longshore men in San Francisco, two-thirds of whom (the 'active' group) were doing particularly heavy work, mainly cargo handling. The death rate from ischaemic heart disease was considerably lower in the active group than in the less active group. The difference was greatest for the youngest age group (35-44 years) in which the active men had a death rate only one-seventh that of the less active men.

Other investigations have suggested that inactivity is associated more with sudden death from myocardial infarction than with morbidity from ischaemic heart disease, and more with occlusive coronary artery disease and myocardial scarring than with mural atheroma. They also indicate that current physical activity may be more important than average activity throughout life. For the relationship between ischaemic heart disease and physical activity two explanations have been suggested. Exertion may lead to an increase in the coronary collateral circulation; or it may prevent intravascular clotting. It has been shown that modified lipid metabolism and acceleration of plasma-clotting time after ingestion of fat is largely abolished by physical activity. Both explanations suggest a possible accommodation between the findings described above and the large body of evidence that relates the incidence of ischaemic heart disease to obesity and the intake of animal fats.

The Modification of Smoking and Other Personal Habits

The relation between personal habits and certain causes of illness and death raises three main questions: whether the evidence is acceptable; if it is, whether effective social action is justified; and if so what form the action should take.

On the first point there is no doubt about the association between, for example, smoking and lung cancer or obesity and ischaemic heart disease or alcohol and road accidents. But some say that, without experimental confirmation, a causal relationship cannot soundly be inferred. We make three comments.

First, it is not easy to conceive of experiments which would remove all doubts. Positive results in the hamster, guinea pig or orang-outang would leave many reservations about their bearing on the aetiology of lung cancer and ischaemic heart disease in man. And human beings cannot ethically be submitted to more exacting tests than those they already undertake voluntarily by smoking and overeating.

Second, experimental findings would be only *relatively* more convincing than the evidence already available. For even planned experiments are open to misinterpretation, and are more conclusive than direct observations only because they can be conducted under more controlled conditions.

Third, inaction stemming from insistence on experimental support for conclusions which are already acceptable to many critical people may result in a large number of unnecessary deaths. In the nineteenth century the association between polluted water and cholera was regarded as sufficient reason for improving water supplies. Had experimental confirmation or even clarification of the nature of infection been required, effective action would have been delayed by many years.

In the case of smoking the evidence is already impressive, and it would be inexcusable to delay action solely on the grounds that one day it may be even stronger. The question remains whether social manipulation of personal habits is justified or likely to be effective.

On the first point the law is already clear. People are not encouraged to kill themselves; and if tobacco caused death in 30 hours instead of 30 years measures of control would be introduced very quickly. It is partly because the effects are delayed, and hence are recognizable by numerical evidence rather than everyday experience, that society takes a different view of the effects of tobacco than of the effects of narcotics.

If an individual is allowed to kill himself, so long as he does it slowly, it is quite another matter to permit others to create the circumstances in which he may do so inadvertently. This, essentially, is the position which results from the sale of cigarettes.

Could social intervention in private habits be effective? Again we may illustrate the possibilities with reference to tobacco. Countries must decide how far they can go in a matter of this kind. We have seen that prohibition of alcohol did not work in the past and most countries have already concluded that prohibition of smoking is out of the question. The reasons that attempts at compulsory control have failed are related to the distaste people have to being forced, as well as to the complex web of factors which determine the smoking behaviour of an individual (figure 17.3); successful efforts to encourage smokers voluntarily to discontinue their habit must take the interrelationships which make up this web into account. The British government has not truly come to terms with the issue. In a democracy, government is representative of the expressed will of society and the courses open to it include: (*a*) raising the retail price of tobacco by raising the taxes on it; (*b*) restricting *by law* the places where it is permissible to smoke in public; (*c*) controlling advertising, which in addition to the familiar pictures on billboards, television and newspapers can take the less direct form of sponsoring sporting and other public events; (*d*) distribution of information about the harmful consequence of smoking on cigarette packets and through the media; (*e*) providing personal assistance to those who want to discontinue smoking. Its performance through the years, regardless of the party in power, has been erratic with respect to the first three, and limited in respect to four and five. All of them are complementary to each other in that they, together with the change in social attitudes to which we have already referred, put pressure on the smoker to stop, offer assistance in doing so, yet leave the final choice to him. Yet other countries have shown how powerful the concerted use of all five can be. The chief reason for official reticence is fiscal. A parallel example of political expediency being placed before health promotion has been the gross over-production of dairy products by the European Common Market.

The approach of society through government to the control of drinking alcohol is similar. Attempts at prohibition through legislation have been more recent than attempts to ban smoking but just as unsuccessful. In the cases of smoking and drinking, the special clinics which offer such treatments as behaviour therapy, drugs, and group support are only likely to be successful in a tiny proportion of all the people who have the habit to excess, namely those who have decided to discontinue, cannot do so unaided and are willing to devote time to succeeding.

Body weight is a good index of health, especially if it is related to height, and as we have seen in economically developed countries, overweight, or obesity, are much commoner problems than pathological thinness due to undernutrition. The government in Britain has helped people to control their weight by influencing patterns of physical activity; it has allocated funds to local governments for the development of leisure centres and sporting facilities, and by the work of the Sports Council, has encouraged adults as well as children regularly to enjoy team and individual sport. A democratic government cannnot prevent overeating, but the British and other governments have when needed encouraged the consumption of wholesome foods, for example by subsidising milk and orange juice for pre-school children and school meals. Farmers also receive subsidies to produce appropriate raw materials.

As has been the case with smoking, health education has also brought about changes in fashion and social norms in the choice of food. In the interests of economy and convenience the baking industry produced bread made from highly purified wheat with preservatives which was sliced and wrapped, but because of evidence that a diet high in roughage is beneficial, public demand for the sliced, wrapped loaf has fallen in favour of bread without additives made from coarsely ground flour. And whereas a decade ago a runner, appropriately clothed, in the public street was a rarity, jogging is now commonplace. It is important to note, however, that although whole-wheat bread and the amenities of the leisure centre are available to everyone, the proportion of those who take advantage of them is much higher in the middle class than in social classes IV and V.

Finally, as the list of proscribed pleasures lengthens, it may be asked why indulgence of habits which give pleasure should be dangerous. Some people prefer sitting to walking; many like tobacco and alcohol; and nearly all enjoy food rich in certain ingredients to which they have become accustomed. Why then can they not relax, smoke, drink and eat, without risking their lives?

The most plausible answer is in terms of selection. Living organisms can adapt to profound changes, given time for genotypes ill-equipped for the new environment to die out, and for those well-equipped to reproduce. But human reproduction is slow, and with the exception of alcohol and in a privileged few, overeating, the adoption of noxious habits to which we have referred has occurred in a very short time, mainly during the twentieth century. Eighty years ago it was exceptional for a man to smoke and no women smoked at all; now almost every second person does. Improved methods of food production and distribution and increased purchasing power have put the temptation to overeat before large numbers of people. And physical activity has been transformed by the introduction of a wide range of mechanical devices especially the motor car. In time the human body could adapt to these as to former changes; but it cannot do so rapidly, and cannot do so at all unless the effects of selection are permitted to operate. If the problem is to be resolved in this way, the death of the susceptible at an early age is the price that must be paid.

Further Reading

Ashton H. and Stepney R. (1982) *Smoking: Psychology and Pharmacology.* Tavistock Publications Ltd., London.

Cleave T. L. and Campbell G. D. (1969) *Diabetes, Coronary Thrombosis and the Saccharine Disease*, 2nd edition. John Wright & Sons Ltd., Bristol.

Editorial (1982) Voluntary agreements do not stop epidemics. *Lancet*, **ii**, 855.

Grant M. (1984) *Same again: a guide to safer drinking*, Penguin Books, Harmondsworth, Middlesex, England.

Health Departments of Great Britain and Northern Ireland (1976) *Promotion and Health: Everybody's Business. An assessment of public and personal health.* HMSO, London.

Hetzel B. S. (1974) *Health and Australian Society.* Penguin Books Australia Ltd., Victoria. Australia.

Morris J. N., Heady J. A., Raffle P. A. B., Roberts C. G. and Parks J. W. (1953) Coronary heart disease and physical activity of work. *Lancet,* **ii**, 1053 and 1111.

Report of the Royal College of Physicians of London (1971) *Smoking and Health Now.* Pitman Medical and Scientific Publishing Co. Ltd., London.

The Surgeon General's Report on Health Promotion and Disease Promotion (1979) *Healthy People.* US Department of Health Education and Welfare, Washington, USA.

Co-ordination of Primary and Secondary Protection

18

The Home

The association between ill-health and adverse living conditions, although perhaps more immediately obvious than that between disease and dirty food or water, is certainly more complex. People who live in unsatisfactory houses are usually poor, and it is difficult to separate the effect of bad housing from the many other adverse environmental influenences associated with poverty. To this must be added the complication of the question posed by Karl Pearson: how much of the high mortality in slum areas is due to bad housing and how much to 'the drifting of physically and mentally inferior sections of the people into these dwellings by a process of selection?'

There are three principal ways in which housing may affect health: first, through the structure of the home, a matter of bricks, or wood or even old petrol cans; second, through the relation between size of the house and the number of people living in it, a matter of overcrowding; and third, through the situation of the house, a matter of neighbourhood conditions and amenities. All are related to society and its values. Although these unhealthy influences are commonly found together, presenting the problem of overcrowding in substandard houses packed closely together in an unfavourable social and physical environment and without social amenities, it will be convenient to consider them separately.

Substandard houses

Badly built, unsound and poorly equipped houses are the direct cause of much ill-health. Without an indoor hot-water supply, dirt and refuse accumulate, vermin are encouraged and the spread of infection is facilitated. When cooking facilities are inadequate and the larder is an unventilated cupboard under the stairs, there is likely to be wasteful buying, an ill-balanced diet and an increased risk of food-borne infection. Uneven floors, steep stairs without handrails, bad lighting and dilapidated furniture and household fittings, lead to accidents in the home, particularly in young children and old people.

Overcrowding

It is easy to understand why overcrowding also causes much ill-health. When large families are living together in one room during the daytime and sleeping several to a bedroom, opportunities for the spread of airborne infection are greatly increased. Young children are particularly vulnerable. Infections are brought into the home from school by older brothers and sisters, and the earlier in infancy the common infections are acquired the more likely they are to prove fatal or to result in chronic ill-health.

Overcrowding may also have harmful psychological effects. When people are living too close together, irritability and frustration due to clashes of temperament and interests are inevitable; lack of privacy makes it impossible to hide these conflicts from children. Overcrowding in the bedroom—children with parents, older children with younger children, brothers with sisters—may lead to emotionally disturbing sexual experiences. The schoolchild has no space for play or for study, and the adolescent is not encouraged to bring friends into the home. The wheel comes full circle when young couples cannot find a house of their own and are forced to spend the formative years of their married lives in the overcrowded houses in which they were reared.

Neighbourhood amenities

The ill effects of living in substandard houses are often augmented by a lack of social and recreational amenities in the neighbourhood. It would be surprising if poor quality houses crowded together in a district short of school accommodation and health centres and devoid of clubs and playing fields did not have an adverse effect on the physical and mental health of those living in them. Two obvious consequences are that adolescents have nowhere to meet except at street corners and children have nowhere to play except on the streets or in derelict houses. The problem of the effect on health of lack of social amenities is not limited to pockets of bad housing in the older parts of our industrial towns. Many of the housing estates built between the wars were designed without a full appreciation of the need for such amenities, and high-rise blocks of flats built since the war have provided a potent cause of social isolation. The same is true of some country cottages which may be primitive, and lacking in mains services such as electricity and water.

Public Control of Housing

The crux of the problem of eliminating bad housing has always been how to provide accommodation at rentals that the average wage earner can afford. The cost of satisfactory housing, like the cost of education and of medical care, puts it beyond the unaided reach of large sections of the population. The rapid increase in population has made it difficult to build enough houses to keep pace with needs; it has also hampered state control of standards and delayed demolition of inadequate old property.

When the population was small and mainly rural there were no great aggregations of urban slum property and the bad living conditions of the poor presented no obvious threat to the health of the well-to-do. But from the middle of the eighteenth century, with the rapid growth of population due to the Industrial Revolution, the situation began to change. Rural labourers poured into the rapidly expanding industrial towns, and squalid clusters of back-to-back, terrace and courtyard houses, without water or sanitation, were thrown up by speculative builders to accommodate them. These houses were probably no worse than the rural hovels the labourers had come from—indeed they may even have been better. But there were far more of them and they were packed more closely together. By the middle of the nineteenth century the evil consequences were obvious to the eye and nose; and the recurrent threat of cholera led to Government action. The Artisans' and Labourers' Dwellings Act (1868) authorized local authorities to repair, or, if necessary, to demolish without compensation, houses 'unfit for human habitation'. This was followed before the end of the century by legislation which empowered them to condemn, demolish and reconstruct whole areas. But, although some of the larger cites, notably Birmingham and Manchester, made good use of their powers to enforce repair of dilapidated houses and to demolish slum property, few new houses were built by local authorities.

Nevertheless, some progress was made. For census purposes overcrowding was for many years measured as the proportion of persons, children being counted as half and infants not counted, living at more than 2 per room in households of less than 5 rooms. By modern standards this is a very inadequate index: a family consisting of a man, his wife and 6 children living in a 3 roomed tenement would not have been classed as overcrowded. In 1891 the percentage of overcrowding in the population was 7.9; by 1911 it had fallen to 5.1. Between 1914 and 1918 building was at a standstill and after the war there was an acute shortage of working-class accommodation. The need was urgent. Objections of subsidized public enterprise were ignored, and substantial exchequer grants were made available for municipal schemes. Although the amount of subsidy and the method by which it has been paid has since varied greatly, the policy of providing financial help from central funds for the building and improvement of working class houses has remained. Of the 4 million built between the wars, 1.5 million were State aided. Since the war considerably more than half the new houses have been built by local authorities, and at the 1951 census 1.1 per cent of the population was 'overcrowded'.

By the 1981 census the criterion for overcrowding, which had been changed to living with more than 2 per room in a small household, was changed again to the more rigid index of 1.5 or more persons per room in a household of any size. At this level 1.3 per cent of the population and 0.6 of households are now defined as being overcrowded. Clearly, although a direct comparison cannot be made with 1951, the state of affairs has been considerably improved over 30 years; nevertheless it still cannot be accepted as being satisfactory.

State subsidies have had two important results: they have increased the rate at which working-class houses are built; and they have substantially raised the standard of these houses. At the beginning of the present century a shared outdoor lavatory was the rule, an indoor water supply was uncommon and a bathroom was unheard of. Today new houses must conform with specified standards of room size, living space and natural lighting; and they must be equipped with satisfactory cooker, sink and larder, and with adequate washing and storage facilities as well as hot and cold water, indoor sanitation and a bathroom. Yet a very substantial proportion of houses is still seriously inadequate. Local authorities have wide powers to inspect in their areas and may order the repair of dilapidated houses and the demolition of those 'unfit for human habitation'. But the cessation of all building and destruction of many houses during the war, immigration since the war, and the still increasing population have seriously hampered the application of these powers.

It is now generally recognized that there must be both public subsidy and public control of standards if the majority of families is to be reasonably housed. There must also be control of the siting of houses and the planning of the neighbourhood in which they are built. Town planning is not a new idea. In the mid nineteenth century Napoleon III did for Paris what Wren in the seventeenth century had hoped to do for London; and the terraces, squares and crescents of Regents Park, Bath and Cheltenham provide good examples of effective planning in the eighteenth century. But these are isolated examples and public control at the national level is a recent innovation and has been taken seriously only since the Town and Country Planning Act, 1947, which has subsequently been frequently updated. The Department of the Environment is now responsible for the central control of planning, and at the local level the County Council for strategic plans, and the District Council for the acceptance or rejection of individual planning applications.

Housing and Health

That there is a close association between poor living conditions and ill-health has been generally accepted and has provided ammunition for more than a hundred years for social reformers who have been able to obtain vigorous support leading to the introduction of successful legislation which has repeatedly been updated. Yet there is little numerical evidence of the precise part played by the various elements of bad housing in the aetiology of disease, disability and death. It is interesting to compare this situation with the general attitude towards evidence connecting tobacco with cancer of the lung and chronic bronchitis. Here the evidence of a close association is statistically unassailable, but a will in society to control the problem has been slower to develop so that legislation has been less radical.

It is easy to demonstrate that people who live in districts where the housing is bad are less healthy than those who live in areas where it is good. At corresponding ages their children are shorter and more likely to suffer from skin infections, to have defective vision and hearing, and to die from pneumonia, enteritis and the common infections of childhood. In adult life they have a higher mortality from tuberculosis, rheumatic heart disease, chronic bronchitis and many other diseases. However, evidence of this type, and there is much of it, does not prove that bad housing is itself indirectly responsible for high mortality. The worst houses are closest together and most overcrowded, and are occupied by the poorest and largest families. The diet of such families is sometimes deficient in quantity and often badly balanced; the wage earners in poor families have the lowest standard of medical care. In effect high mortality rates in slum areas provide evidence, not so much of a relation between ill health and bad housing as a relation between ill-health and poverty, of which a poor standard of housing is an obvious attribute.

Except in respect of accidents in the home, there is probably no clear evidence that substandard housing of itself can affect health directly. It is widely held that cold, damp and insanitary living conditions play a part in promoting chronic and acute rheumatic disease. Acute rheumatism was made notifiable in Sheffield in 1947. Between 1948 and 1950 it was shown to be 3 times more common among unskilled workers than among the professional and administrative classes. But in a special study it was found that there was little difference between patients and controls in respect of standard of housing described in terms of structure, ventilation, light, damp, cleanliness, etc. However, the risk was found to be greater in large than in small families and in schoolchildren than in pre-school children.

The evidence connecting overcrowding and ill-health is rather more convincing, although it is not easy to separate this aspect of the domestic environment from the under-nutrition, and lack of sanitary, washing and cooking facilities often associated with it.

The risk of children contracting lower respiratory infections during the first 2 years of life has been shown to be greater in overcrowded homes, particularly when bedrooms were shared with parents or other children. Children in overcrowded homes also catch measles and whooping cough earlier and are more likely to die from those diseases and as we have seen the case fatality rate from the latter in the first years of life is about 1 per cent (Chapter 16).

The relation between respiratory tuberculosis and overcrowding might be expected to be clear cut. It is not. There is no difficulty in demonstrating that overcrowded areas of large towns have higher notification rates and mortality than less crowded areas; but the relationship is not so obvious in the households of patients. This is not to deny the importance of household contact with an open case in the spread of disease; but the effect of overcrowding *per se* has not been shown to be as important as one might expect.

In conclusion the evidence connecting bad housing and overcrowding with disease is unsatisfactory. But even if it were possible to apportion the precise contribution of insanitary housing and overcrowding to morbidity and mortality from infectious disease and accident, this would probably represent only a small part of the damage done to the mental and physical health of the community by bad living conditions. The improvement in home conditions in the 8 decades of the twentieth century has undoubtedly played a part in lowering national mortality and improving national health.

Some Present Day Problems

In 1949 to Royal Commission on Population recommended that 1 person per room should be the maximum permitted density for any household. In 1981 over 600,000 people in Great Britain were still living at a mean density of over 1.5 persons per room. In addition, 2.8 per cent of households were still without an inside water closet and 1.7 per cent without a fixed bath, albeit a great improvement on 1971. Yet this continuing shortage of accommodation and of household amenities raises the problem of priorities among families on the waiting list as new houses become available. Justice must at least appear to be done, and most local authorities have points schemes which take account of family size, degree of overcrowding, ill-health, state of existing accommodation, war service, length of residence in the area, etc. Health reasons for priority are also recognized: for example the need for a separate bedroom for a member of the family who has respiratory tuberculosis; and ground floor accommodation for a person suffering from advanced cardiac disease or crippling arthritis.

Some families seem incapable of managing the machinery of ordinary family life or of using effectively the health and welfare services available to them. In these families poverty is not so much the cause of trouble as one of its consequences. Perhaps the most characteristic feature of such problem families is the squalor of their home life, which leads to ill-health and premature death of children. From the landlord's point of view they are unsatisfactory tenants and tend to drift into the meanest quarters of the slums; and if rehoused in a new housing estate, they soon turn their new homes into slums. Surveys since the war suggest that about one family in 200 is of this type. Some are social casualties because their bad living conditions are due to chronic ill-heath or death of husband or wife, and with financial help and a little guidance they can be rehabilitated. Most, however, can only be looked upon as socially inadequate; one or both parents is not uncommonly mentally handicapped. Some problem families can be helped a little by substantial outside support and guidance of the type provided by the social services departments of local authorities and voluntary welfare associations; but in spite of social assistance others deteriorate. The ultimate sanction against such families is to remove the children from their parents as 'being in need of care and protection'. But the break-up or segregation of the problem family can never be more than an administrative expedient.

In large cities the rehousing of people from slum clearance areas presents many problems. The choice lies between blocks of flats in the clearance areas, which are usually near the city centre and these have a great attraction for architect and town planner but are much less attractive to the mother with a young family, new estates near the city's edge which take men and women an expensive journey away from traditional inner city employment opportunities, or new satellite towns a long-term policy with its own peculiar difficulties one of which is a high prevalence of mental depression among people who have been moved to a totally new environment, and away from friends and relatives. Wherever the site, the need is not only for new houses, but for a new community with a social life of its own. The provision of employment, shopping and community centres, schools and health centres, playing fields, open spaces, public houses and churches should be as much part of a rehousing scheme as the provision of bathrooms, adequate bedroom space and good facilities for preparing, cooking and storing food. A balanced community should take into account the needs of the young and the old, and of small families and large. It should also make provision for growth and change.

Other current difficulties include: the special and still largely unmet needs of the rapidly increasing number of old people; the extent to which housing shortages hamper the redeployment of labour, so necessary to the national economy when many old industries are dying and new ones being developed; the inadequate provision for large families at one end of the scale and for single people seeking separate accommodation at the other; the special needs of the homeless; and perhaps the most important of all the problem of housing immigrants.

19

Place of Work

In Britain most men and many women spend between 30 and 40 per cent of their waking hours at paid work outside their homes. The jobs they do are extremely varied and expose them to a wide range of environments. Some work places are old, badly lighted, poorly ventilated, inadequately heated, and short of even the basic amenities; others are well appointed with high standards of hygiene and house-keeping and provide excellent health and welfare services. Some occupations make heavy physical demands, others are sedentary; some are associated with well-recognized hazards such as lead, mercury, carbon monoxide, ionizing radiations and asbestos, while many others carry less clearly defined risks of ill-health and accidents; some are intellectually and emotionally satisfying, many are tediously repetitive and uninteresting.

Clearly, the working environment must have a considerable influence on health. The subject is extensive. There are many textbooks, scientific papers and government publications on occupational health, industrial toxicology, industrial psychology, industrial diseases and occupational health services. Even to summarize the wide range of problems involved would be outside the scope of this book and we must limit ourselves to a brief discussion of some of the more important aspects of the subject. First we shall consider the ways in which the working environment may affect health. Then we shall indicate the methods by which adverse influences in that environment may be controlled. And finally we shall review the position of occupational health services in the country.

Work and Health

Harmful influences in the working environment can sometimes reveal their presence in a dramatic and unmistakable manner by causing acute illness or sudden death, as in carbon monoxide poisoning and electric shock, or by giving rise to chronic conditions long recognized as having an occupational aetiology, such as lead poisoning and mercurialism. Sometimes the influence, although direct and specific, is less obvious because of the long latent period between exposure and development of symptoms, as in the production of bladder cancer by exposure to β-naphthylamine and mesothelioma and lung cancer by exposure to asbestos. Sometimes the influence of the working environment is difficult to separate from other known or suspected factors in the aetiology of a disease, for example to distinguish between the parts played by coal dust, smoking habits, childhood illnesses, poor housing and atmospheric pollution in producing an excessive amount of chronic bronchitis among coal miners. There is also the effect—subtle, indirect and difficult to measure—of poor working conditions upon efficiency, sickness absence and accident rates and, with millions unemployed, the effect of lack of work upon health, morale and standard of living.

The physical environment

Heat

In some occupations workers are exposed to extremes of heat, or less commonly, cold, and unless properly protected they may become acutely ill. For example, stokers, foundry workers, miners and others doing heavy work at high temperatures may develop 'heat cramps' due to excessive sweating; workers exposed to low temperatures of refrigerated stores may develop hypothermia, frost-bite or even gangrene. Exposure to such extremes of temperature is uncommon, and when unavoidable the need for protective measures is obvious. But conditions of thermal discomfort far short of the extremes have been shown to lower the quantity and quality of work done and increase accident rates, absenteeism and labour turnover. The sensation of being uncomfortably hot or cold is complex. The radiant temperature of the solid surroundings, the temperature and humidity of the ambient air, ventilation (air movement), physical activity and the type of clothing worn all play their part. Under ordinary conditions air temperatures within the range 16-24°C are considered comfortable by most people doing light or sedentary work. But what is a comfortable temperature for one person may cause discomfort for another, and standards of comfort vary greatly from country to country. In most American hotels air temperatures are at the upper end of the comfort range; in some English hotels they are still at the lower end and sometimes well below it. In industry the question of thermal comfort is complicated by the fact that some occupations are unavoidably associated with high, low or fluctuating temperatures, high humidity or excessive air movement. Summarizing indices have been devised and comfort zones mapped out, but in most places thermal comfort is still sought by a rule of thumb adjustment after complaint, so that uncomfortable working temperatures are probably the cause of much industrial inefficiency.

Light

The effects that inadequate lighting, shadows, flicker, glare and too much contrast have upon fatigue, eyestrain and liability to accidents are well known and are supported by convincing evidence from laboratory experiment and from observations in industry. The need for a good light at working level is generally appreciated, and the intensity and quality of illumination are readily measured. Several occupations with unusual lighting conditions carry special health hazards. Miners who had worked for years at the coal face by the light of flame safety lamps, introduced because of the methane fire risk, used to develop miner's nystagmus, with its overlay of psychoneurotic symptoms. This troublesome and once common condition has disappeared with the improved lighting at the coal face. Acute and painful oedema of the cornea ('arc eye') can appear abruptly 1 or 2 hours after even a momentary exposure to the intense ultra-violet radiation emitted by arc and gas welding apparatus.

Noise

In the nineteenth century it was known that noisy occupations like boiler-making, rivetting and cotton weaving could cause deafness. The refined methods developed for measuring auditory acuity and intensity of noise and its component frequencies have greatly increased knowledge of the harmful effects of the working environment. Intensity (measured in decibels), pitch (measured in Herz Hz) and duration of exposure all need to be taken into account. In general, auditory acuity at the higher frequencies is affected first. Impaired hearing at 4,000 Hz and above can often be detected before a worker himself is conscious of any deafness. However, when the impairment extends downwards into the speech range (below 2,000 Hz) it becomes an obvious social handicap. A given intensity of noise is more damaging if it is concentrated in a narrow band at the higher frequencies than if spread across the frequency range. The threshold level of noise above which hearing damage can be caused is 85-90 decibels (dB). The higher the level the greater the risk of damage and the shorter the exposure needed to cause it—a few minutes exposure to levels above 135 dB(A) can cause severe and irreversible damage to the organ of Corti. Observations in industry suggest that levels below 85 dB(A), although unlikely to damage hearing, may cause irritability and fatigue which lead to lowered output and increased accident rates.

Ionizing radiation

The rapidly expanding use of nuclear reactors to generate electricity and of ionizing radiation in diagnostic and therapeutic medicine has heightened interest in the hazards of occupational exposure to low-level radiation. There are three types of hazard—carcinogenic, teratogenic and genetic, and of these the risk of induction of malignant disease is giving rise to the most concern and the most controversy. The major sources of ionizing radiation to which the general population are exposed are natural background radiation (about 0.1 rem per year) and in a medical setting diagnostic therapeutic radiation (from 0.2-0.4 rem per year). Workers in the nuclear fuel cycle are on average exposed to from 0.3-0.8 rem per year. There is no doubt that low-dose exposure can induce solid malignant neoplasms and leukaemia and it is generally agreed that any extra radiation, however small, above the natural background level will cause an increased incidence of neoplasm. The problem is that these extra malignant neoplasms are indistinguishable from those occurring naturally and estimates of the magnitude of their numbers can be made only by means of extrapolation downwards from the known high level exposure risks derived from studies of survivors of the atom bomb explosions in Japan and of patients who have in the past received high therapeutic exposures, for example for ankylosing spondylitis, or repeated diagnostic exposures, as in the monitoring of pneumothorax treatment for pulmonary tuberculosis and repeated screening for breast cancer, and from animal experiments. More reliable estimates are beginning to emerge from large scale prospective epidemiological studies of workers in the nuclear fuel industry (mining, milling and fuel processing, power reactor operation and reprocessing and research and development). But because of the large populations needed to demonstrate small increases in incidence of even the commonest neoplasms and because of the long latent period which can be 30 years or more between induction and manifestation of the malignancies, such studies are extremely difficult to carry out. However, two points are already clear: solid malignancies are numerically of much greater importance than leukaemia; and carcinogenic effects have already been detected for a working-life exposure to levels well below what are at present promulgated as maximum permissible levels (5 rads per year). Permissible levels are not safe levels.

The psychological environment

Inimical physical environments may produce serious disease such as stoker's cramp, miner's nystagmus and boilermaker's deafness. Today these conditions do not often occur in the United Kingdom. Lesser deviations from physical comfort, however, are still common. Their effect is largely psychological and can be measured only indirectly. We have already mentioned that thermal discomfort, poor lighting and excessive noise appear to influence productivity, absenteeism, accident rates and labour turnover. However, the well-known experiments carried out by Elton Mayo at the Hawthorn works of the Western Electric Company in Chicago between 1924 and 1927 indicated that the relationship between physical conditions at work and psychological well-being is not as straightforward as had previously been thought. A series of improvements in working conditions of a group of workers led to considerable increases in output; but output remained high when the improvements were withdrawn. Mayo concluded that people work better if someone in authority takes an interest in them: job satisfaction is important. Bad working conditions may cause psychoneurotic disturbances; but bad working conditions are often a sign of lack of interest by management and of unsatisfactory relationships within the working group.

Psychological techniques developed in the laboratory are now applied fairly widely in personnel selection and are also used in the study of working practices and of the design of machines and equipment; this is known as the science of ergonomics. People like to know what is going on but often they are not told. Firm decisions based on adequate consultation and communicated clearly are good for morale; incompletely understood rules and contradictory instructions undermine morale.

Diseases of occupations

Frank occupational disease is very much less common today than 100 years ago. The expression 'as mad as a hatter' is evidence of the extremely high risk of mercury poisoning once faced by workers in the felt-hat industry, and many other occupational diseases were common enough to merit demotic names such as knife-grinder's rot, potter's rot and painter's colic. Nevertheless, the old and long-recognized hazards continue to take toll of health and sometimes of life. In 1980 notified industrial diseases included 39 cases of chrome ulceration and 12 of lead poisoning, and many new potentially harmful substances and processes are introduced into industry every year. To uncover new hazards and keep old ones under control there is need for frequent review of national mortality and morbidity data (Chapters 5 and 6) and for continual vigilance by occupational health workers.

A description, however brief, of all major occupational diseases would be out of place here. Although recognition of possible underlying industrial causes of illness is part of clinical medicine, too little attention is still paid by doctors working outside industry to the occupational background of their patients. For example, lead colic is still occasionally treated by appendicectomy, mercurialism dismissed as an idiopathic anxiety state and the occupational origin of many bladder and some lung cancers overlooked. Because the subject is so large we can provide only a short account of the ways in which harmful substances in the working environment may enter or otherwise damage the body because this has important implications for prevention of occupational diseases, and mention only a few of the more important toxic dusts, fumes, vapours and gases encountered in industry.

Portal of entry

Dusts, fumes, vapours and gases occur in great variety as industrial pollutants. Many of them are harmful to health, so it is not surprising that inhalation is the commonest way in which industrial disease is acquired. Some harmful pollutants act as simple asphyxiants: in this category are nitrogen the 'blackdamp' of mines, methane or 'firedamp', and carbon dioxide which is found in fermentation vats and agricultural silos. Others act as chemical asphyxiants: carbon monoxide is very widely produced and used in industry, and hydrogen sulphide 'stink damp' is found in sewers and in mines. Many pollutants damage the respiratory passages: some have an immediately irritant effect, for instance, chlorine is used widely in the alkali industry and in dye works and paper mills, and ammonia is an important by-product of the gas and coke industry; some have an effect which does not become apparent until several hours after exposure, for example, phosgene which has many uses in the chemical industry. Others have a delayed and prolonged effect such as coal pneumoconiosis, which numerically and socially is still an important industrial disease. Some atmospheric pollutants are absorbed from the respiratory passage into the blood, where they act as systemic poisons. This is the way in which lead, mercury, arsenic and cadmium poisoning are usually acquired, and some of the volatile organic compounds in common use in industry are powerful systemic poisons, acting on the central nervous system, blood-forming organs and liver and kidneys, for instance carbon tetrachloride, trichlorethylene, trinitrololuene, benzene, methyl bromide, dichlorethylene and many others.

Some industrial poisons can penetrate the intact skin, but this mode of entry is uncommon. Aniline use in the dye industry, which causes methaemoglobinaemia and liver and kidney damage, and organic phosphorus insecticides can be absorbed in this way.

Occasionally an industrial poison enters the body by ingestion. Food is sometimes eaten in workrooms where lead or arsenic is being used, although this is prohibited by law; and industrial poisons, because they are readily available, are sometimes swallowed with suicidal intent. An often quoted example of disease due to ingestion of materials used at work occurred among girls applying radioactive paint to instrument dials in the United States during the First World War. Some of the girls who had made a habit of using their lips to get a good point on their paint brushes developed aplastic anaemia, necrosis of the jaw and bone cancer.

The prescribed diseases

If persons working in specified occupations develop certain listed diseases they become entitled to benefits under the Social Security Act 1975. These are the 'prescribed diseases'. Apart from pneumoconiosis and dermatitis, industrial disease is now uncommon, but it still occurs often enough for the clinician to bear it in mind when examining adult patients. The Schedule of Prescribed Diseases provides an indication of the continuing importance of industrial diseases and of the occupations with which they are known to be associated. The Schedule is long and complex. Some examples taken from it are given in table 19.1.

Table 19.1 Some examples of prescribed diseases

Disease or injury	Any occupation involving
Poisoning by lead, manganese, phosphorus, arsenic, mercury, carbon bisulphide, benzene, nitro amino or chloro derivatives of benzene, dinitrophenol, tetrachlorethane, tri-cresyl phosphate, triphenyl phosphate, diethylene dioxide (dioxan), methyl bromide, chlorinated naphthalene, nickel carbonyl, oxides of nitrogen.	Use of, handling of, or exposure to fumes, dust or vapour of those substances or their homologues.
Anthrax	Contact with animals infected with anthrax or the handling (including the loading and unloading or transport) of animal products or residues.
Infection by leptospira	(*a*) Work in places which are, or are liable to be infested by rats, field mice or voles or other small mammals. (*b*) Work at dog kennels or the care or handling of dogs. (*c*) Contact with bovine animals or their meat products or pigs or their meat products.
Heat cataract	Exposure to rays from molten red-hot material.
Dystarism, including decompression sickness, barotrauma and osteonecrosis	Subjection to compressed or rarified air or other gases or gaseous mixtures.
Primary neoplasm of the epithelial lining of the urinary tract (renal pelvis, ureter, bladder and urethra) including papilloma carcinoma *in situ* and invasive carcinoma	Exposure to alpha-naphthylamine or beta-naphthylamine, auramine or magenta and certain other compounds.
Non-infective dermatitis, excluding dermatitis due to ionizing particles and electromagnetic radiation	Exposure to dust, liquid or vapour.
Primary malignant neoplasm of the mesothelium (diffuse mesothelioma) of the pleura or of the peritoneum	The working or handling of asbestos or any admixture of asbestos; the manufacture or repair of asbestos textiles or other articles containing or composed of asbestos; the cleaning of any machinery or plant in any of the foregoing operations and of any chambers, fixtures and appli-

Table 19.1 (*cont.*)

Disease or injury	Any occupation involving
	ances for the collection of asbestos dust; substantial exposure to the dust arising from any of the foregoing operations.
Carcinoma of the nasal cavity or associated air sinuses (nasal carcinoma)	(*a*) attendance for work in or about a building where wooden goods are manufactured or repaired. (*b*) attendance for work in or about a building used for the manufacture of footwear or components of footwear made wholly or partly of leather or fibre board; or (*c*) attendance for work at a place used wholly or mainly for the repair of footwear made wholly or partly of leather or fibre board.
Occupational asthma	Exposure to any of the following agents: (*a*) isocyanates (*b*) platinum salts (*c*) fumes or dusts arising from the manufacture, transport or use of hardening agents (including epoxy resin curing agents) based on phthalic anhydride, tetrachlorophthalic anhydride, trimellitic anhydride or triethylene tetramine (*d*) Fumes arising from the use of resin as a soldering flux (*e*) proteolytic enzymes (*f*) animals or insects used for the purposes of research or education or in laboratories (*g*) dusts arising from the sowing, cultivation, harvesting, drying, handling, milling, transport or storage of meal or flour made therefrom.
Pneumoconiosis and byssinosis	Special benefits in relation to a comprehensive list of occupations.
Nickel	Legislation regarding nickel is being changed.

The distinction between 'prescribed' and 'notifiable' industrial diseases is sometimes a source of confusion. The notifiable industrial diseases are as follows:

Lead poisoning	Chrome ulceration
Phosphorus poisoning	Carbon bisulphide poisoning
Manganese poisoning	Aniline poisoning
Arsenical poisoning	Chronic benzene poisoning
Mercurial poisoning	Compressed air illness
Anthrax	Toxic anaemia
Toxic jaundice	Beryllium poisoning
Epitheliomatous ulceration	Cadmium poisoning

All the notifiable diseases are also prescribed diseases but not all the prescribed diseases are notifiable. A doctor who finds that one of his patients has a notifiable disease has a statutory duty to notify the case to the Health and Safety Executive. The notification initiates an investigation of the occurrence with a view to preventing further cases.

Control of Occupational Health Hazards

Our short review of the influence of work on health suggests that control of health hazards in the working environment has two main aspects. The first is the need to protect the worker against dangerous substances, and since the respiratory tract is by far the commonest portal of entry to the body for industrial poisons, this above all requires control of pollution of the atmosphere of the workplace. The second aspect is less precise, but not less important. It is to protect the worker against accident, and to control other aspects of the physical environment, in which he works, particularly exposure to heat, light, noise and ionizing radiation. We shall draw these two aspects of the problem together by considering five basic principles that apply to the control of all occupational hazards. Before stating these principles we may mention two of the aphorisms of Doctor, later Sir Thomas, Legge, appointed in 1898 as the first medical inspector of factories. They are:

1. Until the employer has done everything—and everything means a good deal—the workman can do next to nothing to protect himself although he is naturally willing enough to do his share.
2. If you can bring an influence to bear external to the workman, that is one over which he can exercise no control, you will be successful; if you cannot or do not, you will never be wholly successful.

Legge's aphorisms imply that responsibility for control lies first and foremost with the employer; he can provide primary protection. Secondary protection in the form of devices such as respirators, goggles or use of washing facilities, that depend for their use upon the 'will or whim of the worker to use them' can never be completely effective. With this in mind we can list the first four principles for control of occupational health hazards in order of importance as:

- substitution, the changing of harmful materials and methods for safe ones;
- isolation, the segregation of dangerous processes, to reduce the opportunity for human contact;
- ventilation, that is drawing atmospheric pollutants away from the air workers and breathing.
- personal protection, the provision of protective clothing and appliances for personal use.
- The fifth principle is supervision, without which none of the other principles can be put into practice satisfactorily.

Substitution of materials

The fundamental approach to health hazards is to change harmful materials and methods for safe ones. The most effective method of dealing with an industrial poison is to use a non-toxic substance in its place. Two good historical examples are the substitution of red phosphorus and phosphorus sesquisulphide for white phosphorus in the manufacture of matches, which eradicated phosphorus necrosis of the jaw in workers in match factories, and the replacement of sandstone by carborundum grinding-wheels which played an important part in the control of silicosis. The substitution of wet for dry processes to suppress dust and of quiet for noisy typewriters in large offices to allay irritability are further examples of the application of this important principle.

Substitution is clearly the ideal means of eliminating or controlling a health hazard, but it is often the most difficult to put into practice. To introduce a safe for a dangerous substance may require extensive alterations in an industrial process. There may be no suitable substitute available, and to develop one may involve costly and protracted researches. In such circumstances most firms naturally prefer a less radical approach. However, substitution has the great advantage that in the last resort it can be enforced by prohibiting the manufacture or use of a dangerous material. In this way ill health due to white phosphorus in the match industry, raw lead glazes in the pottery industry and 'silica flour' in foundries was eliminated by statutory prohibition of those substances.

Isolation

If a dangerous process cannot be changed for a safer one, the obvious precaution is to isolate it so that workers do not come into contact with it. This important principle is widely applied throughout industry. Toxic gases, poisonous fluids and harmful dusts are sealed off from the worker in retorts, pipes, ducts, flues, vats, tanks and stills. The complete enclosure of toxic substances may be a necessary part of an industrial process, as in much of the chemical industry, or it may be introduced to avoid waste or prevent explosion. Often it is the cheapest and most effective way of protecting workers against harmful atmospheric pollutants. However, even when toxic gases are completely enclosed, leaks may occur, causing danger for men working in the neighbourhood. Carbon monoxide poisoning is a well recognized occupational hazard for blast furnace workers, and men cleaning and repairing closed systems are also at risk of accidental poisoning. Other applications of the principle include locating dangerous processes and materials in isolated buildings away from the main body of a works, transporting dangerous substances by means of enclosed conveyor belts and gravity feeds, handling radioactive isotopes by remote control, insulating noisy machinery, screening sources of radiant heat and fitting safety guards on dangerous machines.

Ventilation

Good ventilation adds greatly to the physiological and psychological comfort of people working indoors, whatever their occupations; it is essential to the health, and sometimes to the life, of people working in the neighbourhood of industrial processes which produce or use harmful dusts, mists, fumes or gases. In such circumstances good general ventilation, although it may reduce the hazard by diluting the toxic substances, is not enough. As we have seen, total enclosure of a process is the complete solution. But sometimes this is not practicable, and the best safeguard is then a system of local exhaust ventilation to draw the harmful substances away from the air inhaled by workers and to carry it out of the workplace, although this can sometimes produce a health hazard in the neighbourhood of the workplace. When production of a dangerous substance is very localized, as it is in the case of grinding wheels and pneumatic chisels, high velocity ventilation through a small-bore duct with its opening close to the origin of the hazard is the solution. When atmospheric pollutants are produced over a wide area, as in foundries, steelworks and coal mines and in plating, pickling, galvanizing and paint-spraying workshops, the problem of their removal is technically much more difficult and may involve the design and installation of extensive and expensive extraction plant. Every industrial process presents its own problems, and often the atmospheric effluents need to be treated, by such procedures as electrostatic precipitation, filtration or washing, before they can be discharged safely into the outside air. The problem of safe disposal of radioactive wastes is still a matter for debate and public concern.

Personal protection

In a few unusually dangerous working situations none of the above methods of control can be applied. For example, to rescue persons overcome by poisonous gases or to examine, repair or adjust enclosed processes men may have to enter and, for short periods, work in highly toxic atmospheres. The only satisfactory way to control such a dangerous situation is to provide the worker with personal saftey appliances, for example, a self-contained breathing apparatus. In effect, this is an application of the isolation principle by enclosing the worker rather than the toxic process. Except in such uncommon circumstances, protective clothing and appliances should not be the first line of defence against an unhealthy working environment. Although widely used in industry, dust respirators, goggles, helmets, safety shoes, gloves, barrier creams, ear muffs and chemical and fire resistant clothing, should be regarded as no more than an extra precaution after the basic methods of controlling the environmental hazard have been applied. As we have seen they can never be wholly satisfactory, for they depend for their effectiveness upon the cooperation of individual workers who may be careless. The appliances have the further disadvantage that they are often uncomfortable to wear and may interfere with movement, breathing or vision to the extent that they restrict a worker's earning power.

Supervision

The four general principles referred to inevitably depend for their effective application upon supervision of the health of workers in relation to the environments in which they work. This can be carried out satisfactorily only by professionals such as doctors, nurses, engineers, physicists and chemists with a special interest in occupational health. Doctors, occupational health nurses and hygienists should be on the watch for the emergence of new hazards or the reappearance of old ones. Men and women at risk to known poisons should be examined clinically at regular intervals, with appropriate laboratory tests, to ensure that their health is not being impaired. This is known as biological monitoring. Environmental monitoring involves checking the effectiveness of the control of toxic and other hazards at regular intervals by accepted sampling procedures. Codes of safe practice are required and government inspection is necessary to ensure that employers comply with health and safety regulations.

Occupational Health Services

We shall now describe the occupational health services of Britain and comment on their effectiveness. From the time of Robert Owen, many enlightened employers have carried their efforts to provide safe and healthy conditions far beyond statutory requirements. But it is probably true to say that health supervision at work is still one of the less satisfactory features of the country's health services. It is important to distinguish between statutory requirements and voluntary services.

Statutory requirements

Legislation about working conditions has a long history. It began with the Health and Morals of Apprentices Act (1802), which attempted to alleviate the pitiful condition of pauper children who were being sold mainly from poor law institutions to work in the mines and mills of the Midlands and the North. It laid down that apprentices should not work for more than 12 hours a day (Saturdays included), that work rooms should be ventilated and that factory walls should be washed down twice a year. Seventeen years later the Factory Act, 1819, made it illegal to employ children who were less than 9 years-old. From these small beginnings a considerable body of legislation has developed. However, like so much of our social legislation, it has grown up piecemeal and the result sometimes falls short of what is desirable or even clearly necessary. In particular, although the legislation is concerned for the most part only with minimum standards, the machinery devised to operate it is inadequate to ensure that these minimum standards are always observed.

Current statutory provisions for the control of the working environment and the supervision of the health and safety of people at work are chiefly to be found in the Factories Act 1961, the Offices, Shops and Railways Premises Act 1963 and the Health and Safety at Work etc. Act 1974. The Offices, Shops and Railway Premises Act 1963, covers persons working in places other than 'factories' in terms of their general working conditions and the more personal aspects of their health and welfare.

General working conditions

Workplaces must be kept clean and walls washed or painted as prescribed. Workrooms must not be overcrowded and they must be well ventilated, if necessary with local exhaust ventilation to protect workers against the inhalation of injurious atmospheric pollutants, they should be suitably lighted and kept at a reasonable temperature. Appropriate seats must be provided for work that can be done sitting. There must be adequate facilities for accommodating and drying outdoor clothes. Hot and cold water, soap and towels should be provided for washing, and there should be a satisfactory supply of drinking water and a prescribed number of sanitary conveniences.

Personal health and safety

Dangerous machinery must be securely fenced and effectively guarded, and hoists, lifts, cranes and lifting tackle must be sound and properly maintained. Meals must not be taken or meal times spent in rooms where poisons are used. Suitable goggles and other safety appliances must be provided in specified occupations, and special precautions must be taken against gassing and against explosion. First aid boxes of a prescribed standard must be provided and placed in charge of a responsible person with first aid training. Workers in certain occupations are also required to undergo periodic medical examination, for example, lead smelters, vitreous enamellers, tinners, mule spinners, and those working with ionizing radiations and with certain chemicals.

Health and Safety at Work etc. Act 1974

This act is based on the exemplary and forward-looking Report of the Committee of Enquiry on Safety and Health at Work, under the chairmanship of Lord Robens, presented in 1972. The Act is a broad 'enabling' measure and does not go into a great deal of detail; it gives powers to the Secretary of State for Employment, acting through a new Health and Safety Commission, to provide the details through Regulations and Codes of Practice. The Act defines the general duties of employers to ensure the health, safety and welfare at work of employees, to conduct their undertaking so as to safeguard persons not in their employment and other persons, to use the best practicable means for preventing emission into the atmosphere of noxious or offensive substances and for rendering harmless such substances as are emitted. Persons who design, manufacture, import or supply any article for use at work must ensure that it is safe and without risk to health when properly used and they must provide adequate information about it. It is the duty of employees to take reasonable care while working for the health and safety of themselves and others affected by their work and to cooperate with others to enable them to comply with that duty. At the request of trade union safety representatives it is the duty of employers to establish safety committees. The Health and Safety Commission has a full-time independent chairman and nine part-time commissioners. It has taken over responsibility from various government departments for the control of most occupational safety and health matters and, acting through a new Health and Safety Executive, is now responsible for the Employment Medical Advisory Service and a new unified Inspectorate.

Employment Medical Advisory Service

An Employment Medical Advisory Service (EMAS) was established in 1973 to give advice about occupational health problems to employers, employees, trade unions, general practitioners and others. The service is now part of the Health and Safety Executive. The small headquarters staff in London includes a Chief Employment Medical Adviser, a Director of Laboratory Services, a senior adviser in mental health and rehabilitation and a Chief Employment Nursing Officer. At regional levels there are about 100 doctors (Employment Medical Advisers) and 90 Employment Nursing Officers with special knowledge of occupational health problems. The main functions of the service are to provide a central information bank and reference laboratory in relation to occupational health hazards, to investigate and give advice on particular health problems, to advise on the environmental control necessary to minimize general and specific health risks, to undertake epidemiological and laboratory research into new and suspected health hazards and to advise on medical aspects of employment problems, especially those in relation to rehabilitation and to the employment of handicapped young people.

Voluntary services

The large, publicly controlled organisations such as the Coal Board, Steel Corporation, British Railways and London Transport, most of the large, privately owned industries and an increasing number of small firms provide non-statutory occupational health services for their own employees. These services are paid for by the firms themselves and are independent of the statutory services described above and of the National Health Service. The National Health Service itself, the largest of all the publicly controlled employers, in which many jobs are dirty or dangerous or both has been unnecessarily slow to implement the recommendations of the Tonbridge report of 1968. Only now are Health Authorities beginning to establish satisfactory occupational health services for their employees. Occupational health services are essentially preventive in character, and are designed to ensure that the health of workers is not impaired by their working environment and that workers are fit for and fitted to, their work. They also provide first-aid treatment for medical and surgical emergencies and continuing treatment for minor injuries and ailments; some of the larger organizations have set up rehabilitation services, dental, ophthalmic, orthopaedic and chiropody clinics and facilities for radiography and physiotherapy. The establishment in 1978 of a Faculty of Occupational Medicine within the Royal College of Physicians of London has helped to define more clearly standards of post-graduate training, career structures and professional responsibilities for doctors working or wishing to work in the field.

Present position

Two unsatisfactory features of existing occupational health services are their uneven distribution and the inadequacy of laboratory facilities for the examination and investigation of the working environment.

Apart from the advisory and supervisory services provided by the Health and Safety Executive, nearly all occupational health services are non-statutory and are paid for by the firms that provide them. As a result, large, wealthy and enlightened firms provide comprehensive services and small firms (where the worst working conditions often occur) provide little or nothing. In several areas services for groups of small factories are organized on a co-operative basis, for example at Slough, Harlow, Central Middlesex, Dundee, Rochdale, West Bromwich and North Norfolk. But voluntary co-operation to provide non-statutory health and welfare services is not the complete answer to the national problem. Legal sanctions are needed, with a strengthened and enlarged Employment Medical Advisory Service and Inspectorate to help employers to meet their statutory responsibilities.

In Britain laboratory facilities for recognizing and measuring harmful environmental influences at work are seriously deficient. Our services have fallen behind those in the United States and compare unfavourably with those in many European countries. The Government has published many recommendations about threshold limit values (TLV) for toxic substances at place of work. But such recommendations lose much of their point if laboratory arrangements for measuring atmospheric concentration of the toxic substances are inadequate. At present the Health and Safety Executive provides a limited public service, a few large firms employ their own occupational hygienists and occupational hygiene units in certain University Departments in London, Dundee, Manchester and Newcastle offer a problem-solving service for toxic and other environmental hazards.

Further Reading

Schilling R. S. F. (1982) *Occupational health practice*, Butterworth and Co. Ltd., London.

3

Health and Social Services

20

Introduction

Evolution of Health Services

It is useful to recognize four phases in the evolution of our health services. The first is the period before public responsibilities were accepted; the second is that in which public responsibilities developed; the third is the period of the National Health Service as originally planned; and the fourth is one in which there is a National Health Service modified in the light of over 30 years experience. With considerable differences in timing these phases can be recognized in the experience of other countries, although some have not yet entered the third phase of full acceptance of public responsibility for the finance and administration of services, and others may have not contemplated the fourth. That is to say, in most countries the health services provided or planned are still essentially of a traditional kind and nowhere have they been modified to the extent needed to bring them into line with modern requirements.

Phase 1, to 1848. Health services before public responsibility was accepted

It is not strictly true that there was no public responsibility for health services before the mid nineteenth century. Measures for quarantine and for isolation of the infectious had existed for centuries, and the destitute were admitted to county asylums after 1808 and to Poor Law institutions from 1834. But with these exceptions health services were financed by private or voluntary funds and the beginning of public services is usually and reasonably dated from the first Public Health Act of 1848. The history of health services before that time is essentially the history of hospitals and medical practice, discussed in Chapters 21 and 22 respectively.

Phase 2, 1848–1948. The development of public responsibility

The development of public responsibility for medical services in Britain before the introduction of the National Health Service covers a period of exactly 100 years. It began with the introduction of environmental measures in 1848 and ended with acceptance of full responsibility for all preventive and therapeutic services in 1948. Approximately the first half of this period was concerned almost exclusively with control of communicable disease under local health authorities, mainly by environmental measures but including also provision of hospitals for infectious diseases. The year 1906 saw the extension of public services into the field of personal care through the introduction of a school medical service, an extension restricted, however, to preventive medicine. In 1911 public responsibility was extended further into the field of treatment by the National Health Insurance Act. This Act made limited provisions, essentially the services of a general practitioner and certain drugs, to some insured workers but not to their dependents. Finally, in 1948, the government introduced a comprehensive service, available to everyone, and financed mainly by taxation. The second phase is considered more fully in Chapter 23.

Phase 3, 1948–1974. The National Health Service

The National Health Service removed the burden of direct payment for medical services from the large number of people who could ill afford it and in the eyes of the general public this is probably its most considerable achievement. In doing so the Service did not interfere with the relationship between doctor and patient; nor did it prohibit private practice, although as a result of the provision of public services the volume of private work was inevitably reduced.

Indeed if the Service were to be criticized in the light of subsequent experience, the grounds would be, not that it departed from principles essential to the practice of medicine (a criticism sometimes made, particularly by visitors from countries which have not yet accepted a comprehensive public responsibility), but it chose to rely on a structure which had emerged for historical reasons rather than take the opportunity provided by public control to reorganize the services. Apart from shrinkage of private care it made no significant change in the organization of medical practice; the public health service lost its responsibility for hospitals but was otherwise little affected; and while hospitals were brought under a new regional organization which eliminated the long-standing division between voluntary and public hospitals, the relationship of different types of hospitals to one another and to community health and welfare services remained essentially the same. However, while it is easy in retrospect to criticize the original organization of the National Health Service, it is questionable whether on the basis of the experience available in 1948 it would have been possible to do more at that time.

Phase 4, from 1974. The reorganized National Health Service

It was not long after 1948 before it became evident that the traditional pattern of health services which had been incorporated with only minor modifications in the National Health Service was unsatisfactory. Perhaps the most obvious ground for criticism was that although the Ministry of Health (later the Department of Health and Social Security) was responsible for all parts of the Service, local and regional responsibility for general practitioner, hospital and former local government services was divided between three administrative authorities. This led, *inter alia,* to duplication and deficiencies in services, and to an unfortunate division between community and hospital and between preventive and therapeutic medicine. The changes introduced from 1974 were intended to eliminate these divisions, by establishing a unified district, area and regional organization with the responsibility and power to plan comprehensively the health services required by a defined population. In 1982 further modifications were introduced, the most important of which were the abolition of Areas, and the introduction of Authorities in the Districts.

The National Health Service and the changes it has undergone are discussed in Chapter 25.

The Background of Present Day Services

Until the nineteenth century, medical measures comprised no more than the service of doctors to sick patients, and even today, when there has been more than 100 years' experience of preventive medicine, the original concept is still deeply rooted in public and professional consciousness as the essential medical role. This is what brings most students into medicine and it largely determines the character of medical education and the direction of medical science and service. However the traditional concept is beginning to be re-examined, and the present time may prove to be of outstanding importance in the history of medicine as the first in which the requirements for health and the nature of the medical task were seen in perspective. At least three influences are contributing to this reappraisal: the changing character of health problems; the growth of technology; and acceptance of comprehensive public responsibility for provision of medical services.

The change in health problems

If a biologist who had given no special thought to the determinants of human health were invited to express an opinion about them, his reasoning might be along the following lines. Throughout his existence man, like other living things, has been exposed to a high risk of disease and death. In technologically developed countries, this risk has greatly diminished, largely as a result of medical measures, particularly those directed to the prevention and treatment of disease in the individual. In consequence, the health problems of today are different from those of the past; but since medical science will continue to advance, the problems also must be expected to change. Moreover, they will do so in ways which cannot be foreseen, for neither the pace nor the direction of scientific progress can be predicted for more than very short periods.

Such an interpretation would be mistaken both in its emphasis on specific medical measures and in regarding the change in health problems as essentially a continuum. The experience of the past 2 centuries, discussed in Chapters 2 and 3 indicates that the main influences on health are not the prevention and treatment of disease in the individual; and, although health will continue to change, there is nevertheless an important distinction to be made between the problems of the past and those of the foreseeable future. Indeed, the twentieth century may come to be recognized as a watershed separating the infectious diseases which have been predominant during man's evolution from the residual problems which remain when infections are reduced to small proportions. These are particularly congenital handicaps, mental illness, and the disease and disability associated with ageing, problems in which, in general, medical research has tended to be least interested and medical services least successful. Changes in the residual problems are of course inevitable, but it is unlikely that we shall see ever again a change in the spectrum of disease as great as that which resulted from the decline of infections.

The growth of technology

A second influence on thinking about health is the increasing cost of medical services, due largely to the spectacular and, in its financial and administrative implications, alarming advance of technology. Until the late nineteenth century there were few methods of investigating and treating diseases, and even in the first part of the present century, their number was relatively small. In the past few decades, however, there has been an enormous increase in the volume and complexity of technology in medicine and there can be no doubt that it will continue, probably at an increasing rate. The growth of technology is largely responsible for rising costs which result not only from expensive equipment and facilities but from the heavy demands on skilled technical and professional staff. It is not possible to envisage the level of development of technology by the end of the century, but before then it is likely that its complexities and costs will have exposed the inadequacies of the traditional research and service matrix and they have already forced the consideration of economic analysis in medicine which doctors and their patients are only with reluctance contemplating.

Public responsibility

A third influence is acceptance of public responsibility for the finance and administration of health services which in most developed countries is now extensive or complete. For the first time it is both possible and necessary to examine the medical scene as a whole, to consider the balance between research and practice, between prevention and treatment, between care and cure. Medical services can no longer ignore related social services, hospitals cannot function without reference to domiciliary and ambulatory care, and traditional public health is being reshaped in relation to the greatly enlarged public commitment for medical services.

Each of these influences, (changed problems, technological advance, and public responsibility), is important; but it is their coincidence which makes it imperative to reconsider the framework of medical services. The public commitment has come at a time when the outstanding problems are in general more intractable than those they have replaced and when elaborate methods threaten to stretch the resources of even the wealthiest countries. Serious mistakes in organization will be penalized more heavily than in the past, and it is therefore essential to devise a new pattern in accord with the character of the residual health problems and the trend in medical technology.

Limitation of Costs: Health Care Priorities

One of the most formidable problems confronting health services is to find some rational basis of restricting costs which are already high and appear to be potentially unlimited. In England and Wales expenditure on health expressed as a percentage of the Gross National Product has risen from 3.9 to 5.2 between 1950 and 1979; in Sweden over the same period the rise has been from 4.4 to over 10. No country is so wealthy that it can afford to be indifferent to the need to restrict expenditure on health services.

If costs are not to be restricted on an arbitrary basis, there will have to be extensive development in health service accounting and a system of priorities. This raises *four* questions: Are priorities necessary? How can they be reconciled with the obligations of the doctor to his patient? Who should decide priorities? On what basis can they be determined? There is as yet no answer to these questions, which have only recently begun to receive the attention they deserve.

Are priorities necessary?

Reactions to the imposition of charges in the National Health Service many years ago indicated that many people find the whole idea of medical priorities distasteful. They see the need to curtail other public activities, including social services, and recognize that this requires a choice between alternative policies according to their cost and usefulness. Medical services, however, are quite another matter; it is hard to accept suffering from disease due, not to lack of knowledge of prevention or cure, but to insufficient resources to provide essential services. This reaction, though understandable, is based on certain misconceptions which need to be removed if medical priorities are to be considered rationally.

First, it should be recognized that demands for medical expenditure are potentially unlimited, an anomaly to which both the public and doctors contribute in different ways. On the one hand, the public appetite for medical services appears to be insatiable. Just as any child can occupy the attention of as many adults as are willing to look after it, some patients seem able to absorb the time of all the doctors who can be persuaded to see them; and in hospitals, with Parkinsonian logic, patients appear to increase in number to fill the available beds. On the other hand, many doctors are reluctant to consider effectiveness and costs, and vigorously defend their right to make up their minds about what is good for their patients without regard for such tiresome criteria. Not all surgeons who undertake coronary bypass operations are likely to have considered that it would be cheaper, more humane and more effective to invest resources in reducing the risk of developing ischaemic heart disease in the first place and the psychoanalyst has not traditionally inquired whether the results of his therapy are commensurate with the long hours he and his patient spend in communion. All that has been necessary to satisfy public scrutiny or private conscience has been to ensure that a procedure is well intended and has some claim to consideration, at least in the judgement of the doctor who uses it. In such circumstances, it is clearly impossible to set limits on expenditure.

A second source of misunderstanding is the belief that the assignment of priorities in medicine would introduce a new principle. In fact, they are already well established; it never has been possible to do all the things which could usefully be done if there were no limits to resources. And in most countries in Asia, Africa and Latin America the practical possibilities are restricted to a small fraction of those which knowledge would justify. All too often, however, the choice between alternative measures is made on quite inadequate grounds and with little reference to health objectives.

A further misconception is that health depends mainly on treatment of the sick, and that any reduction in the volume of curative services would have disastrous consequences. Interpretation of the reasons for human health as we have seen leads to quite a different conclusion: the most important influences are an adequate diet and avoidance of such environmental hazards as contaminated food, infected water, polluted air and tobacco. If health is to be placed on a different footing from other social goals, concern about restriction of expenditure should not be limited to medicine, but should logically be extended to other social services such as nutrition and housing. There are also no grounds for undue concern about the consequences of some restriction on treatment services. Indeed, it is questionable whether there is any method of treatment of which it could be said confidently that a substantial increase in investment would lead to a commensurate improvement in health in Britain. This claim could already be made for some environmental measures, such as elimination of atmospheric pollution and improved nutrition.

How can priorities be reconciled with the doctor's obligations to his patient?

Two examples will illustrate the difficulty in reconciling the interests of society with the doctor's obligations to his patient. In Britain some 5 in every thousand children are born with a serious malformation of the central nervous system. Those with the most lethal abnormality, anencephalus, are stillborn or die soon after delivery, so that unless some dextrous but misguided surgeon finds the means of prolonging life in the absence of a brain, the problem will not extend beyond birth. Most children with the other common conditions, such as spina bifida and hydrocephalus, also die within a few years, but the proportion surviving can be increased by surgical intervention. However, surgery does not often restore normal functions; most children who survive as a result of it are paralyzed to some degree for the rest of their lives, and the degree of paralysis can usually be predicted at the time of operation. Some are also mentally retarded. If the most active surgical measures were practiced on every viable child with spina bifida, the number surviving but disabled by this condition would be approximately trebled, and a substantial increase in demand for extra care and special education would be required. On the two most important points the malformations of the central nervous system differ from some others, notably those of the heart: operation on a cardiac malformation may restore a child to normal health, moreover even when it is unsuccessful it does not increase the number who survive with a serious handicap.

A very different example of a possible conflict between the aims of society and those of the individual is in the field of family planning. Control of population growth is a necessary condition for human health. Even in technologically advanced countries such as Britain, population size is already too great and, from a public viewpoint, it is looked upon as irresponsible to have a large family. Yet for understandable reasons, family planning operates as a service, not to the community but to individuals, providing them with knowledge and methods that will enable them to have the number of children they desire.

Is it possible to reconcile such diverse private and public ends? No mother would feel safe in bringing her malformed child to a doctor for surgery if she thought his first concern was the public consequence of his action; and the demand for family planning services might perhaps decline if it were known that in the view of the clinic staff, families having more than about 2 children were socially irresponsible. These personal services must therefore maintain a delicate balance between the public and the private, between the natural desire of individuals to have children and the wish of society that its members should be strong and healthy, and their numbers commensurate with resources.

Perhaps the first point to be made is that these are medical issues only to the extent that the doctor provides the information on which the decision is based and is often the agent by whom it is implemented. The primary right of decision is the patient's or, in the case of the malformed child who cannot act for himself, the parents'. This is true when the doctor advises the parents, or even when he is in effect asked to decide for them, as he usually is, for example when a mother is confronted by the impossible choice between short term risk and long term cure from an operation on her child with a malformed heart. In some respects the doctor's position is analogous to that of the barrister who tries to act for his client as his client would act for himself, if he had the requisite knowledge and experience.

The doctor's position is, however, more complicated than that of the barrister in that there are considerable differences of medical opinion about appropriate and justifiable methods of treatment. Since these differences are determined more by religious and moral than by professional convictions, they must be respected. It would surely be wrong to require a doctor to refuse treatment to a patient he believes he can help. What can be asked is that before making his decision the doctor should inform himself about its medical and social consequences. If there are grounds for dissatisfaction with the present position they are that medical opinion is often ill-informed rather than that it is not uniform.

If, however, the doctor is to be free to decide the method of treatment, what can prevent the imposition of an intolerable burden on the medical and social services? The answer, so far as there is one, lies not in directives to the doctor but in the disposition of medical resources. If Freudian psychiatrists are sent to Botswana, they must be expected to practice psychoanalysis. The individual physician has to answer the question 'Shall I refuse to help my patient?' For society as a whole, however, the question takes the more tractable form: 'How best can medical resources be deployed?' It is understandable that a surgeon may find it difficult to refuse to correct a cardiac malformation in a Down's child brought to him for assistance. However, in establishing national priorities in the use of medical manpower, the medical and social consequences should be taken into account and an attempt made not only to consider whether any benefit is likely to be derived by the individual patient, but also to consider whether the resources required could be deployed to the greater benefit of the community elsewhere. Such decisions cannot reasonably be criticized as a denial of life to the handicapped, and if the time ever came when resources were sufficient for all purposes, the formidable problem of medical priorities would no longer arise.

Who should decide priorities?

If the main burden of assessing priorities is to be removed from the practicing doctor, who, on behalf of society, is to take it up? The assessment is best made where major decisions are taken concerning the disposition of resources, and in Britain this may be at national, regional or local level. This discussion will be limited to centrally determined priorities.

The central government department already makes many decisions about priorities. It determines the allocation of resources to different services and regions and tries to influence the pattern of expenditure by issuing firm guidelines about services. For instance in recent years services for the elderly, the mentally ill and the mentally handicapped have been consistently classed as priorities in England and Wales, and there has recently been introduced a system of regional reviews by the Department of Health and Social Security to try to ensure stricter adherence to these recommended priorities. Even within regions the department has a large influence on the way money is spent. Yet in spite of this close supervision of expenditure, there is considerable hesitation in establishing national polices. There is particular reluctance to do anything from the centre that might be interpreted as interference with the doctor's judgement concerning the best treatment for his patient.

With due regard for these reservations, there are nevertheless some issues on which it is inconceivable that a large number of regional and district authorities will all arrive at wise, well informed and, where necessary, consistent policies, and in respect of which it seems essential to consider priorities at the centre. Mechanisms for doing so already exist, but they need to be developed and in some cases modified in relation to particular problems.

On what basis can health care priorities be determined?

This, the last, is perhaps the most difficult of the four issues. All that will be attempted here is a brief comment on two important criteria; effectiveness and efficiency.

Among the first questions to be asked about a medical procedure is whether it is effective for the purpose—prevention, diagnosis or treatment—for which it is employed. This is different from the question of efficiency discussed below, for it asks only whether a procedure is effective, without reference to its costs or the possible alternative uses of the same resources.

There is no doubt about the need to assess the effectiveness of medical methods, both those which may be introduced and many that are already in use. Oliver Wendell Holmes said that if all our drugs were thrown into the Pacific Ocean it would be so much the better for mankind and so much the worse for the fishes. The position is very different today, but there are still a good many procedures of which the best that can be said is that they have not been shown to be effective in the circumstances in which they are employed.

This position is clearly unsatisfactory, but it has this excuse: the problems associated with evaluation of effectiveness in medicine are often quite formidable. In some cases they require not only assessment of a diagnostic or therapeutic method, but also extension of knowledge of the natural history of disease that may require investigation of a large population over many years. In judging the value of screening for cancer of the cervix, for example, it is not enough to show that the recognition of abnormal cells makes it possible to detect carcinoma *in situ*. It is also necessary to know the frequency with which carcinoma *in situ* occurs in the first place and the proportion of those which progress to invasive cancer. For these among other reasons, the assessment of medical priorities requires a considerable extension of research into the effectiveness of medical procedures.

When a procedure is shown to be effective, and logically not before, the question arises whether it deserves to replace alternative methods which are already in use or might be introduced. This takes medical research into the difficult study of efficiency, for which techniques of economic analysis have been developed in other fields of applied science. It is clearly distinguished from the appraisal of effectiveness, being concerned not merely with whether a procedure is useful, but also with the critical question of whether it makes better use of the resources required than the alternatives available.

Such a decision is most readily reached when both costs and benefits can be quantified. In medicine it is conceivable that total costing rather than accounting might be put on a satisfactory numerical basis, although even this is not easy. There have been few attempts to determine the costs of individual medical procedures and there is not yet a consistent basis which takes into consideration the large number of contributing influences commonly involved. For example, hospitals do not dissect the cost of, say, thoracic surgery from other expenditure; nor do they estimate accurately in the field of thoracic surgery the cost of removing a cancerous lung.

But it is the appraisal of benefit which raises the greatest difficulties. Some indices may be of use for specific and limited purposes: for example the duration of stay in hospital and, in the case of working adults, the amount of time lost from work. However, there are important benefits which cannot be quantified in this way. Indeed the goal of reducing all medical benefits to a common quantitative basis is almost certainly illusory, and the final decision between alternatives must usually rest on a value judgement. Nevertheless this judgement should be based on much fuller and more accurate information than in the past, information about costs and benefits, quantified to the extent that this is possible but also amplified by other kinds of evidence.

Further Reading

Abel-Smith B. (1967) *An International Study of Health Expenditure.* World Health Organization, Geneva, Switzerland.

Cochrane A. L. (1972) *Effectiveness and Efficiency.* Oxford University Press for The Nuffield Provincial Hospitals Trust, London.

Hampton J. R. (1983) Is clinical freedom dead? *British Medical Journal* **2**, 1237.

McKeown T. (1965) *Medicine in Modern Society.* George Allen and Unwin Ltd., London.

McLachlan G. (ed.) (1971) *Challenges for Change.* Oxford University Press for the Nuffield Provincial Hospitals Trust, London.

McLachlan G. and McKeown T. (eds.) (1971) *Medical History and Medical Care.* Oxford University Press for the Nuffield Provincial Hospitals Trust, London.

Evolution of Health and Related Services

21

Hospitals

The earliest hospitals were religious institutions concerned mainly with the care of the destitute. Few of them survived the dissolution of the monasteries in the sixteenth century, and for 300 years there was little institutional provision for the sick. In 1700 there were less than a dozen hospitals in the country of which about half were in London. Soon after that date several voluntary hospitals were founded, and large numbers were added during the next 2 centuries.

The voluntary hospitals were secular organizations supported by charity, and in the beginning their purpose was to continue the work of the Church by caring for the sick and needy. However, in the late seventeenth century St. Thomas's Hospital, London began to restrict admissions to short term cases. This practice was soon followed by other hospitals, and it became necessary to find other accommodation for the patients excluded. They comprised the destitute sick, the mentally ill, the infectious, sick children and pregnant women.

Provision gradually came to be made for some of these classes in specialized voluntary hospitals, and this explains the separation of many children's, women's and special hospitals from general hospitals. But three large classes—the mentally ill, the destitute sick and the infectious—were beyond the resources, and to some extent outside the interest, of the voluntary movement. It was therefore necessary to make public provision for them.

The first important public development was the founding of county asylums for pauper lunatics in 1808. In retrospect this can be seen as a significant step, since it separated the hospital care of the mentally ill from general hospitals. In 1889 the asylums were transferred to the new county and county borough councils, which remained responsible until 1948 when the National Health Service Acts placed all hospitals under a common administration.

Another major step in development of public hospitals followed the Poor Law Amendment Act of 1834, which made it necessary for those receiving public assistance to enter a workhouse. It was not intended to provide hospital accommodation; but many destitute people admitted to Poor Law institutions were sick, and this led to the establishment of a second public hospital system, separate from both the voluntary general and the public mental hospitals.

The results could hardly have been more unsatisfactory. The beds in mixed workhouses were unsuitable for the care of the sick. Medical supervision was by badly paid part-time general practitioners, and the nursing by pauper inmates. In 1867 Parliament authorized the construction of infirmaries, designed as hospitals and intended to provide a more acceptable standard of care. Unfortunately the infirmaries soon followed the practice of the voluntary hospitals and began to exclude patients requiring prolonged care. This left the ill-equipped asylums and Poor Law hospitals with most of the work for the mentally ill and the sick poor.

A third division of the public hospital service resulted from concern about infectious disease. The voluntary hospitals did not accept most infectious patients, and stimulated by the appearance of cholera in Britain, Parliament authorized the construction of fever hospitals by local authorities in 1867 after the Epidemiological Society had made a special canvass of informed opinion as to how cholera cases should be managed. From this time there were therefore 4 hospital systems, 1 voluntary and 3 public systems; the latter comprising asylums, later called mental hospitals; Poor Law hospitals for the destitute sick; and hospitals for the infectious. In 1929 the hospital responsibilities of the Poor Law were transferred to the major local authorities, and in 1948 the National Health Service Acts placed all hospitals, voluntary and public, under the Ministry of Health.

This brief account of the early development of hospitals explains the origin of many of their present difficulties. It shows that this most complex of social services was essentially unplanned, and owes its character largely to a series of arbitrary decisions taken by voluntary and public administrations. Even the elementary question of the numbers and types of beds needed to serve a population was never considered seriously. The important issue of the relationship between different types of hospitals was completely ignored. The restrictive policy of the voluntary hospitals, adopted also by the public infirmaries, led to the separate general hospital. The county asylums, founded to care for one of the large classes of patients rejected by the voluntary movement, were the forerunners of the separate mental hospital. And the relegation of the destitute sick to the workhouses brought about the isolation of the chronic hospital.

Hospitals Today

The failure to plan a hospital service is still evident in most countries. Hospitals may have less than 50 beds or more than 2,000; their sites vary in size from a few to several hundred acres. They may be located in industrial, commercial, rural or residential areas. There are large hospitals where there are few people and large numbers of people where there are few hospitals. Teaching hospitals are established with no clearly defined relationship to other hospitals, even to other teaching hospitals in the same area, and the division between the major classes of hospitals—acute, chronic, mental illness and subnormality—are still determined largely by the circumstances in which they developed. There are still no satisfactory answers to fundamental questions concerning hospital size, location and function.

The absence of planning which is evident in the distribution of hospitals is also seen in the use of their sites. Many are too small to provide scope for essential development; and good sites are often spoiled by failure to plan imaginatively, allowing for growth and change of use of facilities.

It can hardly be doubted that the role of hospitals will be more complex in future than in the past. At least three major influences are at work: the increasing sophistication of methods of investigating and treating disease; the complexity of the medical problems which result from improved technology and effective treatment; and the fact that in technologically advanced countries hospitals are becoming the focal point of all medical activities. If hospitals are to meet the many demands on them their development must no longer be determined by ephemeral circumstances but planned with due regard for long-term objectives. Three fundamental issues are their integration, size and relation to welfare services.

Integration of hospital services

We have noted that the separation of the major classes of hospitals resulted from restriction of the work of the voluntary general hospitals, and from division of public responsibility for mental, destitute and infectious patients. The results have been deplorable, both in their effect on the standards of care of patients, and in their far-reaching influence on hospital development. The following have been some of the consequences of fragmentation of responsibility.

(*a*) *Mixing of patients with different needs.* The patients in mental, chronic and acute hospitals are not homogeneous in respect of their medical, nursing and social needs. For example while some elderly patients in mental and chronic hospitals may exhibit the full range of physical and mental illness some of them are indistinguishable clinically from others in general hospitals. Mental hospitals have patients who do not require psychiatric care and chronic hospitals have patients who do. All three classes of hospitals have some patients who should not be in hospital at all.

(*b*) *Division of patients into acute and chronic classes.* The traditional segregation of hospitals gives the erroneous impression that in their need for care patients divide naturally into acute and chronic classes. This impression results from the reluctance of acute hospitals to admit or retain patients who will occupy a bed for more than a few weeks and from the deficient services of mental and chronic hospitals, particularly in the acute phase of illness. With adequate care at all stages of illness including care outside hospital the distribution of duration of stay in hospital would look quite different.

(*c*) *Staffing difficulties.* Probably the most difficult problems confronting many mental and chronic hospitals is that of attracting doctors and nurses in sufficient numbers. It is likely to remain unsolved so long as these hospitals are isolated from the mainstream of medical and nursing interest.

(*d*) *Inflexibility.* It is essential that hospitals should respond to changes in the demands for care and in methods of investigation and treatment. In part this capacity for change is determined by internal construction and site planning; but it is also influenced profoundly by the location of the major divisions of the service. So long as hospitals are isolated from one another they must be inherently inflexible, for it is then much more difficult to convert unwanted facilities to alternative use, and to redeploy staff to different work. Moreover ancient and decaying buildings are unattractive to work in and offer unsuitable accommodation for the patients and for the equipment necessary for their treatment.

(*e*) *Uneconomic construction and operation.* An isolated hospital should be reasonably self-sufficient, since it cannot readily exploit complementary services of other hospitals. This affects both construction and operation: capital costs are likely to be higher, and where a hospital needs its own surgical, radiological, laboratory and other facilities, inadequate demand will almost certainly ensue, use will become inefficient and less effective so that operating costs are inevitably increased.

In order to avoid the disadvantages of fragmentation, efforts have recently been directed towards planning hospitals with the following features:

- All types of patients should be cared for at a common centre in approximately the proportions in which they occur in the related population.
- Patients should be classified according to their medical, nursing and other needs and placed in the facilities most suitable for their care.
- In view of the wide range of patients' needs, the hospital should consist of a number of buildings, with varied size, design, equipment and staff.
- Medical and nursing services should be provided by a common staff.

A hospital centre incorporating these features has been referred to as a balanced hospital community.

The idea of assembling a number of hospital buildings on the same site is not new. Architects and hospital planners have often been attracted by the possibilities of centres providing multiple buildings with some centralized services, and in the period between the two World Wars several were established. Moreover there are places in Britain where, for historical reasons, chronic, mental and general hospitals were built near to one another. But such hospitals did not depart from the traditional view of the role of the hospital, for in spite of their location on the same or adjoining sites the hospitals remained single units, separately staffed and with independent services.

Because it is concerned with all classes of patients, the balanced hospital has its greatest impact on psychiatric, and elderly patients who have suffered most from past deficiencies. On the same site, with a common staff, the standard of care should be capable of being raised to a level long considered obligatory in general hospitals. Moreover, the end of isolation can contribute significantly to a change in public attitudes to mental and chronic illness.

But although the impact of the balanced hospital community is greatest on psychiatric and geriatric care, all parts of the hospital service are affected in some degree. For example, paediatrics requires a close association with obstetrics in investigation of prenatal influences, with general medicine and surgery in exploitation of methods of investigation and treatment, and with psychiatry in consideration of the emotionally disturbed child. Even for general medical and surgical services, which are well developed in many hospitals, there is considerable advantage in proximity, for example in the possibility of immediate transfer of patients who no longer need acute care to a more appropriate unit.

If a hospital is to respond to future requirements it must be designed to allow for growth, change of use and replacement. These are essentially matters for the architect. With a spacious site and imaginative planning it should be possible for a hospital to meet the needs of a defined population over a long period.

Not the least of the advantages of the balanced hospital is the opportunity to improve its appearance. The contemporary hospital is still often a forbidding structure which introduces patients and relatives into an alien world. Particularly for those who are ambulant, and whose stay is measured in months rather than days, the general character of the centre is important. The aim should be a domestic rather than an institutional appearance over a substantial part of the site. It can be achieved by reducing the scale of the buildings, by variation of structure and design, and by separation of hospital facilities by such amenities as shops, restaurants and perhaps recreational clubs which are needed by a considerable resident population of health, technical, and supporting staff.

Hospital size

Many hospitals, including some planned recently, are too small to make economic use of expensive technological methods whose efficient operation requires a large patient flow. Such methods, and the more elaborate ones which will undoubtedly follow, make it desirable either to centralize the services for several hospitals or to build larger hospitals. There are several reasons for preferring the latter approach.

Most hospitals are unable to provide a full range of specialist experience. It has been estimated that 6 physicians and 6 surgeons are needed for this purpose, and when numbers of other types of consultant are increased proportionately, the hospital is capable of serving a population of more than 250,000. It is difficult to predict the number of beds required in a hospital of this kind, working closely with well developed community services, but by present day British standards it would have about 1,2000. Of course, there must be variation in hospital size and function according to the density of population served.

In opposition to the trend towards increased size, it has become clear from experience that the large hospital is often inaccessible for many patients and their families and difficult to manage. The problem of distance is less in most urban areas, and in Britain some 90 per cent of the population are less—usually much less—than 15 to 20 miles from a major hospital. Compromises are needed in rural areas, and they can be of various kinds: hospitals smaller than would, in general, be desirable: greater distances for patients and relatives to travel; and provision of local facilities, possibly for long-stay elderly or psychiatric patients, who ideally should not be separated from their home community.

All large institutions have management problems; but they are not insuperable, and in other fields such as industry and universities they have not been allowed to stand in the way of expansion where this was thought to be justified on other grounds.

Relation between services inside and outside hospitals

For some time it has been evident that many psychiatric, elderly and mentally handicapped patients are in the wrong place. Some are at home or in welfare homes although they need hospital care; others are in acute or psychiatric hospitals when they no longer need their services; still others remain in geriatric and mental handicap hospitals only because they have no home to which they can return.

It is a valid criticism of the National Health Service that it is only now coming to terms with this problem of misplacement of patients, a problem which is due largely to the fact that the respective responsibilities of hospital and non-hospital services have not been clearly defined. It is admittedly not always easy to say whether a patient requires hospital care, for the decision cannot be based on the nature of the disabilities, which are continuously graded from trivial to serious. However the distinction can usually be made by focusing attention on the types of care required, and in such borderline cases it is the need for continuous nursing which makes it desirable for a patient to be in hospital. In practice it is usually not difficult to decide whether a patient's mental or physical condition makes it necessary for him to be under the care of hospital staff.

The Teaching Centre

We shall now consider the bearing of the balanced hospital concept on medical education and the teaching hospital. Some people would say it has no bearing at all. They believe the traditional centre is admirably suited to its three-fold obligation: to provide service of the highest quality; to teach; and to do research.

Patients admitted to teaching hospitals are highly selected, although this is truer of some services than of others. For example geriatrics and psychiatry, are either excluded altogether, or represented by small numbers of beds which bear little relation to the actual size or clinical nature of the problems. Other services, such as those concerned with diseases of the ear, nose and throat may be disproportionately large.

It is not difficult to understand how the restrictions arose; they resulted from grafting the concept of scientific medicine on the tradition of voluntary hospitals. From the time of its rebirth in the eighteenth century, the work of voluntary hospitals was sharply restricted. Those providing voluntary funds were entitled to decide how they should be used, and medical staff receiving little or no remuneration could reasonably expect to determine the nature of the work. Both interests coincided in agreement to leave the State the problems of mental illness, mental handicap infectious disease, and all types of infirmity associated with destitution.

The selectiveness of teaching centres has been accentuated in the twentieth century by the development of scientific medicine. The unexceptionable wish to make medical schools centres of research led inevitably to selection of cases in respect of which knowledge was advancing. They did not include the mentally ill or the chronic sick, who were thus removed from the experience of students and the minds of research workers.

But if the teaching hospital is not characteristic of all hospitals, it is even less representative of medical care as a whole. In the past it had no responsibility for domiciliary services, and was quite divorced from the health work of local authorities. Most medical schools have attempted to remedy these deficiencies by sending students to general practitioners, departments of social service and community health clinics. Nevertheless it is still true that the teaching hospital presents only a restricted view of the institutional care of selected patients.

These restrictions are usually defended on two grounds. First, it is suggested they are needed in order to put before students a high level of clinical practice. And second, for research it is thought desirable to focus attention on diseases of which knowledge is advancing. The limitation of work has, however, three serious disadvantages: one in the bias it imposes on medical education; another in respect of medical organization; and a third in relation to medical research.

It is widely recognized that doctors acquire their concept of practice largely from clinical teachers and often leave the teaching hospital hoping to do the kind of work they saw as students. Since this excludes responsibility for large classes of patients and is based on the most sophisticated methods, it provides an inadequate preparation for many of the realities of practice.

A second objection is that teaching centres are prevented from contributing to thought about the way in which medical knowledge is applied; indeed it is only recently that attempts have been made to include enquiries into the organization of services into the national research programme. Yet the problems raised by the application of medical knowledge are at least as formidable as those associated with its acquisition, and are unlikely to be solved unless taken seriously at teaching centres.

A third disadvantage is that the restrictions limit the scope of research, since they remove important diseases from the observation and experience of the investigator. The slow progress with mental handicap and schizophrenia must be due in part to their exclusion in the past from teaching hospitals. Moreover there are many medical problems which require study of representative patients from known populations. In most teaching centres it is impossible to identify the population from which patients are derived, and the fact that they have reached a teaching centre means they are unlikely to be representative.

To remedy these deficiencies it is necessary for teaching hospitals to accept responsibility for exploring new patterns of practice. They should do so both because they can make an important contribution to the development of services, and because the demonstration of a modern concept of practice is essential to the education of students. This ensures access to all patients from a defined population. But it must also break down the barriers between institutional and domiciliary medical care and between preventive and therapeutic medicine.

We have discussed the advantages of a defined population in which responsibility is accepted for all patients. But teaching hospitals are also engaged in service, teaching and research of a more specialized kind, for which it is necessary to admit a substantial number of selected patients whose homes are scattered over a very wide area beyond the district for which the hospital is primarily responsible. A well planned teaching centre achieves a balance between the two activities: a comprehensive service to a local population; and a service to selected patients drawn from a much wider area. Perhaps the innovation of the District Health Authority with its responsibility for all institutional and non-institutional services of a teaching district will create the right environment.

22

Medical Practice

It is useful to distinguish three periods in the history of medical practice. Until the eighteenth century there were no consultants and practitioners as we now know them, and services were provided by physicians, apothecaries, and barber surgeons. The physician was a professional man, trained in a university and his practice was restricted to a small wealthy clientele. The surgeon was a craftsman, trained by apprenticeship; his work was supposed to be limited to surgical procedures, but many surgeons also practised midwifery, kept shops and dispensed drugs, the charter of the Royal College of Surgeons of England was not granted until 1800. In London where the influence of the Royal College of Physicians was almost all pervading the least considered of the medical workers was the apothecary, a tradesman trained by apprenticeship, who was allowed to charge only for the sale of drugs prescribed by physicians. But by the seventeenth century apothecaries were seeing patients and writing prescriptions and, unacknowledged, they had become the doctors of the ordinary people throughout the provinces.

The second period dates from the eighteenth century when, with the founding of voluntary hospitals, the social distinctions between physician, surgeon and apothecary began to disappear. It became important to a doctor to have a hospital appointment, a new division was established between those who had and those who had not. From this time the status of the surgeon improved, and some apothecaries began to work in hospitals.

The third period began with the 1858 Medical Act which created the General Medical Council. By preparing the way for common recruitment, training and registration of doctors it finally removed the historical distinction between physician, surgeon and apothecary. By 1858 however a new, and from a present day viewpoint more significant, distinction between consultant and general practitioner was well established. It was based, not on substantial differences in training or competence, but on hospital appointments. The British Medical Journal described the country consultant as 'the general practitioner who owes his position to the fact of his holding an appointment in connection with a country hospital.'

We have already discussed the deficiencies of medical services; at the beginning of the century these led to the suggestion that there should be a public medical service. The proposal was not accepted, and the only public provision for the care of the sick outside hospital was through the medical officers employed by the Poor Law. In 1911, however, a Liberal Government, with Lloyd George as Chancellor of the Exchequer, introduced a scheme of National Health Insurance financed by compulsory deductions from wages. This method had been used in Europe from about 1883; but the proposal was criticized in Britain by workers and employers who objected to contributions from wages and profits, and by some doctors who disliked even a limited degree of state control. Nevertheless the National Health Insurance Act had the support of public opinion and of many doctors who were satisfied that under it they would be better off.

The Act provided for insured workers the domiciliary services of a general practitioner and some drugs. It did not include hospital or consultant care, and made no provision for dependants. These deficencies were the main reasons for dissatisfaction with National Health Insurance, and led in 1948 to its replacement by a comprehensive service.

The Organization of Modern Practice

The distinction between consultant and general practitioner is so well established in Britain that it is widely regarded as an inherent feature of medical practice. It is therefore remarkable that the roles of the medical workers are very different in different countries at about the same stage of technological development. As a basis for consideration of the organization of medical practice we shall describe the services in Australia, Britain and the United States of America.

Until about the middle of the present century there was no clear distinction anywhere between general practitioner and consultant. They were not differentiated by training or appointment; and general practitioners often gave a specialist service and vice versa. The reason was that medical knowledge did not justify much specialization. The same arrangements may be found in developing countries today, where one doctor may have to serve a very large population, and occasionally in thinly populated parts of developed countries. However this type of practice has also been retained in certain developed countries. In Australia, for example, major surgery may still be performed by general practitioners.

In the United Kingdom substantial changes in this respect followed the implementation of the National Health Service Act of 1946. Previously specialists, in particular physicians, but also many surgeons, served as general practitioners in the community and offered consultant services in their specialty to the local hospital on an honorary basis. The Act compelled them to make a choice between receiving a salary as a consultant or a general practitioner because the two were administered and funded quite separately (see Chapter 20); there was, however, no objection to a consultant working on a part-time basis and if he wanted to make up his salary to do so by undertaking private practice.

Previously some general practitioners had referred cases to hospital doctors for special treatment or a second opinion; on occasion this was done locally but if the patient could afford it there was often a tendency to send him to the teaching hospital where the general practitioner had trained. It was the rule, however, that the general practitioner managed the case himself in his surgery or the patients' home. This still tends to be the pattern in Australia although there the general practitioner has access to hospital beds. In Britain the result of the change was that the general practitioner now became solely responsible for selecting the patients the consultant is to see, and apart from some emergencies the consultant sees only the patients who are referred to him. This clearly defined system for differentiating *primary* from *secondary* care by referral is peculiarly British, although the distinction between the two levels is made elsewhere. The university teaching centre provides secondary care in line with any other hospital, but it also provides highly specialized care of a nature which requires complex and costly technology and also employs consultants with competence in rare diseases. Cases falling into these two categories are classified as receiving *tertiary* care. They may be referred direct by a general practitioner, but more often are admitted by way of a secondary care or district hospital. Teaching hospitals therefore provide secondary and tertiary care and serve populations of several million spread over large areas of the country.

In the United States medical practice has adopted a different structure. Although the standards of specialization have been carefully controlled at a high level by the American Medical Association, there has been little control over the numbers of specialties, and none at all in the nation at large over the numbers of doctors qualified to practice each. As a consequence the general practitioner has disappeared and the patient is left with a bewildering array of doctors from whom to choose. She must decide for herself whether the pain in her leg is the concern of a neurologist? or a surgeon? if so, orthopaedic or cardiovascular? a rheumatologist? or a psychiatrist? If she is wrong, the specialist she chooses will certainly point her in the right direction, and so in a limited sense make a referral, but the error will have been costly of her money and the doctor's time.

The question arises therefore whether any of the forms of practice exhibited in these countries provides a satisfactory basis for the future relationship between general and consultant practice. In Australia, referral has not gone far enough and services which require specialists are still sometimes in the hands of general practitioners. In Britain, some question whether referral has gone too far, and in the United States specialization has certainly gone too far, so that it is difficult to maintain personal and domiciliary care, and efforts are being made to restore general family practice.

In the light of these considerations we shall examine the role of the consultant and general practitioner.

The Role of the Consultant

The term 'consultant practice' will be used in reference to specialization based on referral of patients. The advance of medical knowledge undoubtedly makes it essential for some doctors to have these conditions for their work, but there are two reasons why they should not be created unless referral as well as specialization is necessary. Referral to a doctor who can be identified by the patient (for example to an obstetrician by a general practitioner who himself does obstetrics), implies differences in breadth of interest and, because it is not possible to acquire deep knowledge and great experience across a broad horizontal field, two levels of competence in the management of narrowly defined problems. Thus in the sense of obtaining advice and treatment for some given clinical problems the patient is asked to go first to the 'less competent' doctor. The alternative would be for her to have direct access to the consultant. This vertical approach has as we have seen been practiced for several decades in the United States, and in the opinion of many has proved unsatisfactory. It has not always been easy to obtain medical advice about simple, common conditions; in many instances a patient cannot at first determine whether his symptoms are in the demesne of say the cardiologist, the gastroenterologist or the nephrologist; and perhaps most important of all, specialist consultants can very rarely be fully cognizant of the immediate personal and social environment of the patient. Therefore in the United States steps have been taken to restore family medicine. In Britain obstetricians have gone a long way to establishing a vertical control of their speciality; but even here a first referral is usually made by the general practitioner even though no intermediary is needed to tell her that her attendant should be trained in obstetrics. On parallel grounds paediatricians are seeking to establish vertical control but this raises more complex issues. One for instance, is that whereas not many general practitioners want to practice obstetrics, most are interested in caring for sick children. In addition to caring for referred patients the consultant has direct access to or controls services involving complex techniques—surgery, anaesthesia, radiotherapy, biochemistry, bacteriology, radiology, etc.—as well as to those of a less technical character where referred work is necessary for expert practice. Perhaps the best example of the latter is psychiatry.

The Role of the General Practitioner

If the consultant is to fulfil the role we have described, the general practitioner must accept responsibility for first contact with the patient, for some services to the patient, and for selection of those who require the work of the consultant. In Britain this has been clarified, the standing of the general practitioner improved and the standards required of him raised by the Royal College of General Practitioners and by the Royal Commission on Medical Education which reported in 1968. Bearing their work in mind let us now consider the services which the practitioner should himself provide.

Personal care

The personal role of the general practitioner has been aptly described as follows: 'The doctor we have in mind, then, is no longer a general practitioner, and by no means always a family practitioner. His essential characteristic, surely, is that he is looking after people as people and not as problems. He is what our grandfathers called 'my medical attendant' or my 'personal physician'; and his function is to meet what is really the primary medical need. A person in difficulties wants in the first place the help of another person on whom he can rely as a friend—someone with knowledge of what is feasible but also with good judgement on what is desirable in the particular circumstances, and an understanding of what the circumstances are. The more complex medicine becomes, the stronger are the reasons why everyone should have a personal doctor who will take continuous responsiblity for him, and knowing how he lives, will keep things in proportion—protecting him, if need be, from the zealous specialist.'

There is widespread support for these views, even where personal medical care is in jeopardy. The reason is not only that most patients prefer to be helped by a doctor they know. It is also that medicine is more than an assembly of specialities, and some doctors should be concerned with the health of individuals in its totality rather than with the study of disease or the application of techniques.

Home care

Care at home has long been a feature of medical practice in Britain. Yet some people believe that it is wasteful of the doctor's and the nurse's time. They suggest that the patient should normally go to his doctor's office or clinic, where there are the necessary equipment and assistance. If too ill to do this he should be admitted to hospital.

One objection to this conclusion is economic. If all who cannot go safely to their doctor are to become in-patients, hospitals will be forced to admit many patients with trivial illnesses. Even more serious would be the transfer to hospitals of patients with a considerable degree of disability or infirmity. In countries where the threat of infectious disease has been greatly reduced, the care of the mentally ill and the aged sick is a prominent part of the medical task. It is very desirable that it should be shared with relatives, who with sufficient medical, nursing and social assistance can often make a large contribution to the care of the disabled at home.

Another reason for domiciliary medical care is that it makes it easier for doctors to accept continuous personal responsibility for their patients. Where home care is not provided the tendency is undoubtedly for the service to become impersonal.

Finally it seems essential for the doctor to be able to influence the patient's domestic environment. Some decisions concerning home arrangements, for example the physical conditions required for the care of an elderly invalid, need to be assessed in the light of medical knowledge. It is very difficult for the doctor to advise on such matters if he never enters the patient's home. And as we have seen the modification of behaviour (bad habits) is a powerful way of preventing disease.

The general practitioner in hospital

An issue about which views change relates to the role of general practitioners in hospital. In some countries they are able to admit and treat their own patients, and many doctors would regard the practice of medicine as unattractive if they could not. In other countries, including Britain, only a minority of general practitioners enter hospital, where they may serve as clinical assistants without independent responsibility.

Several reasons are given why doctors working outside hospital should also have a role inside it. Hospital work provides a good means, perhaps the only means, for a doctor to keep abreast of the rapid advances in medicine which occur during the period of his active work. Moreover the prestige and interest of medicine have been largely focused on hospitals and in the past most doctors prefered to work in them; and where they are prevented from doing so, the future of medical practice outside hospital, and of personal care, is uncertain. Others are that it helps in the provision of continuity of care, and that in their turn the consultants can learn from the general practitioner.

What work should the general practitioner do in hospital? On the one hand it seems unsatisfactory for him to enter merely for the purpose of maintaining contact with consultants. On the other hand the general practitioner should not provide services (such as major surgery) for which specialized training and experience are necessary and if possible he should continue to serve the patients for whom he is personally responsible at home.

Specialization by general practitioners

Opinion is divided on the question whether general practitioners should specialize. In Britain many doctors consider that total family care provides the best basis for their work, and a responsibility for all age groups is scarcely compatible with any significant degree of specialization. Nevertheless, although the suggestion of the Court Committee that some general practitioners should be able to specialize in child health did not receive official government backing, it has some support among general practitioners. But it is by no means uncommon for general practitioners to take a special interest in other fields such as obstetrics, geriatric medicine or psychiatry.

While it is impossible to predict confidently the future organization of practice, it should be recognized that it is not easy for a doctor to maintain competence in the care of all age groups. It will probably become increasingly difficult for him to do so as medical knowledge advances. It is already doubtful whether anyone who gives most of his time to family care can have sufficient experience to deal completely with the occasional unpredictable obstetric emergency.

The general practitioner should bear in mind the influence of the background of personal and social circumstances. For the child, the effects of handicap and illness are largely determined by their influence on his physical and mental development and his education. For the adult they are focused on family responsibilities, particularly reproduction, child care, and employment. For the individual who has retired, loss of income, occupation and other interests have a considerable bearing on the significance of disease and disability, an understanding of which are helpful in the provision of both preventive and therapeutic services.

This organization of practice also suggests a possible basis for the work of the personal doctor in hospital. It would be desirable for him to restrict his hospital role to one of the services with which he was concerned outside. In this way he could often continue to care for his own patients in hospital, transferring them to consultants only for services for which special training and experience are needed. This approach is consistent with the increasing tendency of consultants to restrict their work to a special field of medicine or surgery.

An age-basis is one form of specialization in general practice and many experiments will no doubt be directed towards studying others. We should recognize the limitations of present day arrangements and seek improvements consistent with certain objectives, always bearing in mind the importance of a personal basis for medical care, provision of some services in patients' homes, a hospital role for the domiciliary doctor and unification of personal preventive and therapeutic services.

Services for the Ambulant

The site at which the ambulant patient sees his doctor is important for the future of medical practice. In some countries it is usually the doctor's independent office or surgery; but large numbers of patients are also seen at hospital out-patient departments, or at an intermediate facility such as a group practice surgery, health centre or poly-clinic. Before discussing the merits of these different sites we should consider the features which are desirable in the base for services to the ambulant patient.

- It should be staffed by a number of doctors large enough to make economic use of facilities and ancillary staff. The grouping of doctors in sufficient numbers is also essential to permit some degree of specialization in their work, and to facilitate arrangements for holidays and continuing education.
- It should provide facilities for investigation and treatment which would make it possible to do most of the work for the ambulant.
- It should have nurses, midwives, and health visitors who with the doctor should be willing to work together as a primary care team.
- It should have an appropriate number of receptionists and secretaries.
- It should provide both preventive and therapeutic services.
- It should provide facilities which enable a social worker to join the primary care team.

Judged in the light of these requirements the independent office or surgery is clearly inadequate (although it may be all that is practical in thinly populated areas). It is too small to support enough doctors and ancillary staff or to make economic use of facilities. And although it could conceivably be used for preventive services it is far from ideal for this purpose.

The hospital out-patient department meets, or could be made to meet, all the requirements, and the objections to it are on other grounds. First, it is often too far from the homes of most patients, who cannot be expected to go the same distance for preventive services or minor complaints as for investigation or treatment of serious illness. Second, if all ambulant patients are brought to the hospital, it will be burdened with a great deal of trivial illness and so make extravagant use of its costly resources. And finally, the hospital does not provide a satisfactory environment for all medical activities, particularly for those concerned with prevention of disease. For these reasons it seems desirable to restrict the role of the hospital out-patient department to services for which elaborate facilities are required.

The third possibility is an intermediate facility of the kind known in Britain as a health centre. It was described admirably in 1942 in the proposals of the British Medical Association's Medical Planning Commission, of which Lord Cohen gave the following account ' . . . The BMA's model health centre has a different basis. The building and equipment are to be provided by a statutory authority. Medical care for all insured persons at the centre or in their homes would be provided by GP's of the patient's choice. Private patients are envisaged who would attend at the centre or at the GP's private residence or be visited in their own homes. Depending on the size and nature of the area served, and on special needs (e.g. in factories) the centre will house 6 to 12 practitioners, each of whom will have his own consulting room with a common waiting-room and a small theatre for minor surgery and small X-ray and pathological departments. The centre will have a direct link with a hospital where specialist services (both domiciliary and institutional) would be available and in the hospital might be beds at the disposal of the GP for patients whose domestic circumstances are such that, although specialist treatment is not necessary, treatment away from home is desirable. (Some cottage hospitals now offer this type of service.) This scheme also suggests that the centre should assume responsibility for the antenatal, postnatal, infant welfare and school medical services now rendered by the medical staffs of local authorities. The aims of the centre would be preventive, educational and curative. Each doctor would work at one centre only and each patient would have a choice of centre within reasonable geographical limits and would select a doctor from those working at the centre, provided the doctor was prepared to accept him. A unified system of records could be kept and made available at any other health centre in an area through a card index system at a central bureau. The staff would include principals and assistants; the principals to be paid on the basic salary and *per capita* basis from public funds as already discussed, together with private fees. The sale and purchase of practices would cease . . . '

Although written before the National Health Service was introduced this description meets the requirements referred to above. They are complementary to the hospital out-patient department, and do the work which, because of its character or relative simplicity, is best kept away from hospital. Some are served by consultants as well as personal doctors, so it is necessary to send ambulant patients to hospital only when their investigation or treatment needs facilities which would be both inappropriate and uneconomic at the health centre.

Centres of approximately this type have been advocated widely in Britain since 1920, and two main difficulties have stood in the way of their construction. One has been the reluctance of some practitioners to work in public premises, which were associated in their minds with a salaried service and the other that the cost of health centres originally fell on local authorities, who weighed their merits in relation to other expenditure, mainly unrelated to medicine. However as the number of health centres has increased and as they are proving to be a satisfactory setting for the development of multiprofessional teams they are becoming the main focus of primary and personal medical care.

Further Reading

Cohen H. (1943) A comprehensive health service, *Agenda,* **2**, 25.

Cartwright A. (1967) *Patients and their Doctors.* Routledge and Kegan Paul, London.

Fox T. F. (1960) The personal doctor and his relation to the hospital, *Lancet,* **i**, 743.

Freidson E. (1970) *Profession of Medicine.* Dodd, Mead & Co., New York.

Jefferys M. and Sachs H. (1983) *Rethinking General Practice.* Tavistock Publications Ltd., London.

Pritchard P. (1978) *Manual of Primary Health Care.* Oxford University Press, Oxford.

Royal College of General Practitioners (1965) *Present State and Future Needs of General Practice,* 2nd edition. Royal College of General Practitioners, London.

23

Public Medical Services, 1848–1948

In Chapters 21 and 22 we discussed the evolution of hospitals and medical practice. To complete the account of health services in the period before 1848 when substantial public responsibility was accepted we should refer briefly to measures concerned with the control of the physical environment.

It is customary to trace the origin of environmental control to the efforts of primitive people to clothe, feed, house and protect themselves. Examples closer to modern practice are to be found in Roman civilization: sewers intended primarily for land drainage, but used also for disposal of waste; wells and aqueducts which supplied water; systems of latrines from which excreta were disposed partly by scavengers in carts, and partly by use of the sewers; and the widespread practice of bathing. But these early measures are distinguished from the control exercised later partly by their objectives, which were as much social, aesthetic or economic as hygienic. It is true that the ancient Greeks believed in cleanliness and hygiene but the practices of neither culture rested on a secure foundation.

The earliest measures specifically directed to health were concerned with the isolation of the infectious. From ancient times attempts had been made to segregate lepers, but with this exception it was not until the fourteenth century that even the most rudimentary public health regulations were introduced. They followed the catastrophe of the Black Death (1348), and were extended in the next 3 centuries as the plague recurred. Essentially these measures consisted of notification and isolation of infected persons, disposal of infected articles such as clothing (chiefly by burning), and identification and evacuation of the houses of those infected. They were also concerned with the quarantine of individuals who might be suffering from plague, a measure adopted by the City of Ragusa (Dubrovnik) in 1377 and later practised widely elsewhere.

Quarantine was first used in London in 1580 to prevent the landing of sailors and goods at the time of an epidemic of plague in Lisbon.

The measures used before the eighteenth century are notable both for their nature and for their limitations. It is surprising that some were of a very practical kind, for ideas about infection and its spread had advanced little from the time of Hippocrates. It is perhaps equally remarkable that once it was recognized that houses and clothing might contribute to the spread of disease, it was not also seen that bad living conditions were everywhere associated with high death rates. Two possible explanations can be suggested. First, attention was fixed primarily on epidemic disease, to which all classes of society were exposed, rather than on the endemic infections which were more conspicuously related to living conditions. And also there were two theories about the cause of epidemics themselves, both misleading. One was that they were due to changes in the atmosphere referred to as general epidemic constitutions or miasmas (some thought these derived from the spontaneous generation of "poison"); the other that they were all due to contagion—the touching of the healthy by the sick. Neither school considered cleanliness, control of housing or clothing, purity of food and water to be of importance.

The eighteenth century

During the eighteenth century there was a considerable advance in recognition of the significance of the environment, supported by a demonstration of the effectiveness of its control in prevention of two diseases, scurvy and lead poisoning. The last recorded death from endemic plague in England was in 1671; but in 1719 an outbreak reached Marseilles, and an English physician, Richard Mead, was asked to suggest measures for its prevention. His report, *Short Discourse on Pestilential Contagion*, was widely read. Mead did not reject the view that infection resulted from corruption of the atmosphere, but he believed that the risk of the disease existed only in the immediate neighbourhood of the infected person. He therefore recommended a very stringent application of the traditional measures: isolation and quarantine. But he also prescribed much wider changes in the total environment—better housing, cleanliness, ventilation, disinfection and control of nuisances, and in doing so was some 200 years ahead of his time.

The significance of the environment was further emphasized by a number of investigations of living conditions. Pringle, an army surgeon, became interested in the relation between bad hygiene in barracks and army hospitals and the spread of infection. He correctly concluded that 'gaol fever', 'hospital fever' and 'ship fever' were the same disease, later identified as typhus, and observed the influence of insanitary conditions on the spread of dysentery. In *Observation on Diseases of the Army* (1752) he recommended improvements in hygiene, diet and clothing, and later attempted to have these principles applied to civilian hospitals and gaols. A similar series of enquiries and recommendations for the Navy were reported by Lind in his *Essay on the Most Effectual Means of Preserving the Health of Seamen* in 1757, and by Blane in *Observations on the Diseases of Seamen* in 1785.

The examination of association between living conditions and disease was not restricted to the services. It had long been recognized that prisons and hospitals, like ships and army camps, were centres in which and from which infectious diseases spread rapidly. In 1773 Howard, a well-to-do country gentleman influenced by the writings of Pringle and Lind, undertook a Winter's Journey no less poignant than the one that Schubert set to music in the last year of his life. He visited many prisons in England, and devoted his remaining years to an intensive study of conditions in prisons at home and abroad. He showed the association between insanitary conditions and disease, and pointed to the need for reform.

In each of the enquiries to which we have referred the evidence about the association between environment and disease was of an indirect kind. It was essentially the observation that infection and insanitary conditions tended to be found together; it did not amount to a demonstration that improvement in any specific feature of the environment resulted in prevention of a specific disease. Many people, among them some doctors, remained unconvinced.

Such a position became distinctly less tenable after two experiments in preventive medicine. The first was the demonstration that scurvy could be prevented by eating fresh fruit. This possibility had been suggested at a much earlier date, but it was put beyond reasonable doubt in 1748 by Lind, whose book *Treatise on Scurvy* was largely responsible for the decision that the Royal Navy should provide an adequate supply of lemon juice for ships at sea. The second experiment showed that a form of colic which was endemic in Devon was attributable to lead poisoning. As early as 1739 it had been observed that colic was sometimes associated with cider drinking, but it was not until 1767 that Baker demonstrated irrefutably that the illness was caused by lead absorbed by the acid cider from the vats and presses in which it was made.

The nineteenth century

From the outset of the nineteenth century the effects of the industrial revolution became marked. The new factories required labour, and as many people required work there was a rapid movement of population from the country to the towns. By the mid-century half the population of London had been born outside the town, and in Manchester, Liverpool and Glasgow the proportion of country folk was even higher.

One result was a deterioration in working conditions. There was no strong central or local authority with powers to control the location of industries and to impose standards of building practice. Town planning was unheard of, and factories were built without regard for the health of those who had to work in them. Conditions of employment were for all practical purposes uncontrolled. There was no factory inspectorate, no Ministry of Labour or Department of the Environment and there were few trade unions. If we wish to be reminded that our claim to progressive social policies is of very recent origin, it is only necessary to recall that 150 years ago it was possible to exploit paupers; to use women and children for much of the underground work in mines; to force children of 6 to do manual work for 14-15 hours a day for 6 days a week, and to whip whem if they faltered; and to expose workers to the risk of industrial disease or accident without obligation to compensate them or their dependants should they fall sick or die.

The domestic environment was also bad. Houses at best of poor design and indifferent quality were hastily erected, and are still to be seen in the slum property of industrial towns. In the literature of the nineteenth century there are many descriptions of urban life such as the following by Engels* of 1844.

'Passing along a rough back, among stakes and washing lines, one penetrates into this chaos of small one-storied, one-roomed huts, in most of which there is no artificial floor; kitchen, living and sleeping room all in one . . . Everywhere before the doors residue and offal; that any sort of pavement lay underneath could not be seen but only felt, here and there, with the feet. This whole collection of cattlesheds for human beings was surrounded on two sides by houses and a factory, and on the third by the river, and beside the narrow stair up the bank, a narrow doorway alone led out into another almost equally ill-built, ill-kept labyrinth of

* Engels F. (1892) *The condition of the Working Class in England in 1844* pp. 51 and 53-4. George Allen & Unwin, London.

dwellings . . . Everything which here arouses horror and indignation is of recent origin, belongs to the *industrial epoch*. The couple of hundred houses, which belong to the Old Manchester have been long since abandoned by their original inhabitants, the industrial epoch alone has crammed into them the swarms of workers whom they now shelter; the industrial epoch alone has built up every spot between these old houses to win a covering for the masses whom it has conjured hither from the agricultural districts and from Ireland.'

The effects of industrialization were superimposed upon hygienic conditions which were already bad. In spite of the advocacy of Mead, Pringle, Lind and others there had been no substantial improvement during the eighteenth century. Methods of supplying water and of disposing of sewage and waste were still primitive, partly because of lack of technical knowledge, and partly because of the absence of public authorities having enough power to be effective. Water for drinking purposes was obtained from rivers and streams which were frequently polluted; open ditches and gutters served as sewers and emptied into rivers; indeed it was not unusual for householders to dispose of their waste by opening a window and emptying it into the street.

It is scarcely surprising that some people find it hard to believe that mortality did not increase in the early nineteenth century. It is not a matter on which we can be dogmatic, and we have reviewed the evidence, such as it is, in an earlier chapter. We suggested that the undoubted deterioration of the domestic and working environments was counter-balanced by improved nutrition and increased opportunities for employment. The extent of the movement from the country indicates that for many people the choice was between employment in the towns and none at all. Today it is possible to believe the workers are attracted from rural areas by the supposed glamour of town life, but it is hardly credible that any sane person went to industrial areas in the early nineteenth century unless driven by sheer necessity.

The Introduction of Environmental Services, 1848

At the beginning of the nineteenth century there was virtually no effective public control of water supplies, sewage disposal, housing or foodstuffs. By 1875 all these features of the environment had been subjects of Acts of Parliament. The reasons for introduction of legislation at this time was undoubtedly complex. The period was one of profound social change, of which universal male suffrage (1884) and compulsory education (1870) are notable examples. But some things are believed to have had a special bearing on the pace of legislation concerned with the environment and health.

One was an advance in understanding of the significance of the environment. Even after the demonstrations of Lind, Pringle and Baker in the eighteenth century, many people remained unconvinced. This position became almost untenable after the publication in 1842 of a *Report on the Sanitary Conditions of the Labouring Population of Great Britain*. This document, largely the work of Edwin Chadwick, presented the results of an investigation into the relation between environmental conditions and ill-health. By present standards much of the evidence would be regarded as inadequate, but there was a lot of it, and it all pointed in the same direction. Its most significant conclusion was: 'That the primary and most important measures, and at the same time the most practical, and within the recognized province of public administration, are drainage, the removal of all refuse from habitations, streets and roads, and the improvement of the supplies of water.'

Public concern about the environment was also sharpened by experience of infectious disease. Again it was not the prevailing endemic level of mortality which caused alarm, but the new threat of cholera. This disease, which had a case fatality rate close to 100 per cent, although prevalent in the East, had been uncommon in Western Europe and unknown in England until the nineteenth century. It appeared in four major epidemics: 1830-2; 1848-9; 1854; 1865-6. The preventive measures where inadequate, in part because of reluctance to invest in sewerage, but more particularly because of resistance from the water companies and their spokesmen in Parliament to ensure that their product was wholesome; widespread public concern greatly strengthened the hands of those who were pressing the government to act. There are analogies between the problems of controlling cholera and typhoid in the nineteenth century and diseases caused by smoking today.

We need not trace in detail the history of environmental medicine in the second half of the nineteenth century. The first imporant measure was the Public Health Act of 1848. Its provisions were essentially to provide legal support for those local authorities which wished to control the environment or take other steps toward the promotion of the public health; London was excluded at that time. It was not until the Act of

1875 that control of certain essential features of the environment was enforced. These were: water supply, sewage disposal; control of slaughtering of animals; parks and open spaces; isolation hospitals; and a beginning of control of housing. It should be remembered that these changes were introduced with no clear understanding of the nature of infectious disease. Indeed Edwin Chadwick, the most ardent advocate of reform, denied the contagious nature of infection, and throughout his life held the view that it was due to miasma or corruption of the atmosphere.

In the same period there was also a notable improvement in circumstances of employment. The first serious attempt at control of working conditions was the Factory Act of 1833, which restricted daily hours of employment of young children (to 9 hours for children under 9 years, and to 12 hours for children aged 11-18) and introduced factory inspectors. It was not until 1842 that Parliament prohibited underground employment of women and girls, and of boys under 10.

The effectiveness of environmental measures was of course greatly strengthened when Pasteur, working first on the nature of fermentation and later on diseases of silkworms, established the bacterial origin of an infectious disease of insects. The causal organism of a human disease (anthrax) was first identified by Koch in 1876, and from this time Pasteur, Koch and their followers rapidly laid the foundations of the new science of bacteriology.

In time bacteriology did much more than provide a rational explanation for the success of administrative measures previously taken. It showed how infection is spread, including the unsuspected existence of 'carriers'; it made it possible to diagnose infectious disease with much greater precision; and soon it led to protection against infection by means of immunization.

Although environmental services have improved progressively during the twentieth century, the work of controlling the disease which stems from the physical environment is still far from complete. Among the features whose adverse influence on health is still conspicuous in England and Wales are atmospheric pollution; indifferent housing, diet, working conditions; and road traffic.

The effect of atmospheric pollution is evident in relation to mortality from almost all respiratory diseases, particularly chronic bronchitis and lung cancer. Indeed at the present time in Britain the advantage of rural over urban health, in so far as it is indicated by mortality statistics, is greatest in respect of respiratory disease (see table 6.3). It seems probable, therefore, that further control of atmospheric pollution is one of the most important measures now available to public authorities.

The relation of housing to health, although less easily identified in national mortality statistics, can scarcely be doubted. There is evidence of an effect of crowding on mental illness and on physical illness, particularly from infectious disease and accidents. Further improvements in housing can therefore be expected to make a significant contribution to health.

Although gross nutritional deficiency occurs rarely in Britain today, there are three sections of the population whose health may be jeopardized by lack of food. They are old people, the late children of large families and those of immigrants. It is among the elderly that poor nutrition is most common, and in spite of the resources provided by retirement pensions and Social Security their diet is sometimes inadequate and inappropriate. Some malnutrition in children is attributable to the fact that the largest families are, in general, the poorest. The late children are exposed to infectious diseases, conveyed by their brothers and sisters, at a time when family resources are at a minimum. There problems are also concentrated among immigrant groups.

During the present century most of the crude toxic hazards of occupation—mercury, lead, arsenic and phosphorus—have been eliminated or controlled. Nevertheless the standardized mortality ratios indicate that there remain substantial risks associated with certain forms of employment. Some of them are attributable to low income, but others reflect the effects of the working environment. One of the most obvious adverse features is the industrial atmosphere, which is still responsible for much chronic bronchitis and all pneumoconiosis. Another is the high risk of industrial injury. It seems reasonable to believe that in time such risks will be eliminated, but there will remain the possibility that some of the many new organic compounds which are constantly being introduced into industry will prove to be toxic, and constant vigilance will be needed to control them.

The risks to health associated with road traffic (which possibly include lead poisoning from exhaust fumes) are already formidable and are likely to increase. All that need be said about them here is that they will not be reduced without a more radical solution of the traffic problem than any so far applied.

The Introduction of Personal Health Services, 1907

We have reviewed the circumstances which brought a public medical service into existence during the second half of the nineteenth century. By 1900 it comprised local authority environmental and hospital services for the mentally ill and the infectious and Poor Law hospital services. The only public provision for patients outside hospital was a limited form of general practitioner service for the destitute. All others had to make and pay for their own arrangements for treatment.

Pioneer maternal and child welfare clinics had been established in Paris and London in the 1890s, but it was not until 1915 that a prenatal centre was established (in Edinburgh) from which nurses made visits to pregnant women. This was part of a new phase in the evolution of the public service, the creation of health services concerned with the individual. It had a significant influence on later developments and we must consider the way in which it came about. In broad terms, it resulted from widespread concern about health, particularly of children, and from recognition of the inadequacy of the existing medical services.

By the end of the nineteenth century the improvement in health in England and Wales had been considerable. Mortality had declined continuously for 30 years, and the reduction was large enough more than to offset the effect on the growth of population of a coincident decline of the birth rate. But it was a disturbing feature of the trend that there had been no improvement in mortality in the youngest age group in which the risks of death were still very high. Infant mortality was 154 per 1,000 live births in 1900, a good deal lower than in the eighteenth century, but about the same as in 1870. The reason for this is even now not altogether clear. But public opinion was no longer content to accept a high infant death rate as inevitable and had come to believe in the practicability of preventive measures.

Another reason for concern about health was the amount of poverty which remained after more than 50 years of progress. This was demonstrated in two investigations of social conditions, one by Charles Booth in London and the other by Seebohm Rowntree in York. At an earlier period the results might have been dismissed as unrelated to health, but by the end of the nineteenth century the effect of poverty on health was generally admitted, and Simon, the Medical Officer of the Privy Council, referred to it as 'among the worst of sanitary evils'.

Evidence of a more direct kind was provided by the results of inspection of recruits for the Army. In the years 1901-02, 40 per cent were unfit for service, the commonest reason being poor physical development, defective vision and heart disease. Reports concerning the health and physical condition of schoolchildren and of adolescents seeking employment in factories were equally disturbing.

An Inter-Departmental Committee on Physical Deterioration dealt widely with public health, and its Report discussed subjects as different as atmospheric pollution, stillbirth registration and the employment of women. It contained two recommendations which were particularly important in relation to the future personal health services: that schoolchildren should be medically inspected at regular intervals; and that school feeding should be undertaken by local authorities.

At this time the only general public medical service outside hospitals was the one provided under the Poor Law, which made available to the destitute the part time services of poorly paid general practitioners. Other people had to pay for their medical care, and many did so by voluntary insurance or through friendly societies. It was widely recognized that these arrangements were quite inadequate, and that extension of the public medical service was required. It proved much more difficult to agree about the nature of the extension. Clearly the Poor Law was an unsatisfactory authority to administer medical services, but the kind of organization which should be created was for many years the subject of dispute. Broadly there were two proposals, and the service which eventually emerged was a compromise between them.

The first proposal was that there should be a unified state medical service, based on public health principles, and organized in local areas. This was recommended to the Royal Commission on the Poor Law (1905-09) by the heads of the four Government medical departments, who undoubtedly expressed the views of most doctors in the public service.

The alternative proposal was that the additional public medical services should be provided by doctors in private practice. According to the medico-political committee of the British Medical Association (1909) 'the most satisfactory provision for the treatment of children whose parents cannot afford to pay for it is to place them under the care of private practitioners, who should be adequately remunerated out of public funds independently of the Poor Law'. This was the view of doctors in private practice, and there were indications that at that time many of them would have been prepared to accept a salary for part-time public service.

The full implementation of either of these proposals might have prevented a division between preventive and therapeutic personal services. For the medical staff of progressive public health authorities were then extensively engaged in treatment as well as prevention of disease, and had both been sanctioned by Parliament it is very probable that a unified service would have grown up, no doubt with serious effects upon private practice. Alternatively, had general practitioners been permitted to undertake the work in schools, and later in child welfare clinics, it is also possible that division might have been avoided. In this case the attitude of doctors to local authority administration and payment by salary might later have been different from what it was. The Education Act, 1907, and the Maternity and Child Welfare Act, 1918, effected a compromise, by assigning the preventive personal services to public health authorities, while curtailing treatment they could offer in deference to the wishes of private doctors.

The School Medical Service, the first personal health service under local authorities, was introduced in 1907. Almost from the beginning it comprised the features which have remained virtually unchanged to the present time: provision of free food; medical inspections; ascertainment of the handicapped; and treatment. At the outset the treatment of defects discovered in schoolchildren was considered to be a matter for parents to arrange; but it was soon evident that this was quite unsatisfactory, and school clinics were established, mainly for the treatment of minor ailments.

The growth of maternal and child welfare, the second personal health service, was slower than that of the School Medical Service and it was not well established until after the First World War. Until then the service was largely voluntary, and its adequacy varied considerably according to the enterprise and means of local authorities. The Maternity and Child Welfare Act 1918 established a public service which also has retained its character with remarkably little change until the present time. Its main activities were provision of food (no longer available), routine inspection, advice to mothers and—in a restricted form—treatment.

National Health Insurance, 1911

The assignment of personal health services to local authorities, and their restriction essentially to preventive measures, had two important consequences. It made prevention of disease a public responsibility and left treatment as a private one; and it associated the preventive personal health services with environmental medicine and separated them from the services provided by general practitioners and hospitals.

Public responsibility for health services had been extended further by the National Health Insurance Act of 1911 (Chapter 23). Although schemes of this type had existed on the continent of Europe from the late nineteenth century, the Act was a new departure in Britain and was initally resisted by the medical profession. The essential features of the new service were as follows.

(*a*) It was financed by employer and employee on the insurance principle.
(*b*) It applied compulsorily to a restricted class of employed persons and did not even cover their dependants.
(*c*) It offered limited benefits—treatment by a general practitioner but not by a consultant or hospital.
(*d*) It was administered locally by Insurance Committees which were quite separate from the local authorities.

This modest beginning was of considerable significance in the history of health services as a whole. It extended public responsibility into therapeutic services, for the first time on a substantial scale. However the responsibility was not assigned to the existing public health authorities under local government, but was placed under a new organization and this perpetuated the division between preventive and therapeutic medicine.

The Background of the National Health Service

Costs of medical care

The most important reason for introduction of a comprehensive health service was undoubtedly the difficulty many people found in paying for treatment. In 1938 the benefits provided under National Health Insurance were available to about 20 million insured workers; rather more than half the population had to meet their own costs or seek assistance through the Poor Law. All hospital treatment had to be paid for according to the means of patients, which were assessed. Many people protected themselves against the risk of hospital expenditure, through voluntary contributory schemes whose rapid growth in the years between the wars reflected the extent of the need.

The combination of public and private finance was unsatisfactory. In principle it was open to anyone in need to appeal to the Poor Law; in practice this safeguard was far from adequate, either because patients were not poor enough to qualify for public assistance, or because they preferred not to be treated rather than apply. The main grounds for criticism of the pre-war medical services were therefore that many patients were inadequately treated, or were placed in financial difficulty by the costs of treatment.

Difficulties of hospitals

Other significant influences were the problems which confronted hospitals. At the outbreak of war rather fewer than half the hospitals and one-third of the beds were under voluntary bodies; the remainder were under local authorities. (These estimates do not include mental hospitals.) Both systems had their difficulties. Most voluntary hospitals were too small; more than 500 of the 700 general hospitals had fewer than 100 beds. Many were inadequate in design, staff and equipment; yet because of limited finance it was not possible to remedy the deficiencies, and the technological revolution, to be accelerated by the war, was just beginning. Indeed the voluntary hospitals, originally supported by charitable funds, had become increasingly dependent upon payments made by patients, either directly or through insurance schemes.

The difficulties of the public hospitals were equally serious. They were transferred to local authorities in 1929 at the beginning of a time of extreme financial difficulty, and it was not always possible to allocate to them the money they required. Inevitably therefore standards varied according to the wealth and initiative of local authorities. Moreover the intention to make hospitals a public health responsibility was far from being realized, and in 1939 almost half the public beds were still administered under the Poor Law. These beds were filled with the mixed population which had long been the responsibility of the Poor Law Authorities, and conditions had not been improved materially by the change in administration.

But the problem of the pre-war hospital service was not merely that there were too few beds and too many unsatisfactory beds. It was also that improvement was prejudiced by the existence of two separate systems of administration.

Uneven distribution of staff

Another difficulty of the pre-war medical services was the uneven distribution of staff between different areas and between different parts of the service. In deciding where to work doctors and nurses are naturally influenced by local circumstances. Although some devote their lives to the care of the deprived, most for personal reasons choose pleasant places, and for professional reasons prefer posts where facilities are good. Before 1946 most consultants and nurses favoured general, particularly voluntary, hospitals, and general practitioners the wealthier parts of the country. In consequence many public hospitals were inadequately staffed, and there were too few practitioners in the less attractive industrial and rural areas.

It should not be thought that these circumstances which led to a comprehensive health service were peculiar to Britain. How to make medical resources available to everyone is an international problem. Moreover it has recently become more acute, both because modern methods of investigation and treatment have greatly increased the costs of medical care, and because it is now widely accepted that no one should become ill or remain ill for lack of any service which it is possible to provide.

Further Reading

Baker G. (1767) *Essay concerning the cause of endemial lead poisoning in Devonshire.* Delta Omega, London (reprinted 1958).

Booth C. (1902) *Life and Labour of the People in London.* Macmillan, London.

Engels F. (1892) *The Condition of the Working Class in England in 1844.* George Allen and Unwin Ltd., London.

Rosen G. (1958) *A History of Public Health.* MD Publications Inc., New York.

Rowntree B. S. (1901) *Poverty, a Study of Town Life.* Macmillan, London.

Simon J. (1897) *English Sanitary Institutions*, 2nd edition. Smith, Elder & Co., London.

24

Social Security Services

Although the risks of epidemic infectious diseases have been shared by all classes of society, it has long been evident that people who are sick are often poor. It has not always been recognized that a considerable proportion of them are sick because they are poor. Until the nineteenth century is was possible to believe that the sick poor were in some way intrinsically inferior, and that an improvement in their circumstances would have little effect on their health, and perhaps only a temporary effect on their poverty. In preferring £5 he would be happy to spend, to £10 he would be unhappy to save, Mr Doolittle in Shaw's *Pygmalion* would have been regarded by some people as typical of a class for which little could be done in respect of health or wealth by public action.

We have seen that the association between poverty and disease began to be recognized during the eighteenth century; but it was not until the publication of Chadwick's *Report on the Condition of the Labouring Classes* in 1842 that the significance of bad living conditions began to be accepted and not until the identification of bacteria after 1871 that the relationship came to be understood.

It is not difficult to see why the effect of the environment on health should have been noted first in relation to infectious disease, since it was the threat of infection which led to concern about living conditions. In the present century, however, it has been shown that the effect is by no means so restricted. For example, some nutritional disorders are clearly due to a deficient or ill-balanced diet; and carcinoma of the stomach is an example of a non-infectious illness which is much more common among the poor of the world than among the well-to-do.

In medicine concern with the social security services which prevent or relieve poverty is twofold. In the first place, knowing that these services are important to health, doctors have a general interest in their adequacy, and should have something to say about the priority they merit on medical grounds. Secondly, since many patients are ignorant about these services, some knowledge of them is a desirable part of the equipment of the practicing doctor.

The social security services will be more intelligible if we consider first the causes of poverty, and the ways in which it can be relieved. The common circumstances in which an individual may require assistance are sickness, disablement (whether temporary or permanent), unemployment, old age, pregnancy, death of a wage earner, inadequate earnings, improvidence and idleness. Although the significance of these causes of poverty has been different at different periods, four have always been particularly important: sickness; unemployment; inadequate earnings; and old age.

The methods of financing relief of destitution are charity, voluntary insurance through guilds, sick clubs, commercial insurance, compulsory insurance financed by employer or employee, and either local or central taxation. In the past assistance was first from charity and later voluntary insurance also, but in the present century the trend has been towards increasing reliance on compulsory insurance and taxation.

History of Services for the Relief of Need

The problem which has plagued reformers for as long as there has been public concern with destitution has been to relieve distress without encouraging idleness, to assist an individual when he needs help without diminishing his own efforts to help himself. This dilemma was reflected in the social legislation of 3½ centuries. At some times the paramount consideration was the relief of need, at others the fear of idleness, but the trend has been towards more concern about distress and less about idleness. Nevertheless the problem still exists, although we now prefer to speak of it in terms of security and incentive. The change in terminology is itself significant.

The earliest social services were provided by religious orders, augmented in medieval times by the manor houses and by merchant and craft guilds. Many monasteries kept a small hospice or almshouse where poor travellers could get food and temporary shelter, and some provided more permanent care for the sick or weak. In villages feudal lords generally accepted the obligation of caring for their own retainers; in towns merchant and craft guilds practised voluntary mutual aid, while some boroughs provided charities to relieve needy residents of long standing and good character. With the decay of the feudal system and the dissolution of the monasteries many of these social obligations disappeared, and for a considerable period little was done to relieve distress. During the sixteenth century vagrancy and destitution increased so much that it became imperative to deal with them; statutes forbidding vagrancy were common and beggars and wanderers were sometimes beaten or placed in the stocks. Unfortunately the problem is not one of the past, for vagrants are similarly treated in many developing countries today. By the middle of the century attempts were made to put the poor to work on materials supplied by merchants. Officers of the parishes tried to collect voluntary contributions for the relief of deserving poor, and in a few towns for example London and Norwich the principle of a compulsory levy for the relief of the destitute had been accepted.

The Poor Law

Public relief of the poor in England dates from 1601, when the Elizabethan Poor Law Act was passed. It gave to the service a distinctive character which endured for more than 3 centuries. First, the Poor Law provided a local service, administered by unpaid Justices of the Peace and financed by a compulsory parish levy; central direction was weak, and the adequacy of the service varied greatly from one parish to another. Second, the character of the service was in general very harsh; relief was given only in cases of extreme need, and for a considerable period was restricted to residents of long standing. Third, assistance was subject to a test of means (or lack of them) of the applicant and his family. The first Poor Law Act stated 'It shall be the duty of the father, grandfather, mother, grandmother, husband, or child of a poor, old, blind, lame, or impotent person or other poor person, not able to work, if possessed of sufficient means, to relieve and maintain that person.' The test of means was very searching, and it had to be shown that both the applicant and his relatives had exhausted their resources.

Throughout the seventeenth and eighteenth centuries the administration of the Poor Law was virtually unchanged. It became somewhat more severe in the early nineteenth century when the economic consequences of the Napoleonic Wars placed a severe strain on the available resources. In 1832 a Royal Commission investigated the administration of poor relief, and its report resulted in the introduction of the Poor Law Amendment Act of 1834. Responsibility was transferred from the Justices of the Peace to locally elected Boards of Guardians. The Act attempted to deter applicants, by insuring that relief should not place the recipients in circumstances as favourable as those of the lowest paid labourers, and by requiring recipients to enter an institution. From the early eighteenth century it had been the practice in some areas to make admission to a house of correction or workhouse a condition of assistance. The extension of this practice after 1834 led to the rapid growth of the workhouse system; it also had the unexpected result of establishing an important branch of the hospital service under the Poor Law Authorities.

There was no substantial change in the character of the Poor Law in the later years of the nineteenth century, and at the beginning of the twentieth it was still the instrument of a harsh social policy. Its operation was criticized by the Royal Commission on the Poor Law established in 1905, and a Minority Report of the Commission, largely the work of Sidney and Beatrice Webb, recommended its abolition. In the years that followed other services were introduced which to some extent replaced the Poor Law, or attempted to make up for its deficiencies. It was not until 1948, however, when the National Assistance Act was passed, that the Poor Law was finally abolished.

Workmen's compensation (1897)

For almost 300 years the Poor Law was the only public service concerned directly or indirectly with the relief of need. The introduction of the Workmen's Compensation Act of 1897 was significant, not only because it introduced the first complementary service, but also because in conception it departed from principles embodied in the Poor Law. Before 1897 it was possible for a worker to obtain compensation for industrial injury or sickness only by proving negligence on the part of his employer; his claim was treated in the same manner as any other claim for negligence, and was not strengthened much by the fact that he was employed. After the 1897 Act the employer was considered to be liable for the results of industrial injury, and it was unnecessary to prove that he had been negligent. In the beginning this principle applied only to specific hazards in a small group of dangerous trades, but in 1906 it was extended to almost every occupation. We should note that the Workmen's Compensation Act provided no public financial or medical assistance to the sick or injured worker; it merely conferred legal rights on him or his dependants, and left them to enforce those rights as best they could by agreement or at law. Even so, the Act was a departure from long established principles in its recognition of some degree of responsibility of an employer for his workers.

Non–contributory Pensions (1908)

A characteristic feature of the Poor Law was its insistence that the recipient of relief should first demonstrate his need. The first departure from this principle was the scheme of old age pensions introduced in 1908. The Old Age Pensions Act provided for a fixed weekly sum to be paid to persons of either sex aged 70 years or more, if they fulfilled certain requirements. These included not only qualifications in respect of nationality and residence, but also the demonstration that the applicant had not failed to work according to his ability, opportunity and need. Once an individual had been accepted, however, the payment was made as of right, and was not subject to the discretion of a public officer. The Act thus made separate provision for an important group of applicants among aged people, and was the first step towards the break-up of the Poor Law.

National Insurance (1911)

The Poor Law and old age pensions were financed by local and central taxation respectively. The National Health Insurance Act of 1911 introduced for the first time in Britain a public service financed in part by insurance contributions. The service included both health insurance and unemployment insurance.

The National Health Insurance Scheme embraced both the limited range of medical services referred to in Chapter 20, and a weekly sum paid to insured persons who were sick or disabled. Like the medical services, the benefits were restricted to the insured person and in the event of his death were not at first available to his dependants. In 1925, however, an Act of Parliament provided pensions for widows, dependent children and orphans of insured persons, and for insured persons at the age of 65. These new pensions were grafted on to the existing scheme of National Health Insurance.

Unlike health insurance, unemployment insurance in the beginning applied to only a limited section of the working population, to persons in a group of industries with a high level of seasonal unemployment. But the general level of unemployment was so high in the years after the First World War that it was necessary to extend the scope of the Act, and by the mid thirties it included the greater part of the working population. The scheme provided a weekly benefit to be paid for a limited period to eligible unemployed workers.

Like old age pensions, the benefit provided under national insurance was paid as of right, subject only to a record of satisfactory contributions, and to that extent was an improvement upon the Poor Law. Nevertheless there were grounds for serious criticism. In the first place, the level of benefit was not fixed according to basic needs, or adjusted in relation to rising prices. Secondly, it took no account of the size of the family, nor, until 1925, of the needs of dependants after the death of the insured person. And finally, the amount of benefit available in cases of sickness and injury was substantially reduced after a limited period of receipt of benefit.

It will be evident that both the unemployment and health insurance arrangements under the 1911 Act had features which were a distinct advance beyond the provisions of the Poor Law, as well as limitations which made them less than a comprehensive solution of the problem of need.

The Assistance Board

The last major step which preceded the final abolition of the Poor Law was the creation of the Assistance Board in 1934. An Act of Parliament took from the Poor Law responsibility for relief of the unemployed, and transferred it to a new administrative body supported by national funds. The significance of this development can be stated briefly.

In the inter-war years mounting unemployment had made it necessary to extend the scope of unemployment insurance. Even so, many men exhausted their right to insurance benefit, which as we have noted was available only for a limited time, and inevitably turned to the Poor Law for assistance. By this time there had been considerable improvements in the policy and administration of the Poor Law: the workhouse system had been abandoned; scales of relief were more generous than formerly; and in 1929 the basis of local administration had been improved by transfer of the functions of the Boards of Guardians to the Public Assistance Committee of local authorities. Even so, arrangements were still far from satisfactory. Relief was subject to the discretion of the relieving officer and the means test was applied stringently. The incidence of unemployment varied throughout the country and inevitably the demand for unemployment relief often fell most heavily on the poorest local authorities. In 1930 a Royal Commission reviewed the problem of unemployment insurance, and its report was followed by the creation of the Unemployment Assistance Board. It had a dual purpose: to remove from the unemployed the obligation of appealing to the Poor Law and to support the finances of sorely-pressed local authorities. In 1940 it was renamed the Assistance Board, and took from the Poor Law the further task of providing relief for aged persons in need of supplement to their pensions. It later became the principal organ of the central government for making allowances to civilians in financial need because of the war. It was not until 1948, however, that it finally took over the remaining responsibilites of the Poor Law.

The Beveridge Report

In 1941 a committee was appointed by the war time coalition Government 'to undertake, with special reference to the interrelation of the schemes, a survey of the existing national schemes of social insurance and allied services, including workmen's compensation, and to make recommendations'. The results were published in the Beveridge Report. It was a document of historic importance, not only because it provided a basis for the social legislation which followed, but also because it attempted for the first time to deal comprehensively with the problem of poverty.

We have traced the evolution of the public social services concerned with relief of need and have seen that with the exception of the Poor Law they were introduced after the Workmen's Compensation Act of 1897. At the time of preparation of the Beveridge Plan, the main schemes in existence were the Poor Law (1601), workmen's compensation (1897), pensions (1908), sickness and unemployed insurance (1911), and unemployment assistance (1934). The chief criticisms of these arrangements were that they were costly and difficult to administer, and that they left serious deficiencies. The Beveridge Plan aimed to simplify procedures and reduce administrative costs.

The Plan was not, however, devised only with regard to existing deficiencies and administrative convenience. It attempted to direct the public social security services according to certain principles. One was that relief of need should be only one facet of a social policy concerned with the five giants: Want, Disease, Ignorance, Squalor and Idleness. The other principle was that the social contract between the individual and the state should be based on the idea of security for service. It was intended that the individual should work and contribute when he could, and that when he was unable to work—because of sickness, injury, unemployment, old age or death—the state should provide for him and his dependants. It should be noted that in spite of its humane objectives the Plan had by no means lost sight of incentives. It made service and contribution a condition of benefit; and the scale of benefit was intended to provide no more than the necessities of life. Indeed the Beveridge Report was the first serious attempt to solve on a national scale the ancient problem to which we have referred: to relieve distress without encouraging idleness.

The method suggested in the Report was a compulsory insurance scheme with these features: a flat rate of benefit; a flat rate of contribution; unification of administrative responsibility; adequacy of benefit; all workers, employed and self-employed, to be included.

The crucial feature was adequacy of benefit. The intention was to provide an amount of money, adjusted according to the number in a family, which would be sufficient to meet essential requirements. It was envisaged that the problem of want would thus be dealt with by insurance, and the need for other methods of assistance would be reduced.

Present Day Health and Related Services

25

Organization of Health Services

The National Health Service 1948

In Chapters 20 and 23 we discussed the background of the National Health Service (NHS) in the period preceding its introduction in 1948. We noted that at that time the health services comprised essentially the following elements: two hospital systems, one voluntary and the other public; environmental and personal health services under local authorities; and general practitioner services financed partly by national health insurance and partly by private payments.

There are several ways in which this organization might have been adapted to meet the needs of a comprehensive service. All three elements might have been brought together under local authorities, and this arrangement was indeed proposed in a White Paper which preceded the Act. However this approach was strongly and effectively resisted by doctors, both general practitioners and consultants, who were opposed to administration of health services by local government.

Theoretically it would also have been possible to create a new regional administration for hospitals and consultants and to bring general practitioner services under local authorities. In view of the opposition of doctors in private practice such an approach was not considered seriously. A third possibility would have been to leave the environmental services with local authorities but to transfer their responsibilities for personal health to new local or regional bodies which would also be concerned with general practitioner and hospital services. This approach was later adopted in the revision of 1974, but in 1948 it would have been resisted strongly by local authorities, with their 40 years of experience in administering personal health services.

The decisions finally incorporated in the NHS were to leave local authority health services relatively unchanged except for the transfer of their hospital responsibility, and to create two new and separate administrations, one for general practitioner and the other for hospital and consultant services. This meant that while centrally a single government department (the Ministry of Health) was responsible for the NHS, local and regional responsibility was divided between three authorities, one elected and two appointed. In a little more detail the administration was as follows.

Central administration

The Minister of Health was responsible to Parliament for all the work of the National Health Service. However it should be noted that several other government departments had responsibilities for health activities which remained outside the NHS, particularly: the Ministry of Education for the health of school children; the Ministry of Labour for the health of workers; the Home Office for the care of deprived children and the control of dangerous drugs; the Board of Control for lunacy and mental deficiency; and the Privy Council for medical research. However in the discussion of the NHS and its later revision we shall be concerned only with the responsibilities of the Ministry of Health which was expanded to absorb the Ministry of Pensions and the Board of Control and to assume other responsibilities and become the Department of Health and Social Security in 1968. The Secretary of State for Health and Social Security became a member of the Cabinet.

Hospital and specialist services

The National Health Service Act of 1946 brought all hospital and consultant services under public control and created a new basis for their administration. England and Wales were divided into 14 Regions, in each of which a Regional Hospital Board (in Wales and Welsh Hospital Board) was made responsible for planning and administering hospital and specialist services, except those in teaching hospitals which were administered separately by Boards of Governors directly responsible to the Minister of Health. In Scotland, where tradition had been different, both teaching and non-teaching hospitals were administered by 5 Regional Hospital Boards. In Northern Ireland, also, the combined responsibility was assigned to the Northern Ireland Hospitals Authority.

Local authority services

The Act transferred the local authorities' hospitals to Regional Hospital Boards but left environmental and personal health services essentially unchanged. In some respects their responsibilities were extended, for example to include an ambulance service and the care and after-care of certain sick and handicapped persons. The Act also made local authorities responsible for providing, equipping and staffing health centres.

General medical and dental services

General medical and dental services, pharmaceutical services and supplementary ophthalmic services concerned with sight testing and the supply of spectacles were administered by Local Executive Councils (LECs) which among other things assumed responsibilities of the Insurance committee (Chapter 23). The areas for which they were responsible were those of local health authorities, but the administrations were quite separate. The chief responsibility of the LECs was the organization of general practitioner services.

Finance and private practice

The new service was financed mainly by taxation and only marginally by insurance contributions. Consultants were remunerated by salary, either on a full time or a part time basis, according to the number of weekly sessions. Because most general practitioners objected to a salaried service, their payment was through a *per capita* fee for each patient on their lists, together with a number of allowances and fees for service.

In this context it should be mentioned that the service allowed doctors to choose their patients and patients to choose their doctors. The only barrier it raised to private practice was to offer an alternative service which was publicly financed.

The National Health Service in Perspective

The most obvious achievement of the Service was to make medical care readily available to all and to remove the burden of direct payment from everyone, a matter of special importance to the large number of people who could ill afford it. Many of the fears expressed about the public service proved to be groundless. It did not victimize doctors or public; it did not stifle initiative; it did not disturb the relationship between doctor and patient. The limitations were of a subtler kind and were rooted in the tradition of health services.

In retrospect, it can be seen that the National Health Service continued to use with only minor changes the framework of services which had evolved in the preceding century. Perhaps the most fundamental weakness of tradition was that it divided local responsibility. There was no single authority with the duty and power to plan comprehensively for the local population, making the best use of resources according to a well-judged scheme of priorities; the framework of services divided hospital from domiciliary care and preventive from therapeutic medicine. Inevitably there were deficiencies, particularly in the domiciliary and community services and in the care of the elderly, the disabled, the mentally ill and the mentally handicapped. There were also duplications, for example in maternal and child health services which were divided among local authorities, general practitioners and hospitals.

Fragmentation and its consequences were reviewed in 1964 by a national committee which recommended, in the Porritt Report, unification of local health services. This idea was discussed for several years and finally implemented in 1974. The reorganization should be recognized as an event of great importance, for it was the first attempt in Britain, and among the first anywhere, to recast the framework of services which had evolved, uncoordinated, in previous centuries.

The Reorganized National Health Service in England, 1974

The services which were brought together in the reorganization of the NHS in 1974 England were therefore:

(*a*) The hospital and specialist services previously administered by the Regional Hospital Boards, Hospital Management Committees and Boards of Governors of Teaching Hospitals.
(*b*) The family practitioner services, administered by the Local Executive Councils.
(*c*) The personal health services, administered by local authorities through their health committees. These included ambulance services; epidemiological work; family planning; health centres; health visiting; home nursing and midwifery; maternal and child health care; medical,

nursing and supplementary arrangements for the prevention of illness, care and after-care; and vaccination and immunization.

(*d*) The school health service, administered by the local education authorities.

The NHS became responsible for the inspection and registration of private nursing homes. It was also required to provide school health, child guidance and health education services, but it was recognized that in these cases local authorities should be concerned with related activities which require joint planning.

Two very important services continued as responsibilities of local authorities and are therefore outside the NHS. These were the personal social services (to be discussed in Chapter 26) and environmental health, which is interpreted to include: measures for prevention of the spread of communicable disease other than immunization, some epidemiological investigation and treatment; powers relating to food safety and hygiene, port health and the diseases of animals which affect human health; public health aspects of environmental services; and enforcement of requirements about environmental conditions at work places.

Responsibility for the health of persons in relation to their employment remained with the Department of Employment. The provision of treatment and care of people who suffer injury or ill health through their employment is of course a responsibility of the health authorities.

The service in Wales 1974-1982 was closely similar to that in England. Those in Northern Ireland and Scotland were not, and differed from each other. Their present structures are described below (pp. 289, 300, 302).

Restructured National Health Service in England, 1982

Although the restructuring of 1982 followed naturally from the reorganization of 1974, a series of events precipitated it. First, a Royal Commission on the National Health Service had been established which was charged among other things to resolve:

- contention about pay, which had developed between the government and the medical profession, particularly pay for work during unsociable hours
- a general feeling of dissatisfaction that existed about the three tier system (region, area and district) which administered the Service
- the extraordinarily cumbersome series of committees and advisory

bodies which had to be involved if the doctors or nurses were to be consulted about service developments or administrative change

- the ineffectiveness of the planning system of which much had been hoped.

The new structure, which was introduced in 1982 and is already coming to be looked upon as an improvement on the old, left the Regions unchanged, but created District Health Authorities. Multidistrict area health authorities were disbanded and single district areas became districts. These changes were not introduced without considerable human suffering. Health authority staff, lay, medical, and nursing alike, in all districts and many areas found for the second time in 8 years that their job was to be dissolved, and many of them chose the option of early retirement rather than compete once more for appointment with younger men and women.

Other prices which have been paid have been the loss in most cases of geographical coterminosity between a health authority and a local authority. Frequently previous collaborative arrangements had been imperfect, but they had always been better than what has so far been offered by the majority of new district health authorities and the local authorities. Another casualty it would seem is what would have been a newly achieved integration of the Family Practitioner Committees (FPC) with other parts of the health service and with local government. Between 1974 and 1982 the area of responsibility of each FPC was coterminous with an Area Health Authority (AHA), and so bore a parallel relationship to local government. Now that the AHA has been disbanded, there is no simple way, should it be desired, that FPCs can be integrated with the rest of the NHS. Many thinking people look upon this isolation of the administration of general practice, especially at a time when pressure is being brought to create an effective and fully integrated primary care team including nurses and health visitors (employed by the district health authority) and social workers (employed by local authorities), as a retrograde step.

Prior to restructuring, there were 90 Area Health Authorities in the National Health Service in England and Wales, the majority of which had more than one District; now there are 192 District Health Authorities grouped in the 14 regions of England and Wales.

The framework of the new organization is illustrated in figure 25.1 and discussed in more detail below.

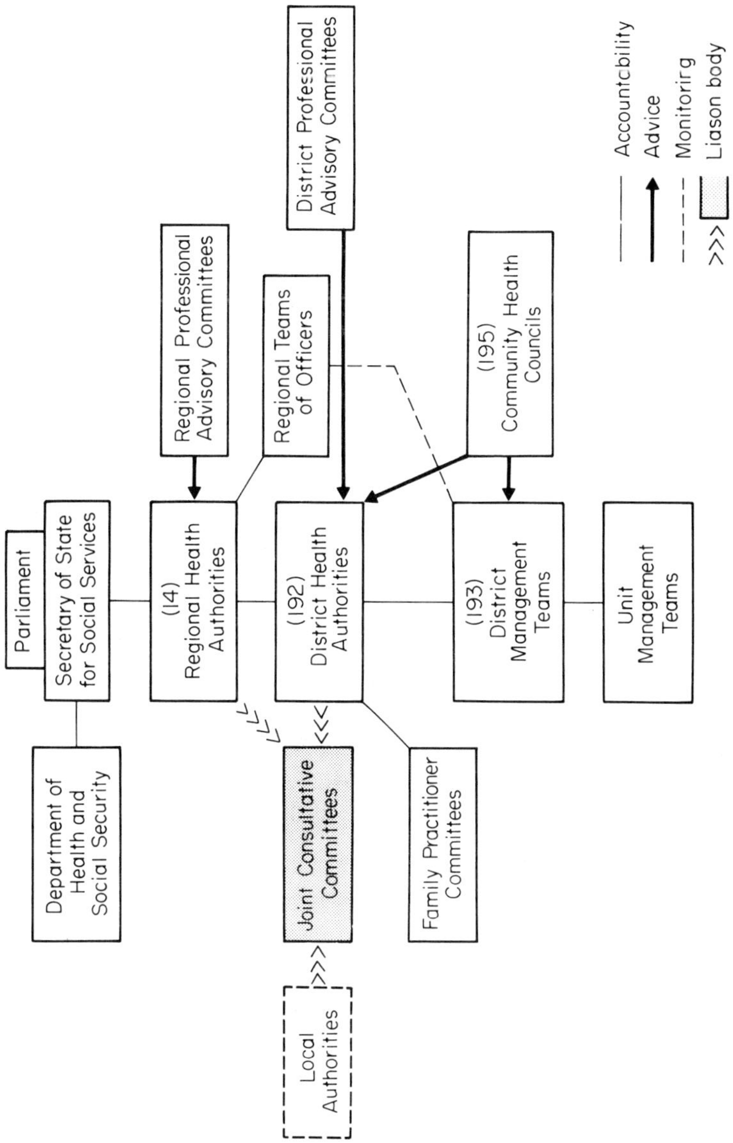

Figure 25.1. Organization of Health Services in England.

Central organization

The Secretary of State is responsible to Parliament for national policies related to health and for the administration of the NHS in fulfilling these responsibilities he is assisted by the Department of Health and Social Security (DHSS), and is concerned with:

- Establishing national policies and priorities which influence the magnitude, nature and balance of services to be provided.
- Agreeing with regions and districts the objectives and plans developed in the light of national policies.
- Allocating resources to enable health authorities to put their plans into effect. A national formula based on the work of the Resource Allocation Working Party (RAWP) is used which is an estimate of need based on population size and structure. (It should be noted that since family practitioner services are provided separately they are therefore not included in regional and district budgets).
- Developing resources essential to the services. This requires specialist work on such matters as personnel (DHSS has specific responsibilities in relation to recruitment and training of skilled staff) capital development, finance, property and supply.
- Other functions best organized centrally. They include: certain types of research and preparation of some national statistics, purchase of some equipment or supplies; supervision of superannuation schemes. The microbiological service related to communicable disease is administered centrally by the Public Health Laboratory Service Board on behalf of the Secretary of State and recently the PHLS Communicable Disease Surveillance Centre has taken over the responsibilities for infectious disease which were formerly those of the DHSS.

The DHSS has some responsibilities apart from the National Health Service, particularly the personal social services and social security. It is also concerned with licensing of medicines, the control of food safety and hygiene, and acts as the production authority for the medical supply industry.

Regional Health Authorities

Regional Health Authorities (RHAs) are responsible for administration of 14 regions whose boundaries in general correspond to those of the

14 planning regions formerly used for the hospital service. They serve populations varying from 2 to 5 million. The Chairman of the RHA and its members are appointed by the Secretary of State after consultation with interested organizations including the universities, the main local authorities and the main health professions. The responsibilities of the RHA comprise several activities—planning, co-ordination and supervision, executive functions and some other miscellaneous matters.

Planning

The RHA is concerned with strategic plans and priorities derived from a review of needs identified by District Health Authorities (DHAs); in this role it is guided by national policies. It is also responsible for identification and provision through the DHAs of services that need a regional approach, for example, the arrangements for tertiary specialities such as neurology, neurosurgery, radiotherapy and some types of laboratory investigation. These arrangements affect the deployment of medical, dental and scientific staff. Finally, the RHA has a special responsibility, with the universities, for service facilities needed to support undergraduate and postgraduate medical and dental education, as well as research.

Co-ordination and supervision

The RHA has to review district plans, to ensure that they are adequate and attainable, consistent with national and regional policies and co-ordinated with the work of local authorities. The Regional Authority is particularly concerned where the needs of a district have to be met in part outside its boundaries, for example by a hospital. Using local adaptations of the RAWP formula and on the basis of the plans agreed with the DHAs, the RHA is responsible for allocating resources and monitoring subsequent performance.

The RHA is also concerned with co-ordination of services between adjacent DHAs, for example emergency cover, siting and use of ambulance stations and training.

Executive functions

These include the design and construction of new buildings and works. The more important projects are undertaken directly by the RHA;

other building work is delegated to DHAs with regional guidance and approval. Responsibility for operation and maintenance is also delegated to the districts.

Other services

These include a blood transfusion service and sponsorship of some research projects, for example in epidemiology, requiring regional resources. The region is also responsible for purchase of some—mainly expensive—equipment such as diagnostic imagers; for the computation of statistics; and for the provision of selected training facilities.

Regional Officers

The RHA is advised by a Regional Team of Officers (RTO). They are responsible for advising on such matters as the preparation of a 10 year regional strategic plan, guidelines on priorities and available resources, allocation of resources to districts and reviews of DHAs performance. However the Regional Officers are not directly responsible for their counterparts in the district administrations.

In 1984 the Secretary of State, Norman Fowler, decided that each Region should appoint one of the Regional Team of Officers or, exceptionally, another person to the newly designated post of Regional General Manager (RGM). The purpose of the change (which enjoys only qualified support within the medical and nursing professions) is to focus the Region's choice of priorities more sharply and to lead the Regional Team of Officers to swifter decision making and more incisive action. Figure 25.1 does not incorporate this innovation the effect of which on organisational structure is expected to vary from Authority to Authority.

District Health Authorities

There are 192 District Health Authorities (DHAs), between 8 and 22 per region. Most serve populations of 150,000-300,000 (average 245,000), though the range is considerable: 90,000 to 860,000. The Chairman of each DHA is appointed by the Secretary of State after consultation with the Chairman of the RHA. There are usually 16-18 DHA members, appointed by the corresponding local authorities, by the University, and by the RHA after consultation with the main health professions and other organizations. The functions of the DHA comprise both planning and operation of services. Planning and development of services is undertaken in co-operation with the RHA and corresponding local authorities. It requires appraisal of existing services and identification of their deficiencies, and is conducted within national and regional guidelines (see Chapter 27).

District Officers

Like the RHA, the DHA is advised by a team of officers, the district management team (DMT). With the introduction of general managers in 1984 team leadership was assumed by a District General Manager (DGM) whose role is analogous to that of the RGM. Up to that time the DMT had comprised the District Administrator, District Medical Officer, District Nursing Officer and District Treasurer, together with a representative consultant and general practitioner each elected by their peers. The team had shared responsibility for overall management of the district, although the individual officers had had clearly defined responsibilities for the management of particular elements of the service. Their shared responsibilities included advising the Authority on formulating policies, choosing priorities and planning the development of its services. Correspondingly, they were responsible for ensuring that the Authority's decisions were implemented.

Under the new arrangements the DGM carries ultimate responsibility and is accountable to the DHA for the overall management of the district. The individual chief officers are accountable to the DGM for their respective management responsibilities, but give their professional advice directly to the DHA. Figure 25.1 does not incorporate this innovation, the organizational effect of which is likely to vary from the expansion to the disbandment of DMTs.

Community physicians

In the 1974 reorganization of the NHS the term 'community physician' was introduced to describe medical specialists, most of whom had been employed formerly by local health authorities as medical officers of health, and by Regional Hospital Boards as medical administrators. However, their role has been modified considerably in the reorganized service and they now work in posts at regional and district level.

The community physician has three main functions. First, as a specialist he is expected to provide information for clinical colleagues and to advise on alternative approaches to care, taking account of the relation between health and local authority services. Second, as a manager, he is concerned with planning of services, with provision and interpretation of information, with evaluation of services and with preventive measures and the promotion of health (for example in relation to immunization, screening and health education). Third, he has a special role in relation to local authorities, particularly in respect of advice, collaboration and liaison in four areas: environmental health, child and school health, housing and personal social services especially as the latter two apply to elderly, mentally ill, mentally handicapped or physically handicapped people.

Most community physicians at regional and district level work as specialists in community medicine (SCMs). The District Medical Officer (DMO) has already been referred to as a member of the District Management Team. In addition he manages the non-medical staff of the district department of community medicine such as information scientists, and co-ordinates the activities of SCMs who like himself are of consultant status. The Regional Medical Officer (RMO) performs an analogous role at region and in addition monitors the performance of the DMO and his specialist colleagues at district. The training and professional standards of the specialty are the responsibility of the Faculty of Community Medicine of the Royal Colleges of Physicians which was founded in 1972.

Units of managment

As a result of the 1982 re-structuring, management below district level is conducted by units of management. DHAs have been given free rein to organize these on a geographical basis, or based upon hospital units, the community services, or the management of a particular care group, such as the elderly or the mentally handicapped. Most DHAs have established between 3 and 6 units. Each is run by a team which until the introduction of general managers in 1984 comprised a unit administrator directly accountable to the district administrator, a director of nursing services directly accountable to the district nursing officer and one or more representatives of the medical staff working in the unit. In addition community services unit management teams generally admit a representative of general practice, and there may be representation of other interests such as clinical psychology or occupational therapy in the mental health unit teams, for example.

National policy encourages the delegation of decision making, together with managerial and financial control, from district to unit level, and from unit teams as near as possible to the point at which care is given. Conversely, managerial accountability upwards is increasingly taking the form of reporting achievements against agreed targets of performance. The 1984 changes are intended to lead to the appointment of Unit General Managers (UGMs) accountable to DGMs. These appointments are specifically intended, *inter alia*, to improve clinician's accountability for their use of resources.

Joint Consultative Committees

There is a considerable overlap in the interests of health and local authorities, particularly in relation to the care of children, elderly, physically disabled, and mentally ill or mentally handicapped people. In order to make balanced provision for the populations they serve, each health authority and its corresponding local authorities are required to nominate authority members to serve on a Joint Consultative Committee whose function is to advise on the planning and operation of services in spheres of common interest.

Professional advisory arrangements

At each level of the health service, arrangements are made to enable professional staff to influence the process of management. At unit and district level, the consultant medical staff are generally organized into speciality based Medical Divisions which co-ordinate their views through a Medical Staff Committee or a Medical Executive Committee for transmission to the unit or district team. Nursing and the other professions have corresponding arrangements for formulating advice about policy, priorities and the functioning of services. Analogous committees exist at Regional level, while nationally the Central Health Services Council for England and Wales is appointed by the Secretary of State and has standing committees dealing with various professional interests (medical, dental, nursing, ophthalmic and pharmaceutical) and specialist committees dealing with matters like immunization policy and practice.

Family Practitioner Services

The 1974 reorganization of health services did not change the status of general medical and dental practitioners, ophthalmic medical practitioners, opticians and pharmacists; all of them continue, as before, to provide services as independent contractors. So while it was hoped that general practitioners would develop and in some cases modify their work to make it an integral part of a comprehensive service, the Health Authorities have no responsibility or power to bring this about.

The DHAs are responsible however for developments where general practitioner services involve other parts of the service. These have included planning and development of health centres, plans for contractor services in new towns or redevelopment areas and arrangements for nurses and other skilled staff employed by the DHA to work with general practitioners. The DHA in turn has to ensure that its plans affecting contractor services are acceptable to general practitioners.

Family Practitioner Committee

The contracts involving general practitioners are administered by Family Practitioner Committees set up by the DHAs. They are responsible for contracts with practitioners, administration of terms of service (including remuneration schemes) and statutory disciplinary arrangements. Half the members are professionals appointed by the local professional committees and the remainder are appointed by the DHAs and local authorities. It is envisaged that the FPCs will become separate authorities directly accountable to the Secretary of State.

In the light of these arrangements we may summarize the relation of the management of the National Health Service to the doctors providing clinical services. The health authorities are responsible for providing all the general and clinical facilities and back-up services for the hospital doctor's day to day work, but the way he uses these in the care of his patient is entirely a matter for his own judgement. This considerable power of his to commit resources in the interests of his patients is known as his clinical freedom and is exercised by all doctors; conversely, we have noted that the main purpose of introducing general managers at unit level is to hold clinicians more closely to account for their use of resources. In the case of general practitioner services, however, health authorities have no direct responsibility, except as we have seen in the construction of health centres, as well as in relation to those parts of the work of the general practitioner which impinge on other services.

Community Health Councils

One of the most important issues raised by the organization of health services is the role the public should play in their evolution and management. At the beginning of this chapter it was noted that in its original form the NHS left personal health services with local authorities but created separate administrative systems for hospital and general practitioner services. In unifying the services, the 1974 revision transferred the personal health services to newly created health authorities. This finally took from local authorities responsibility for personal health care, with which they had been associated in various ways for about a hundred years. There remain many critics of this decision, particularly among those who consider that health services should be administered, as they are in Finland for example, by elected local authorities directly accountable to the public who provide the finance.

In the reorganized service the views of the consumer were to be represented by the Community Health Councils. There is a Council in each district (two DHAs have two each) and its role is to represent to the DHA, with whom it must meet every year, the interests of the public. In order to do this it has power to secure information about the services, to visit hospitals and other institutions, and to have access to the DHA and its officers. The DHA in turn is expected to consult the Council about developments, particularly those, such as closure of hospitals or change of use of facilities, in which the public is likely to be particularly concerned. Apart from such lines of communication and influence, the Councils have no direct responsibility for the planning and administration of services.

Finance

The financial arrangements for the reorganized services are essentially the same as that of the original NHS: the costs are still met mainly from taxation, from money voted by Parliament for health services. The DHSS makes capital and revenue allocations to the RHAs which in turn allocate funds to DHAs. Payments to general medical practitioners, it is important to note, are funded separately by the Department and not through the RHAs. The NHS also recognizes the special financial needs of 'teaching districts', that is for those which have substantial facilities used for medical and dental education and research.

The RHA receives from the Department a specific identified allowance for teaching and research and it is the responsibility of the RHA to use these funds to ensure thai facilities related to teaching and research are adequate in the teaching districts.

Perhaps the chief variation in the earlier financial arrangements was the relief to local authority expenditure which resulted from the transfer of responsibility for their personal health services to the new unified administration.

Arrangements for London

It was necessary to make special arrangements for London, where there were features affecting the planning and administration of health services. Among these features were the established pattern of local government, the types and distribution of hospitals, with a large number of separate undergraduate and postgraduate teaching hospitals, and the fact that general practitioner services were administered through Family Practitioner Committees over areas much wider than the individual London boroughs.

In London there are 4 RHAs, each of which inevitably contains teaching districts, and each of which has a sizeable rural hinterland. The DHAs do not always conform to borough boundaries. An ambulance service continues, as formerly, to be administered as a single service for the whole of Greater London. The planning of teaching hospitals, especially postgraduate hospitals, presents particular problems in London. Special Health Authorities (SHAs) were created in the 1982 restructuring to manage a number of the postgraduate hospitals; most other teaching hospitals are likely to be greatly affected by current arrangements to amalgamate most of the capital's medical schools in pairs.

The Organization of Health Services in Other Parts of the United Kingdom

In general, the aims of the unification of health services in 1974 and of their restructuring in 1982 were common to all parts of the United Kingdom. Nevertheless there is some variation in the pattern of administration, determined both by the tradition of services in each country, and by the smaller size of the populations which required some modification of the organization described for England. In Northern Ireland there is the important difference that health and social services are administered by the same authority.

Wales

Although the administrative structure of the health service in Wales is similar to that in England, it differs in a number of respects.

It was considered unnecessary in a country with less than three million inhabitants to interpose a regional health authority between the DHAs and the Welsh Office (the central government department). Consequently there is no RHA and the Welsh Office is responsible for strategic planning within the Principality and for monitoring the performance of the 9 DHAs. Professional advice is available to the Secretary of State for Wales from committees representative of the main health professions in Wales and from the Welsh Council, as well as from bodies advisory to the Secretary of State for Social Services.

In all main areas of planning and decision making there is a substantial delegation of responsibility to DHAs. But a special body—the Welsh Health Technical Organization—is responsible for certain specialised and technical supporting tasks. These include the design and execution of major capital works, the systematic evaluation of contracting arrangements for supplies, and a computer-based central management information service.

Unlike most of England, the boundaries of the DHAs are coterminous with those of the local authorities, the exception being the county of Dyfed in which there are 2 DHAs.

Scotland

Health services in Scotland were reorganized under the National Health Service (Scotland) Act, 1972, and at the time of writing are being further modified (figure 25.2). The principles behind the reorganization were essentially the same as in England but there are some differences in the administration of the services.

Central administration

The health services are the responsibility of the Secretary of State for Scotland. He is advised on the planning and development of the service

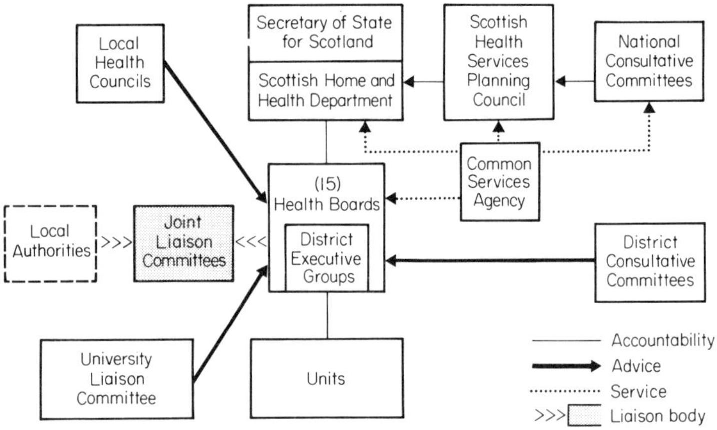

Figure 25.2. Organization of Health Services in Scotland.

by a Health Services Planning Council, with members appointed by each health board (see below), by each university with a medical school and by the Secretary of State for Scotland. The Planning Council in turn is advised by National Consultative Committees composed of representatives of the various professions in the Health Service who contribute to planning as it relates to their professional contribution to health care. There is also a Common Services Agency whose function is to provide the Departments and Health Boards with a number of important services which are necessary throughout Scotland and are more effectively administered nationally. These include the ambulance service; the blood transfusion service; the planning and execution of major building projects; and central functions in relation to information and research, health education and monitoring patterns of communicable disease.

District administration

Scotland is divided into geographical areas each of which is the responsibility of a Health Board. The population within Board geographical areas varies from 1,000,000 to 15,000 in some parts of the mainland and on the Islands. Boards are directly responsible to the Home and Health Department, which provides the finance for the development and maintenance of an integrated health service. In Scotland the Health Board is the authority with which general practitioners have a contractual relationship. The chief officers of the Health Board function as a District Executive Group. Health Boards collaborate with local authorities through community physicians (community medicine specialists) and Joint Liaison Committees.

Every Health Board is required to establish a Local Health Council or Councils. The role of the Councils is analogous to that of the Community Health Councils in England; that is to say, they have no executive powers, but represent the interests of the public by commenting on the adequacy of local health services.

Differences which should be noted in the organization of health services in Scotland (compared with England) are:

(*a*) the responsibilities of the Regional and District Health Authorities in England are combined in the Health Boards and
(*b*) general practitioner services are financed and administered by the Health Boards rather than by a separate body, the Family Practitioner Committee, but receive their finance directly from the central Department.

Northern Ireland

In Northern Ireland major policy decisions are made by the Department of Health and Social Services of Northern Ireland under The Health and Personal Services (Northern Ireland) Order 1972 (figure 25.3). The services are administered within this policy by four Health and Social Services Boards covering the Eastern, Northern, Western and Southern districts of the province. These are bounded by local government district boundaries and include several local government districts in each health district.

Members of the Health and Social Services Boards are appointed by the Minister. Some are nominated by the Local Government District Councils; others are professional people such as doctors, nurses and social workers, appointed after consultation with the professional organizations; and the remainder include businessmen, trade unionists, and members chosen from the universities and colleges and voluntary organizations dealing with health and social problems.

Each Board is served by four main committees a Health Services Committee, a Social Services Committee, a Policy and Resources Committee and an Administrative Services Committee.

Most of the work of the Boards is delegated to professional officers who constitute the District Executive Team. This consists of a Chief

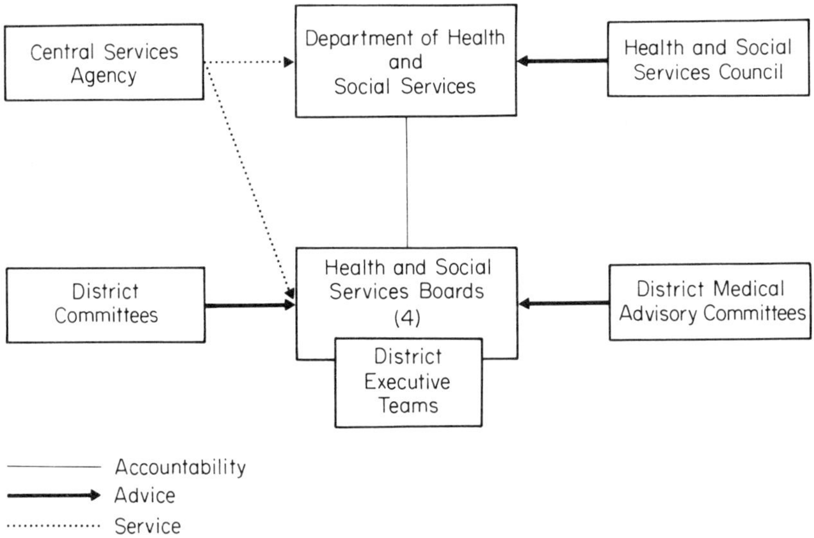

Figure 25.3. Organization of Health Services in Northern Ireland.

Administrative Officer, a Chief Administrative Medical Officer, a Chief Administrative Nursing Officer, the Director of Social Services and the Chairman of the District Medical Advisory Committee. The latter committee represents all the specialities and general practice in the area.

Thus in Northern Ireland, unlike the rest of the United Kingdom, the Health and Personal Social Services have been integrated and there is no need for separate liaison arrangements. This has many advantages in the treatment and prevention of conditions in which the social and medical aspects are closely interwoven, for example, alcoholism and other addictions, self-poisoning, mental illness and mental handicap. It should be noted, however, that centrally the Northern Ireland Office is responsible for children taken into care and for adoption.

The equivalent in Northern Ireland of Community Health Councils in England and Wales are District Committees which represent consumer interests. These committees are appointed by the Health and Social Services Board and members include local government councillors and representatives of local voluntary organizations. They have no executive power but have the right to visit hospitals, hostels, and homes for children and the elderly to assess the quality of the services provided and make recommendations.

There are a number of central advisory committees whose chairmen, along with the chairmen of the Boards, constitute a Health and Social Services Council to advise the Minister. Another central body with important functions is the Central Services Agency. It is responsible for payments to general practitioners, dentists and pharmacists and opticians; for the selection and appointment of consultants and other senior hospital staff on behalf of the Boards; for legal services; and for central contracts for supplies.

General practitioners continue as independent contractors but, like Scotland, their contracts are with the Boards.

Further Reading

Report of the Resource Allocation Working Party (1976) *Sharing Resources for Health in England*. HMSO, London.

26

Organization of Personal Social Services

Post War Social Services

Relief of need

The discussion in Chapter 24 of the evolution of social security services related to health was focussed on services directed to the relief of need. Beveridge had recommended that these services should be financed in future mainly by insurance, and he envisaged that if the levels of benefit were adequate there would be less need than formerly for public assistance of other kinds. Parliament attempted to implement these proposals by passing four Acts: The National Insurance Act, 1946; the National Insurance (Industrial Injuries) Act, 1946; the National Assistance Act, 1948; and the Family Allowances Act, 1945. The first three were concerned with insurance and assistance, and the fourth made provision for payments to families according to the number of children. The object of the last was to relieve the burden in large families where the stress of poverty and ill-health was sometimes severe.

In one important respect post war developments departed from Beveridge's proposals: the levels of benefit paid under national insurance were never adequate and it was therefore necessary to rely heavily on assistance. The reason for this was largely outside the control of the government; it was due mainly to the rise in the post war cost of living and, to a lesser extent, to the granting of retirement benefit to persons who had contributed for only a short period. Inflation, and the resultant difficulties, have continued to the present day, so that there is still the imbalance between insurance and assistance which Beveridge hoped to avoid.

Personal social services

Personal social services provided by the state originated in the Poor Law, which, under its general responsibilities for the destitute, made provision for, *inter alia*, orphaned and deprived children, the mentally ill, the mentally subnormal and the aged poor. However, with the gradual dissolution and final repeal of the Poor Law these responsibilities were transferred to other departments of the local authority and the process was completed in 1948. In that year the Children's Act required local authorities to appoint a Children's Officer and to establish a Children's Committee with the duty of caring for deprived children. A later Act extended these obligations and provided the basis for preventive action which would 'promote the welfare of children by diminishing the need to receive children into or keep them in care'. The National Assistance Act, 1948, by taking from the Poor Law responsibility for financial assistance to those in need, provided the basis for the welfare services of local authorities, which included accommodation and other services for the elderly, the physically handicapped and the homeless.

Another group of personal social services developed under local authorities in association with their health services. As early as 1918 the Maternity and Child Welfare Act empowered local authorities to employ home helps for mothers in the lying-in period and during the Second World War this service was extended to other classes such as the sick and infirm. Local authorities had acquired responsibilities for the mentally ill and mentally handicapped and these were increased considerably in the post war period. Their duties under the National Health Service to prevent illness and provide care and after care also involved them in extensive social services, particularly in relation to the infectious, the chronic sick and problem families.

Yet another class of local authority social services evolved in conjunction with education, for example enforcement of school attendance, special educational facilities for handicapped pupils, provision of free meals and child guidance. Finally we should refer to the considerable welfare functions developed by housing departments in their work on slum clearance, redevelopment and rehousing.

The Seebohm Committee

The local authority and allied personal social services were reviewed by a government committee which published its recommendations in 1968.

At that time the services were divided between the children's welfare, health, education and housing departments of local authorities. The Committee concluded that the services were deficient in quality and quantity, and as examples they cited the waiting lists for day and residential care for the mentally ill, the mentally and physically handicapped and the aged. The services were also thought to be poorly coordinated and difficult of access by the public. The Committee attributed these deficiencies mainly to lack of resources and to the division of responsibility for the social services between several departments of local authorities.

The solution for these difficulties suggested by the Seebohm Committee was unification of the social services in a comprehensive social services department. The services proposed for inclusion were:

(*a*) the services provided by children's departments;
(*b*) the welfare services provided under the National Assistance Act, 1948;
(*c*) educational welfare and child guidance services;
(*d*) the home help service, mental health social work services, other social work services and day nurseries, provided by local health departments;
(*e*) certain social welfare work undertaken by some housing departments.

The Reorganized Personal Social Services

The personal social services were reorganized under the Local Authority Social Services Act, 1970, which gave effect to three of the recommendations listed above—(*a*), (*b*) and (*d*). The Act made no reference to the welfare services provided by the education and housing departments, as these are not statutory services and no legislation was necessary. In the case of the child guidance service, so many agencies—health, education and children's—were concerned, that it was felt that any legislation would be unnecessarily complicated. Local authorities were required to unify the services under a Social Services Committee and to appoint a Director with responsibility for administration of the following services:

Services for children and mothers

In general these services are responsible for promotion of the welfare of children and in some cases, mothers. The work includes responsibility for children who cannot be cared for in their own homes and are said to be 'taken into care' (orphans, deserted children, some children suffering from mental disorder, etc.); arrangements for adoption; protection and care of the young in relation to criminal proceedings; provision of day care of children under 5 years, including day nurseries and child minding; care (including residential care) of unsupported mothers.

Services for old people

These are services concerned mainly with the provision of care for older people, either in the community or in residential establishments. They include the home help service, meals on wheels and the provision of old people's homes. They are also concerned with protection of property when people are removed to hospital and with defraying of funeral expenses of those who die with no finances to cover the cost of burial.

Services for mentally ill and mentally handicapped people

The services promote the welfare of persons suffering from mental disorder and for this purpose the Act grouped together, perhaps unwisely, mental illness and mental handicap. The services include the separate provision of residential accommodation and making arrangements for training and employment. They also cover responsibility for the welfare of the mentally disordered in hospital.

Services for physically handicapped people

The services are concerned with the welfare of persons who are blind, deaf, or otherwise physically handicapped. They include provision of facilities for training and employment of the disabled.

The reorganization of health and social services described in this and the preceding chapter has separated the administrations of the two services in the United Kingdom, except in Northern Ireland where they are under the same authority. Social services have been unified under local authorities; health services, including personal health services, have been placed under the National Health Service. In Chapter 25, we considered the reasons, largely rooted in history, why health services were not placed under local authorities. The Seebohm Committee, after reviewing various alternatives, came to the conclusion that it was desirable to create a comprehensive social services department under local government.

The grounds which influenced the Seebohm Committee in this decision did not persuade all medical people. Some were particularly concerned about the separation of responsibility for health from that of welfare of the elderly and physically handicapped people, whose medical and social needs are intimately related, if not inseparable. There was criticism of the decision to separate from health services the social services for mentally ill and mentally handicapped people, whose social and medical needs are also closely associated. However the Committee concluded that these objections were outweighed by the advantages which would result from a unified social services department, and this conclusion was accepted in the reorganization of the services in Great Britain. In Northern Ireland, as we have seen, responsibility for personal social services is undertaken by the unified Health and Social Services Board.

The social worker

In the years prior to 1970, some social workers had specialized to become medical social workers, psychiatric social workers etc. In the Local Authority Social Services Act of that year, however, on the recommendation of the Seebohm Committee, an improved career structure was provided for them all, but specialization was abandoned. The wisdom of some aspects of this Act is still in question.

Voluntary agencies

When the National Health Service was first introduced it was considered appropriate that the state should accept responsibility of meeting the needs for health services and social support for everyone with the exception of patients who chose to pay for private medical care. Barbara Castle, Secretary of State in the Labour government of the early 1970s, reversed this policy, and since then the importance of voluntary agencies, which frequently had been small, and local, has steadily been enhanced. These fall into two broad groups, which to some extent overlap. One provides care, or funds research such as the British Heart Foundation or Age Concern and the other consists of self-help groups, like Alcoholics Anonymous and the Schizophrenia Fellowship. There are many others.

Further Reading

Central Office for Information (1977) *Social Services in Britain*, Reference Pamphlet 3. HMSO, London.

Townsend P. and Davidson N. (1982) *Inequalities in Health*. Penguin Books Ltd., Harmondsworth, Middlesex.

27

Planning Health

Introduction

All planning has three principal components:

- considering the ways in which the future could be an improvement on the present;
- working out changes which would be necessary to bring about the desired improvement and which have priority within the resources likely to be available;
- deciding how the chosen changes should be implemented.

Health planning was first attempted by the Soviet Union. During its first decade it was ridiculed by Western governments of the day, but was adopted by almost all of them 25 to 30 years later during the period of social reconstruction which followed the Second World War. In the NHS its purpose was considered to be: 'to make subject to calculation what was previously left to chance, to organize what was previously unorganized, to replace spontaneous adjustments with deliberate control'.

Health planning at national level

Measures undertaken by society to promote health, to prevent illness, to treat the sick, and to provide rehabilitation for the disabled and continuing care for its most handicapped or frail members currently absorb between 5 and 10 per cent of the gross national product of each of the advanced industrial countries.

Such levels of expenditure have come about as a result of a vast increase in resources devoted to health care in these countries in the years since the Second World War. In the USA, for example, expenditure on health care increased from 4.5 per cent of the Gross National Product (GNP) in 1950 to 9.0 per cent in 1979; in Canada from 2.9 per cent to 7.2 per cent and in the United Kingdom from 3.9 per cent to 5.2 per cent over the same period. These changes in the investment of resources have enabled the world's richest countries to take advantage of the concurrent progress in biomedical research which has produced a whole new range of effective drugs and high-technology medical equipment. The benefits derived by particular groups of patients from these advances have been immense. In particular, standards of care of the acutely sick have steadily improved; maternal and perinatal mortality have been very greatly reduced; and disablement from a number of chronic conditions has become capable of alleviation or delay, for example degenerative disease of the hip, ischaemic heart disease, and Parkinson's disease.

Such progress has been accompanied by an emphasis on the development of hospitals rather than care in the wider community, and with a bias towards curative medicine rather than prevention of illness and the promotion of health. With the encouragement of doctors society has demanded hospitals capable of exploiting the new high technology, and the politicians have responded by providing the necessary funds. New techniques and costly apparatus have been constantly introduced, usually with inadequate assessment of their relative benefits.

This high-technology approach has been directed more towards the health problems which have presented to doctors in their consulting rooms, than to trying to prevent such problems from arising in the first place. Expenditure on health promotion and disease prevention has received a miniscule proportion of the expanding health budgets; people have embraced a new faith—belief in the health professional and his technological wizardry, at the expense of knowledge about their own health and self-confidence in looking after themselves. Moreover, technological medicine has brought in its train a host of unintended illness: hospital infections; accidents in the use of dangerous diagnostic and therapeutic techniques; and the adverse effects of drugs. It is very questionable whether further investment in curative medicine would provide good value in terms of reduced premature mortality, serious morbidity and long-term disablement, compared with the alternative of investing in prevention.

And yet, bowled along by public expectations, governments continue to provide more of the same, so that 'hi-tech' begets 'hi-tech'. This process has been compounded by the narrow definition of government departmental responsibilities in most advanced industrial countries. Health ministries are seen as responsible for curing illness. The interrelationships which exist between the promotion and maintenance of health and:

- the prevention of poverty and unemployment,
- educational investment and attainment,
- fulfilment of individual potential,
- community development,
- the safety of industrial processes,
- agricultural policies,
- the home environment,
- and transport policies and provision,

are generally overlooked, systematically ignored, or even denied. For example, the simple implications of implementing a policy for controlling the prevalence of tobacco-related illness are often denounced by government. The usual rationalization is a curiously incomplete concept of individual freedom, which can be regarded as no more than a political fig leaf for fiscal discomfort, commercial lobbying, both (or worse). Similarly, there has been, and in many countries still is, a failure to consider the ill-effects on health that many industrial processes have placed upon health care systems; quite apart from ignoring the consequent human suffering, their costs have not been offset against the benefits derived from the industry. Likewise, the deterioration of health caused by unemployment and poverty creates a burden which health care systems can only mitigate. Prevention lies at the heart of government's social values and consequently should heavily concern its economic policies.

In addition to these problems, it is necessary to consider those brought about by demographic and social change. As we have seen, the late effects of variations in the birth rate in the twentieth century, together with a steady improvement over 3 centuries of standards of nutrition and general livelihood, have combined to increase the proportion of elderly people in the population. We have also seen that the diseases of infancy and childhood are steadily being replaced by the more intractable diseases of old age. In most advanced industrial countries, the absolute numbers of very elderly people are increasing while those to whom they have chiefly looked for help and social support—those in late middle-age and the younger elderly—are starting to decrease in number. At the same time, family stability is decreasing significantly, creating insecure conditions for children and leaving some people in loneliness, while the trend towards women working outside the home is changing the role of the family in providing care for the aged and disabled, as well as for children. The nature of much post-war housing redevelopment, both in its location and design, has contributed to social isolation and fragmentation of the care and support which families and communities have previously provided.

The role of national government in health planning thus far exceeds the simple allocation of a specific proportion of the national wealth to running or supporting health services. It is greater than deciding upon the distribution of that wealth between the different parts of the country, or even between different parts of the service (primary or secondary; acute or long-term). It includes the components set out at the beginning of the Chapter, and in all is no less than:

- formulating ways in which the future health of the people could be better than the present;
- working out the changes in all relevant government policies that would be necessary to bring about the desired improvement;
- selecting priorities which could be afforded within the resources they are prepared to make available for health;
- deciding how these priorities can be implemented;
- implementing programmes to meet the priorities.

Such comprehensive planning of health should involve many government departments and is largely absent in the advanced industrialized countries, where health planning is usually narrowly defined in terms of the health care services. However, both the constantly rising costs and diminishing marginal benefits of high technology medicine, and of the missed opportunities for health promotion and disease prevention, are now gradually being recognized and starting to make their mark on government policies.

Planning in the National Health Service in the United Kingdom

Until its reorganization in 1974, the National Health Service had no formal planning system. Apart from planning rationalization and redevelopment of hospitals (begun in 1962), Regional Hospital Boards, and the then Ministries of Health, found themselves called upon to react to problems and crises as they occurred. The planning system was introduced to force the health authorities to think ahead and to consider the optimum way of fulfilling locally the objectives and priorities which are laid down by the Health Departments on behalf of Parliament.

The national objectives and priorities are brought fully up-to-date every few years and communicated to the Regional Health Authorities. The minor changes which are made from year to year, together with the the following year's resource allocations, and outline resource assumptions for future years, are made known to the Regions on an annual basis. The Regions in turn provide the District Health Authorities with information about their resource expectations and guidance on policies and priorities. This is done in two distinct cycles, the 5 year *strategic* planning cycle and the annual *operational* planning cycle.

Strategic planning in England

Because of the length of time it takes to plan, build and commission health buildings (especially large hospitals), or to replace a long established hospital-based service by a service in the community, or to recruit, train, and deploy staff, or indeed to measure the health of a community, health authorities are required to establish a 10 year framework for the development of their services.

The process is initiated by the DHSS and Parliament which issue up-to-date national objectives and priorities couched in very broad terms, and publish information about resources they expect to be available for the first 5 years of the 10 year period.

Regions use the guidance which they receive from the DHSS as a basis for preparing strategic planning guidelines for the district health authorities. The manner in which this is done varies from region to region, but the elements of the process are generally as follows. Each region forms teams to embrace the main areas of health services such as children's services, services for the elderly, services for people with mental handicap and so on. These teams comprise members of all the relevant health professions together with senior planning and management officers, to include the spread of professional and geographic interests across the region. Their task is to relate the DHSS guidelines to local circumstances in their region and take into account the progress made by districts in implementing the existing Ten Year Regional Strategic Plan. The work of each team results in the drafting of Regional Strategic Guidelines in broad terms for each main service area. These are then brought together in a common framework by regional planners for submission by the Regional Team of Officers to the Regional Health Authority for approval. Once approved, the Regional guidelines are issued to districts to provide the basis for policy for strategic planning at district level.

The way planning is done varies considerably from district to district. District Health Authorities may choose to issue the guidelines to their planning teams with observations on local applicability provided by district officers, or may turn to the planning teams for their interpretation of the regional guidelines. In either case, the District Health Authority is responsible for issuing to its planning teams outline guidance for their work which is in keeping with regional policy.

The composition of planning teams also varies greatly from district to district. Before 1982, it was a responsibility of community physicians to convene them, and this practice has continued in most districts. Other members of the team comprise the appropriate unit management team, clinicians and other health professionals from relevant disciplines and specialities, appropriate local authority staff when joint planning is involved, representatives of voluntary organizations, and planning, information and finance staff. They are accountable for their work to the District Management Team (and to local authority managers where joint planning is involved).

A typical district generally has teams covering each of the main fields which require joint management and planning with the local authority:

- children
- the elderly
- mental handicap
- mental illness
- physical handicap and chronic disablement

as well as teams based solely on the health service such as:

- acute services
- maternity

In addition, there are usually arrangements for co-ordinating the planning of non-medical clinical services (such as occupational therapy, physiotherapy, speech therapy) and the non-clinical support services (such as transport and catering).

The arrangements shown in table 27.1 for mental illness illustrate the membership of a typical joint team.

Table 27.1 Possible arrangements for mental illness joint planning

National Health Service	
District Officer Mental Health Unit Management Team	: community physician : administrator : director of nursing services : consultant psychiatrist : clinical psychologist
Local Government	
Social Services Department	: senior manager : head mental health social worker*
Housing Department	: senior manager
Voluntary Organizations	
Local Mental Welfare Association Other Voluntary Associations	: representatives
N.H.S. *or* Local Government	
	: planning officer : information support : finance officer

* Usually a member of unit management team.

The process of strategic planning

The intention of a planning team is not to propose an unobtainable ideal, but to set out priorities for the most effective use of given resources in terms of agreed and clearly described objectives over carefully stipulated periods of time. The planning process therefore proceeds in a series of related steps.

(*a*) Explicit definition of the objectives which are set for the 10 year periods. The description of an objective is couched in terms of the patient groups in greatest need within the district; the elements of service most in need of more resources; and the diseases which most require preventive measures or a treatment programme. All of these components are, of course, inter-related.

(*b*) As a result of this detailed analysis of the problems, possible policy options for attaining the objectives are reviewed.

(*c*) These options are then considered in the light of available resources, and other possible constraints, and an explicit choice is made from amongst them.

(*d*) Programmes are evolved in broad terms to achieve the objective which relates to the chosen problem. Not only is a statement made of what is to be achieved, but details are set out of how long it will take to reach various stages along the way.

(*e*) Means of evaluating achievements as they relate to the objective are included so that, if necessary, modifications can be made.

(*f*) The team programmes are considered by the District Management Team, and plans which involve the local authority are amalgamated with them to form a draft strategic plan which is submitted to the District Health Authority for approval.

Uses of strategic plans

Strategic plans:

- provide the framework for the annual operational planning cycle, (which is described below) because they advise district health authorities of programmes of service development to be implemented together with the timescale for implementation;
- provide Regional Health Authorities with the basis for agreeing with each district a reasonable rate of progress towards achieving national and regional policy objectives and for monitoring the congruence between each year's operational planning proposals and the reaching of longer-term targets;
- at a higher level provide DHSS with a rational framework for judging how effectively Regions are moving towards the attainment of national policies and priorities.

Although they are concerned with a 10 year period, strategic plans are generally modified after 3 years, in the light of evaluation of progress and of changing circumstances, and are completely revised after 5 years for a further 10 year period.

The operational planning process in England

On the basis of the District Strategic Plan and up-to-date Regional guidance, the District Health Authorities issue local planning guidelines each year and the District Management Teams call on their planning teams to prepare operational plans covering the next 2 financial years. The plans must demonstrate how the strategic plan's objectives can be fulfilled by developing a timetable on a year-on-year basis towards the 10 year goals. The plans must also demonstrate that the evidence obtained from the evaluation of existing programmes is being taken into account. Operational Programmes are necessarily detailed, in contrast to the broad programmes of the strategic plans, and they contain individual proposals for staff, equipment, minor building works and supporting requirements.

When the operational plans are approved by the District Health Authority, the proposed operational programme for the forthcoming year is funded and implemented, while the forward plan is sent for consultation to relevant Community Health Councils, Local Authorities and neighbouring health authorities. The following year, the results of consulation are taken into account when the forward plan is developed into an operational programme.

Appraisal

The National Health Acts of 1973 and 1977 set out that the purpose of the National Health Service is 'to secure improvement:

- in the physical and mental health of the people . . .
  and
- in the prevention, diagnosis and treatment of illness'.

A planning system, was introduced in an attempt to replace disjointed incremental changes with a rational comprehensive approach to health service development. After almost 10 years of operation of the planning system, perhaps the most damaging evidence that it is failing to fulfil these ideals and purposes lies in the continued increase in the share of NHS resources devoted to high technology medicine, even though care of children, of the elderly, of the mentally handicapped and of the mentally ill have been national priorities throughout its period of operation.

Numerous reasons have been advanced for this failure. The organization of the NHS into multi-district areas has been blamed. There is some evidence that the former single district areas were better able to achieve their priorities between 1974 and 1982 than their multi-district counterparts. The disruption caused to planning between 1979, when proposals were first published for restructuring the NHS, and 1984, when the process was complete, undoubtedly delayed the development of skills and the accumulation of experience in this recently introduced field of NHS endeavour.

Blame has also been attributed to the newness of rational comprehensive planning to the NHS and the inadequacy of staff responsible for the task, both in terms of numbers and experience. Controls on management staff expenditure continue to limit the number of staff which can be devoted to planning; the restructuring in 1982 carried some of the most experienced planning staff into more senior positions (which in the longer term ought to bring considerable benefits); the development of planning skills within the NHS is still at a rudimentary stage compared with other public and private enterprises of lesser size and complexity.

It has also been suggested that perhaps the NHS will never be susceptible to rational planning; in particular because the medical staff involved in high technology medicine have control over the limited additional resources available to the NHS in a manner which the planning system is unable to challenge. Credence is lent to this view by difficulties in managing hospital pharmaceutical budgets; the existence of numerous 'creeping' developments, arising out of clinical freedom, and the extent to which press, politicians and some clinicians resort to waving shrouds when 'essential' developments are threatened.

Finally, attention has been drawn to the differing philosophies, funding arrangements and planning cycles of health and local authorities which are said to render almost impossible the successful joint planning of comprehensive services. Here again the restructuring of the NHS in 1982 disrupted organizational and individual roles and relationships which had developed over a number of years.

Annual reviews

The continuing failure of the NHS to implement workable programmes which would lead to national priorities being met was a major contributory factor in the introduction of annual reviews of performance by the DHSS in 1982 and of general managers in 1984. Reviews entail health ministers and senior civil servants annually assessing with Regional

Chairmen and Regional Teams of Officers the progress made by each region towards national policy objectives. Regions in turn review progress in districts, and in each case a plan of action is agreed for achievement by the following year. It remains to be seen whether this can contribute to the implementation of policy, and also the extent to which it will co-exist successfully with the planning system. In theory, at least, authorities with well-developed and workable planning arrangements ought to be best able to cope with the extra burden which undoubtedly derives from annual review, though they would be least in need of it. One benefit of the review system which was not advanced by ministers when they established it, is that they should now be much better placed to learn from the health authorities the consequences of continuing failure to define national objectives in health and a national strategy for achieving them; a failure which as we have seen undermines the optimal use of the limited resources which are available to the NHS.

Further Reading

Glennerston H., Korman N. and Marsten-Wilson F. (1983) *Planning for Priority Groups.* Martin Robertson, Oxford.

Klein R. (1983) *The Politics of the National Health Service.* Longman Inc., New York.

O'Neill P. (1983) *Health Crisis 2000*—World Health Organization. William Heinemann, London.

28

Maternal and Child Health Services

Maternal health

The health needs of a pregnant woman can be stated simply as her wish for a fulfilling experience for herself safely concluded by the delivery of a healthy infant. First, she should have a medical examination early in pregnancy to ensure that her general health is good, and another some time after delivery to determine whether it has subsequently been in any way impaired. Second, at regular intervals during pregnancy, labour and the puerperium she requires the help and advice of a skilled attendant. And third, at any stage, she should have immediate access to specialist hospital services if the need arises.

But although these requirements are easily summarized it is by no means obvious how they are best met. Organized obstetric services are of comparatively recent origin and they are still not entirely satisfactory. It will be easier to understand their present organization if we consider first the way in which they have evolved.

Evolution of Maternity Services

Until the nineteenth century midwifery was almost exclusively the province of women. From that time an increasing proportion of pregnant women who could afford to do so paid a doctor to attend them, but the large majority continued to be delivered by midwives over whose activities no control was exercised; they had no recognized training, no representative organization, and except in the case of the few hospital-trained midwives their standard of practice was very low. Charles Dickens's Sairey Gamp was the prototype, with her request for refreshment 'to be brought regular and draw'd mild'. The foundation of the Midwives'

Institute (1881) and the passing of the first Midwives' Act (1902) marked the beginning of standardized training and regulated practice.

Except for the few who worked 'on the district' surrounding a teaching hospital, all midwives earned their living by private practice. The rapid extension of hospital midwifery and the decline of the birth rate put many out of business, and after the introduction of a wholetime salaried municipal midwife service in 1936, few private midwives remained. From this time domiciliary midwifery became for all practical purposes a local authority monopoly.

Hospital obstetrics

The founding of the Rotunda Hospital in Dublin in 1745 and the establishment of a few lying-in beds in London teaching hospitals mark the beginning of medical interest in obstetrics. But for the next 150 years the growth of hospital maternity services was slow compared with the remarkable expansion of other hospital facilities. The reason is not far to seek: the maternal death rate in lying-in hospitals was so high, mostly from sepsis, that few women chose to be confined there. In the Maternité of Paris, for example, maternal mortality between 1861 and 1864 was 124 per 1,000 births. This is hardly surprising when it is remembered that midwife pupils attended normal labours and fever cases alike, and doctors often went to women in labour from the postmortem room and surgery without removing their top-hats and frock-coats or washing their hands.

By the end of the nineteenth century, it became clear that puerperal fever was often spread by doctor and midwife and could be prevented by cleanliness and routine disinfection of the hands. At the same time anaesthesia and antiseptic techniques were making obstetrical interference less disastrous. For the first time mortality rates in hospitals began to bear comparison with those at home. The proportion of confinements in hospital has continued to increase. It was 30 per cent in the nineteen-twenties, 60 per cent in the nineteen-fifties and is now over 90 per cent.

General practitioner obstetrics

Although medical obstetric specialists were well established in most large towns by the beginning of the nineteenth century, the practice of midwifery by doctors was still frowned upon by the Royal Colleges. In 1827 the President of the Royal College of Physicians wrote to Sir Robert Peel the Prime Minister that the practice of midwifery was 'an act foreign to the habits of gentlemen of enlarged academic education'. There was, however, an increasing demand from well-to-do women for doctors to attend them, and in 1868 the General Medical Council insisted that medical students must conduct 20 labours before sitting their final examination. Since the Medical Act of 1886 qualification in midwifery as well as in surgery and medicine has been required for registration.

A considerable barrier to an efficient maternity service was the cost of medical care. The National Health Insurance Act of 1911 made no provision for maternity, other than the payment of a small cash benefit to the woman insured in her own right. In 1918 the principle was accepted of fees paid from the public funds (recovered if possible from the patient) to medical practitioners called in by midwives in emergencies. Within the National Health Service there are now no financial barriers.

Antenatal clinics

The need for regular antenatal supervision is today generally accepted but 50 years ago it was unheard of. As hospital practice expanded, antenatal clinics slowly became a feature of hospitals with lying-in beds. They served partly as supervisory centres for 'booked' cases and partly as clinics to which outside doctors could refer patients for a consultant opinion. At the same time local authorities began to set up voluntary supervisory centres, staffed by their own doctors. The two services developed side by side, but made little contact with one another.

Maternity services before the National Health Service

The diverse origins of the maternity services explain their complicated pattern before the introduction of the National Health Service. About half the confinements in England and Wales were in voluntary or municipal hospitals, but criteria for hospital admission were not at all clearly defined. The hospital usually accepted responsibility for antenatal supervision of its booked cases, but occasionally part of the supervision was provided by the patient's general practitioner or in the district antenatal clinic.

The other half of the confinements were at home, attended by municipal midwives. The midwife accepted responsibility for antenatal care, working in close cooperation with local authority doctors and health visitors at the district antenatal clinic. These women were referred to hospital or to their own general practitioner should the clinic doctor discover any contraindication to domiciliary delivery during the antenatal period. If difficulty arose during labour or the puerperium, a local general practitioner was called and his fee paid by the local authority according to a scale fixed by the Ministry of Health.

A small proportion of women arranged for their general practitioner to attend them at home or in a private nursing home. In such cases a municipal or private midwife usually assisted the doctor. He accepted responsibility for antenatal supervision, but sometimes the patient also attended a local authority clinic. If an emergency arose during confinement, a consultant obstetrician was called in.

Maternity services under the National Health Service

The National Health Service effected two immediate changes in maternity services: local authorities lost their maternity hospitals to Regional Hospital Boards and women became entitled without charge to a maternity medical service if they decided to have their babies at home. There were also two important long-term effects: local authorities are no longer concerned with antenatal care or domiciliary midwifery and hospital delivery, often in a short-stay unit, has become the accepted norm. Women booked for hospital delivery receive a first comprehensive antenatal examination at the hospital and then, if there are no abnormalities, their general practitioners and community midwives usually provide antenatal care until about the thirtysecond week. From then until delivery they attend the hospital antenatal clinic. Many women choose to attend the hospital antenatal clinic throughout their pregnancy. A small proportion of women elect to receive their antenatal care from general practitioner obstetricians and are delivered in general practitioner maternity units.

Two other important and related developments should be mentioned: the changing attitude towards abortion and the growth of family planning and birth control services. The Abortion Act (1967) introduced legal termination of pregnancy into the United Kingdom, with the provision that two doctors must agree that the mental or physical health of the mother would be seriously affected by the birth of the child. Under the National Health Service (Family Planning) Act, 1967, local authorities were given power to provide contraceptive advice for women on medical or social grounds, and in 1974 contraceptives were made available on prescription as a regular part of the Health Service.

Appraisal of Obstetric Services

Achievement

From contemporary records of hospital and private practice, and from what is known of maternal mortality in developing countries today, it seems probable that 150 years ago at least 10 women died in childbirth for every 1,000 births. When puerperal fever assumed epidemic proportions mortality sometimes increased tenfold to 10 per cent. By the end of the nineteenth century the level had fallen to below 5 per 1,000 in England and Wales, but from that time it did not decline much until the mid-thirties. The rate then fell rapidly, and it is now less than 0.2 per 1,000 total births (figure 28.1).

The reason for the trend of maternal mortality in the nineteenth and early part of the twentieth centuries is not clear. The decline since 1935 can be attributed first to the control of sepsis by chemotherapy and antibiotics, second to the control of haemorrhage associated with the introduction of a reliable blood transfusion service and third to a fall in mortality from toxaemia, partly explained by better antenatal care (figure 28.2). Toxaemia is now virtually the only cause in England and Wales. Although a great deal has been achieved, confidential enquiries into maternal deaths indicate that even at their present low level about half of them are associated with an 'avoidable factor'. This does not necessarily mean that in all these cases death could have been prevented. But it does imply that some aspect of the mother's care fell short of what should be expected from a comprehensive maternity service. For example haemorrhage is largely preventable, and deaths from toxaemia are often attributable to poor antenatal care. As the number of maternal deaths from all causes has declined, induced abortion has become relatively more important. The Abortion Act (1967) has brought about a substantial decrease in deaths from illegal operations and a small increase in deaths from legal abortion.

The assessment of the quality of maternity care is most readily made in terms of the failure of the fetus or newborn child to survive, and the most useful indication is perinatal mortality. This index groups together stillbirths and deaths in the first week of life, both of which can be

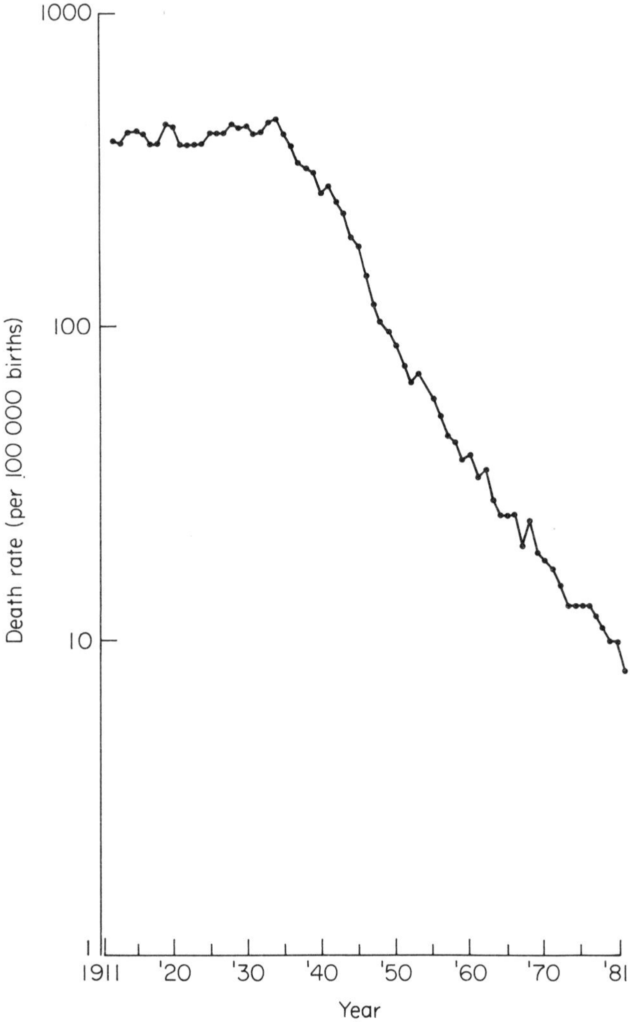

Figure 28.1. Maternal mortality rate England and Wales 1911-1981.

attributed broadly to influences operating before and during delivery. Figure 28.3 shows the trend of perinatal mortality in England and Wales since 1928, when stillbirths were first registered, and compares it with the trend of mortality in the first month and the first year of life.

The fall in death rate in the post-neonatal period has been steepest and that during the first week of life has been least. This is only in part attributable to advances in medical knowledge of obstetrics as specific as

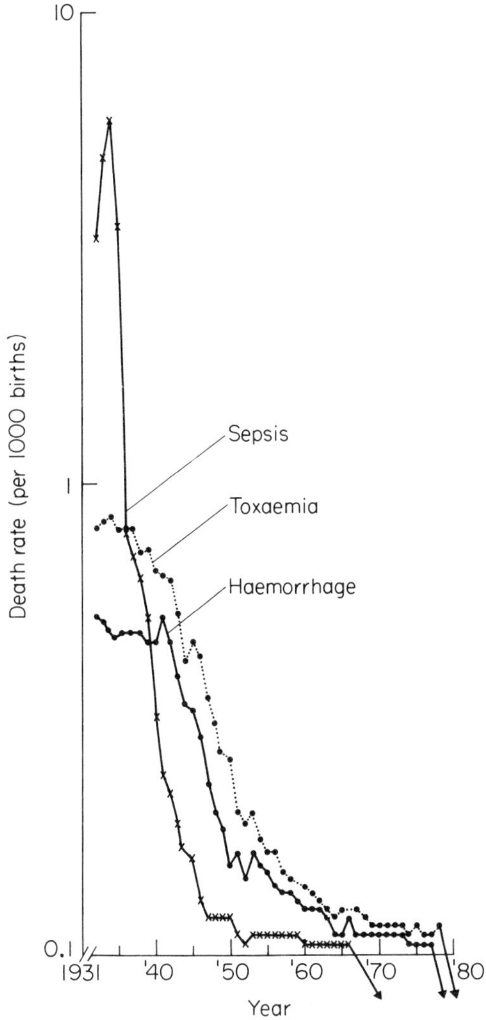

Figure 28.2. Maternal mortality rates due to sepsis, toxaemia and haemorrhage, England and Wales 1930-1980.

those which largely explain the decline of maternal mortality, but improvements in antenatal care and obstetric services have certainly made an important contribution.

Hospital or home confinement

There are wide differences of opinion about the desirability of conducting a substantial proportion of deliveries at home. In Sweden and

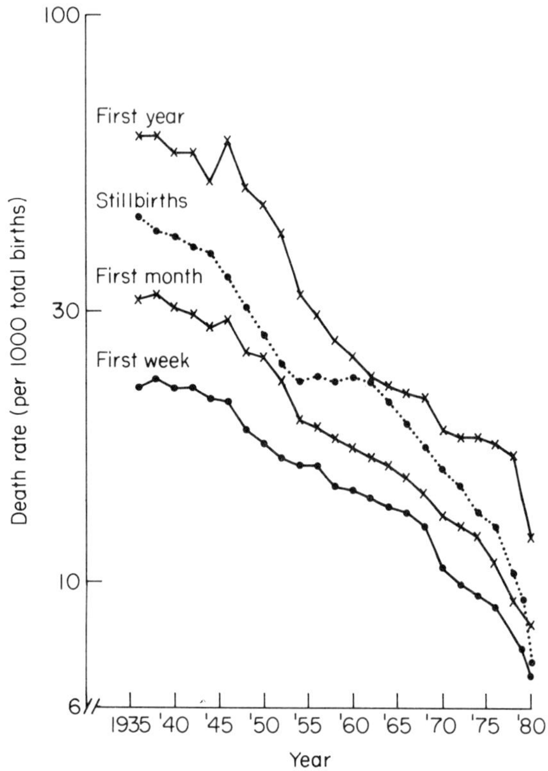

Figure 28.3. Death rate at birth and by end of first week, first month and first year 1935-1980.

the United States almost all doctors favour institutional delivery, and in New York, for example, 98 per cent of births are in hospital (the remaining 2 per cent are said to be in taxis).

Experience in countries such as England and the Netherlands shows that given good antenatal care, reasonable home conditions, well-trained midwives, carefully selected patients and an efficient emergency service, domiciliary delivery is compatible with relatively low perinatal and maternal mortality rates. Yet there are grounds for believing that these rates might be even lower if all deliveries were in hospital. For when perinatal mortality is low further reduction depends on the skilful handling of problems which are technically complex and sometimes cannot be anticipated. The need cannot be met entirely by emergency measures in the home, nor by hasty transfer of a mother or new born child to hospital. It is mainly for this reason that most experienced obstetricians favour hospital confinement and also why we are moving rapidly towards a time when almost all deliveries are likely to be conducted in short-stay specialist or general practitioner obstetric units. Although a maternity hospital is the safest place for the mother and her baby during and immediately after labour, some mothers prefer to be delivered at home and a good home is undoubtedly the best place for a normal baby after the first few hours. The time when mother and child should be transferred from hospital to home is a matter for individual assessment, but in the majority of cases the transfer can be made within 12 to 48 hours. An increasing proportion of hospital obstetric beds are occupied for only 48 hours (short-stay units), and the small number of women who are cared for in general practitioner maternity units usually return home within 12 hours. The success of this practice is dependant on good support at home from the family, the doctor, the midwife, and later the health visitor.

The general practitioner obstetrician

Under the National Health Service a woman may, without charge, book her own doctor to attend her during her confinement, and if he does not undertake midwifery she may choose a 'general-practitioner-obstetrician' from the local obstetric list. When the Act was framed it was intended that admission to the obstetric list should be granted only to practitioners who had shown a special interest in midwifery, by having held a resident, postgraduate appointment in obstetrics, or by having dealt with a certain number of midwifery cases in their own practices, but these requirements have not been strictly observed. Although the doctor engaged by a patient accepts full responsibility for the management of pregnancy, labour and puerperium, in practice the midwife is still the normal attendant at birth. However, in case of difficulty she has on call a medical attendant who should know the patient.

Antenatal supervision

In 1946 at least 80 per cent of women confined at home attended local authority antenatal clinics; today women rely on their general practitioner and the maternity hospital for antenatal supervision. The maternity medical service was intended to be an addition to facilities already available, not a substitute for them. Close supervision is required if the complications of pregnancy and labour are to be discovered early enough to avoid unnecessary morbidity and mortality. Most doctors recognize this but by no means all see their patients fortnightly until the 36th week and then weekly until they are confined, as was the practice in local authority clinics. Moreover many services were more easily provided at a clinic than they are at a general practitioner's surgery, and clinics offered an excellent opportunity for instruction in preparation for childbirth, and for contact with the health visitor who would visit the home after the birth. The growing tendency for practitioners to practise in groups and from health centres makes it easier to provide a high standard of antenatal care.

Child Health Services

One fifth of the population of Britain is under the age of 16. In the rest of this chapter we are concerned with the special health needs of this important sector of the population and the health services that have evolved to meet those needs. From the point of view of needs, three age periods can be distinguished: the neonatal period; the post neonatal period (from the end of the first month to the end of the first year); and the rest of childhood through adolescence to school leaving.

We have already seen that most of the problems arising in the neonatal period are related to prenatal and intranatal influences (Chapter 3). The principal causes of death and disability are immaturity, malformation and birth injury. Prevention of these conditions, so far as they are preventable, lies largely in the province of maternal care and the maternity services, but the care of affected infants who survive into childhood calls for coordination of paediatric, general practice, nursing, social and educational services in hospital and community.

The post neonatal death rate remained very high until the beginning of the twentieth century, since when it has declined dramatically. Most deaths were due to gastroenteritis, bronchitis and pneumonia, malnutrition, tuberculosis and the common infections of childhood which as we have seen are measles, whooping cough, diphtheria and scarlet fever. These causes of death are particularly susceptible to control by manipulation of adverse physical and social environments such as bad feeding, lack of cleanliness, insanitary housing, overcrowding, maternal inefficiency, as well as low standards of medical care; and the evolution of services to effect that manipulation has been largely responsible for the decline of the death rate. Infant deaths have become the subject of confidential enquiries of the type previously undertaken only for maternal deaths. Retrospective enquiries are not easy to interpret, but the results indicate that there is still considerable scope for further reduction in the post neonatal death rate, mainly by continuing to raise the standards of care of low birthweight and sick new born babies and by paying more attention to the total situation of such infants in the post neonatal period—their vulnerability to infection, and the adequacy of their parents and of the home environment. In particular, doctors, nurses and social workers need always to bear in mind the rapidity with which an ailing infant's condition can change for the worse.

From about the end of the first year children enter an extended period during which the risk of dying is extremely low. But although mortality is low, morbidity is comparatively high. Upper respiratory and bowel infections are common, and it is at this time that most of the common infections of childhood are contracted. By the age of 15, about four-fifths of children have had chickenpox, and before immunization was generally available, three-quarters had had measles and whooping cough. Rickets, bone and joint tuberculosis, rheumatic fever and diphtheria, all at one time common, are now rare, but accidents in the home and on the streets remain an important cause of morbidity and sometimes of permanent handicap. The period of childhood is also characterized by rapid growth and development and in the late years by the physical, psychological and social manifestations of adolescence. Health needs are determined by these characteristics. Children need a diet adequate to meet the demands of rapid growth, protection against infection and physical injury, a background conducive to normal social and emotional development, and surveillance to detect and where possible treat and correct congenital and acquired disabilities, with appropriate educational and social services in support.

With the reorganization of the National Health Service in 1974, school health services were transferred from local authorities to area health authorities. This for the first time placed all child health services within one administrative framework and the principle was retained at restructuring in 1982 when responsibility was assumed by district health authorities. However, because of the way in which services for children evolved and because the responsiblity for educational and social services still rests with local authorities, it will be convenient to consider separately services for preschool children and services for school children.

Preschool Children

Hospital and general practitioner paediatrics

Hospital interest in diseases of children is even more recent than in obstetrics. The provision of special hospitals for such children began as a voluntary movement in the middle of the nineteenth century; Great Ormond Street Hospital was founded in 1852 and it and other children's hospitals remained largely voluntary concerns until the National Health Service. Many workhouse inmates were young children, but until well into the twentieth century special accommodation for children in public hospitals was limited to fever hospitals. Paediatrics is now a well developed specialty and most of the children in district general hospitals are gathered together in children's departments with appropriate facilities such as open visiting, sleeping accommodation for parents, day rooms and play areas. Like other well developed specialities it is already fragmenting into sub-specialties—perinatal paediatrics, developmental paediatrics, paediatric cardiology, gastroenterology, neurology, oncology, haematology and others.

During the nineteenth and early part of the twentieth centuries, deficiencies in medical education and lack of financial incentive kept the standard of general practitioner paediatrics at a low level. Academic instruction in paediatrics was first given by obstetricians, and it was not until the second half of the nineteenth century that medical schools began to show any real interest in the subject. The first chair was established in 1906 at King's College Hospital, London, and it was said in London that the only thing most doctors knew about the care of children was Dr. Still's telephone number. It was not until after the Second World War that universities moved towards putting the subject on an equal footing with medicine, surgery and midwifery in the final examination.

The National Health Insurance Act of 1911 provided the first public domiciliary medical service outside the Poor Law, but it made no arrangements for the children of insured workers. Some doctors accepted children in sick clubs, and for a few pence per week contracted to provide medicine and advice when needed. Nevertheless the medical care of preschool children remained most unsatisfactory until the National Health Service made available without charge a general practitioner service for every child.

Local authority services

When local authorities entered the field of personal health services at the beginning of the century in response to public concern about the inadequacy of provisions for the care of children, the voluntary infant welfare movement comprised three main activities:

- Home visiting for the purpose of advising recently confined mothers on the feeding, clothing and general care of their children. This was the British contribution to the infant welfare movement and the origin of the Health Visiting Service. It began in Manchester in 1862, first on a voluntary basis and later as a salaried service.
- Consultation clinics, introduced in France ('consultations de nourissons'), for medical supervision of children which were in effect the first child welfare centres, precursors of child health clinics.
- Distribution through milk depots ('gouttes de lait') of cheap, safe milk to mothers not able to breast feed their babies, also first developed in France.

These features were gradually adopted and developed by local authorities. From them evolved the child welfare service which local Health Authorities provided under the National Health Service, the responsibility for which now rests with District Health Authorities.

(*a*) *Health visiting*

In the past there was great variation in the qualifications and experience of health visitors, who at different times and in different places have been voluntary 'lady visitors', working class women with families of their own who had undergone a short course of instruction, sanitary inspectors, midwives, nurses and even doctors. Today only state registered nurses with training in midwifery are accepted for the 12 months full time training which leads to the Certificate in Health Visiting.

The health visitor calls on the mother within a few days of her return home from hospital, or, in the case of early discharge or home delivery, as soon as possible after the midwife has left. She has no legal right of entry but is rarely refused admission. After the first visit she encourages the mother to attend a child health clinic, but she visits the home again from time to time as she thinks necessary. Although she is a trained nurse, she does not undertake sick-nursing duties, except occasionally in rural areas. Her province is to advise and educate the mother with regard to such matters as maintenance of breast feeding, preparation of artificial feeds, weaning and protection of the child against infection and accident. In short she is concerned with the control of the domestic environment to reduce the risks of death and disability. Although health visitors still have an important role in the care of expectant and nursing mothers and of children under 5 years of age, their field of interest has been extended greatly by the National Health Service and by general practitioner attachment schemes. Many now work closely with general practitioners as members of the primary care team and give advice about health problems affecting other members of the family, particularly the elderly, the sick and the handicapped.

(*b*) *Child health clinics*

The original purpose of child welfare centres was to follow up the progress of preschool children under medical and health visitor supervision. From the beginning many centres provided food for mothers and children at reduced rates; free in necessitous cases. Later cod liver oil and for some years orange juice were also dispensed. Since the closing of the Ministry of Food after the Second World War local health authorities have accepted responsibility for the distribution of National Dried Milk and vitamin supplements. Proprietary foods are still often available at wholesale prices on the recommendation of the doctor, and the distribution of food is considered by some to provide an important incentive for attendance.

Child health clinics are now the focal point for medical consultation and for advice and education about all matters related to the health of young children. They provide facilities for screening for defects of vision and hearing, assessment of child development and early diagnosis and assessment of physical and mental handicaps.

Most of the doctors who work in the centres are women. They are known as clinical medical officers and many are whole time members of the staff of the District Health Authority. Others attend on a sessional basis, in which case they may be also in general practice or in hospital paediatric practice, and they usually have postgraduate experience in developmental paediatrics, child psychiatry and clinical paediatrics. When a child first attends a centre, usually between 2 and 6 weeks of age, it is examined by the doctor. Subsequent examinations, at 6 months and then approximately at each birthday up to the age of 4, are tending to become a responsibility shared between doctor and health visitor. The health visitor assumes the role of observer in the early detection of handicaps and is often made responsible for screening tests. In this respect the attachment of health visitors to group general practices, especially in health centres, has great advantages for communications and access to records. Some general practitioners, especially those working in groups, assume in liaison with their primary care team, responsibility for most of the tasks discharged by the clinical medical officer.

Appraisal of services for preschool children

The development of child welfare centres with their three services—health education, medical examination and food distribution—coincided with a rapid decline in child mortality, but in the same period there were other changes likely to improve the health of children, for example, a decrease in mean family size, improvement in the standard of living, and, more recently, the introduction of effective therapy. We must therefore rely on a commonsense appraisal of each type of service.

There can be little doubt that the instruction of an uninformed mother by an experienced health visitor or doctor is valuable. Breast feeding, bowel-training, preparation of artificial foods, and weaning are not matters in which it is possible to rely either on a mother's instinctive good sense, or necessarily on the advice given by friends or relatives. A few women in favourable circumstances used to receive professional instruction from other sources, mainly from private doctors, but most women obtained it from welfare centres or not at all. However, much of the traditional advisory work of doctors in health clinics can now be done equally well by the health visitor. Indeed the conditions for which medical advice is given are those with which the health visitor has been trained to deal, and does deal when no doctor is available.

The initial medical examination is a different matter. This demands more knowledge of developmental paediatrics and a wider knowledge of congenital defects and clinical medicine than the health visitor can command. Subsequent surveillance of young children's developmental and health progress can probably be left to health visitors provided they have facilities for early referral to clinical medical officers with their special interest in and knowledge of child health. Such doctors in their turn need the backing of comprehensive multidisciplinary assessment centres for handicapped children of the type that health districts are now establishing.

The importance of the contribution that the distribution of dried milk and vitamin supplements from welfare centres has made to the health of young children is not in doubt. However, it is to be hoped that in the future the reputation of child health clinics will rest on the high quality of their work, and it is difficult to see how the sale of infant foods does anything to enhance that reputation and this should be organized as a separate activity.

The personal health services of local authorities were introduced because of concern about the health of children at a time when infectious disease was predominant. When 1 child in 10 was dying from an infection in the first year of life, the most urgent requirement was to protect those who were normal at birth from the deleterious effects of the postnatal environment. Children died mainly because they were underfed and because they were infected at a vulnerable age in overcrowded and insanitary homes. It was in such circumstances that the domiciliary services for children developed, with the health visitor as the key worker. Her job was not to nurse the sick child, but to attempt to prevent sickness by advice and assistance to the mother.

In decaying and depressed areas of cities there are still underprivileged children and families who have to be made aware of and persuaded to use available services. However, with higher standards of living, a better educated population and comprehensive medical services, the health of the normal child has become more secure and the problems of children who are physically or mentally handicapped have become relatively more important.

The health visitor is well placed to support the doctor in the early ascertainment of handicaps because she is the only health worker who sees all children soon after birth and at intervals during early life. Her experience in dealing with the health problems of mothers and young children is unrivalled. Now that the earlier objectives of her work have been largely achieved, the policy of attaching health visitors to groups of general practitioners is a natural development, with a shift in emphasis from an advisory role to one focussed on ascertaining and helping the sick and handicapped of all ages.

School Children

Local authority services

Compulsory education was introduced in 1870, but widespread malnutrition interfered with the proper use of this facility and in 1906 an Education Act permitted the new local education authorities to provide milk and meals to elementary school children who were unable by reason of lack of food to take full advantage of the education provided for them. At about the same time the Interdepartmental Committee on Physical Deterioration recommended that 'a systematized inspection of school children should be imposed as public duty on every school authority' and this led to another Education Act in 1907 which laid the foundations for a school health service. Regular medical inspections soon revealed a substantial amount of untreated illness and disability among the children, and local education authorities began to provide treatment in clinics, first for minor ailments such as skin conditions and later for ophthalmological, orthopaedic and other conditions. Medical inspections also helped to identify children with serious physical and mental handicaps who needed special educational treatment.

(*a*) *Milk and meals*

The provision of milk and meals by local education authorities was for a long time an inadequate and unattractive service subject to a means test. The upheaval of the war of 1939-45 changed its character—many mothers were out at work and the need to maintain the health of children led to a great expansion of the service and freed it of its association with poverty. Free milk is now provided for children at nursery schools, for handicapped pupils and, where there are medical reasons, for junior school pupils. The uptake of school meals has fallen since government permitted the abolition of subsidies by local education authorities and there is a movement towards providing cafeteria, free-choice meals for older pupils. There is growing concern about the effect of this change on childrens' nutritional habits and their health in later life. It is a sign of our affluent times that medical interest in the nutrition of school children has moved from the problems of under nutrition to those of obesity and dental caries.

(*b*) *Medical inspections*

School inspections were introduced to identify previously unrecognized defects in children, to supervise their treatment and to ensure that serious defects impeded educational progress as little as possible. They provided, in fact, a screening programme for school children long before screening became fashionable. With the developments in the preschool services, a National Health Service and a growing interest in developmental paediatrics most of the defects likely to interfere with education are now discovered and well-documented before school entry, but the surveillance of preschool children is still not sufficiently comprehensive for the school entry medical examination to be dispensed with. At that examination a child's medical history, physical growth, vision, hearing, speech, motor function and intellectual, social and emotional development are reassessed in the learning situation. Subsequent examinations are much more selective—special examinations at the request of parents, teacher, school nurse or health visitor. The role of the school nurse was at one time limited to receptionist and inspector of personal cleanliness at the routine medical examinations. It now includes undertaking tests of visual and auditory acuity and of physical and neuromotor development.

(*c*) *School clinics*

Under the Education Act of 1944 local education authorities were required to provide, free of cost to parents, all forms of treatment, except domiciliary treatment, for pupils attending maintained schools. This treatment was provided in minor ailment clinics and specialist clinics. The clinics offered treatment for a wide range of conditions, especially those which were ophthalmic, orthopaedic, and otolaryngological, and many special services such as speech therapy, child guidance, remedial exercises, and orthoptic services. Formerly the clinics were staffed and maintained by local education authorities but under the National Health Service they became the responsibility first of Regional Hospital Boards and now of District Health Authorities. There is a growing tendency to transfer the specialist services from the clinics to hospital out-patients departments.

(*d*) *Handicapped children*

Seriously handicapped children often have special educational needs and sometimes those needs can be met satisfactorily only by special education arrangements. It is the statutory duty of Local Education Authorities under the Education Act 1981 to identify all children with learning difficulties (not just those with serious handicaps) as early in their lives as possible and to make arrangements to meet their needs. Whenever practicable this should be in ordinary schools, even though they may be taught in special classes. (Chapers 29 and 30).

Appraisal of School Health Services

Over the past century mortality rates have declined more for children than for any other age group. They have fallen to the extent that in 1981 the death rate for children aged 5-14 was less than one-thirtieth of the rate in 1841-50. Almost all of this improvement is due to the decline of mortality from infectious disease attributable mainly to a rising standard of living, control of unhygienic living conditions and, latterly, immunization programmes.

The general health of children has also improved a great deal, although this is not so well documented, despite the routine recording for more than 60 years of defects found at routine school medical inspections. There has certainly been a remarkable increase in the age specific height and weight of children and a steady decrease in the mean age at onset of menstruation in girls. On the average children aged 12 years are 12 cms taller and 6 kg heavier than children of the same age 70 years ago and girls begin to menstruate 3 years earlier than they did at the beginning of the century. Skin, eye and ear infections are much less common and rickets and bone and joint tuberculosis have become extremely rare conditions in indigenous Britons, although they are found in immigrants from the tropics. It is impossible to assess reliably the contribution of the school health services to this improvement in health, but it is probably safe to assume that they have been less important than the rising standard of living, improvement in environmental services and introduction of immunization procedures. Even the provision of milk and meals at school can have had no very great effect before the Second World War, for the milk in schools scheme was not introduced until 1934 and in 1938 only 4 per cent of children were taking school meals. Since then, however, school meals, and for several decades the treatment of major and minor ailments and disabilities and the medical surveillance of handicapped children in relation to their educational progress, are likely to have made an important contribution.

Routine school inspections, school dinners and school medical officers of the old type are now an anachronism and are fast disappearing. But there is no question about the continuing need for the following:

- Surveillance of the physical growth and the educational, social and emotional development of all children attending school;
- Identification of children with physical or mental disabilities which may affect their ability to learn in the ordinary school situation;
- Continued medical surveillance of children with physical and mental disorders which may have important implications for their educational and psychological development;
- Advice for teachers to help them to interpret the educational significance of what doctors and other health professionals may know about particular children;
- A multidisciplinary consultation service for children with educational problems that may have underlying physical, social or psychological causes and for adolescents with difficulties in relation to psychosexual adjustment, drug taking and other health matters;
- Maintenance of immunization programmes for school children;
- An advisory service on health education programmes in schools.

Further Reading

Confidential Enquiry into Postneonatal Deaths 1964-66 (1970) DHSS Reports on Public Health and Medical Subjects No. 125. HMSO, London.

Report on Confidential Enquiries into Maternal Deaths in England and Wales, 1976-1978 (1982). DHSS Reports on Health and Social Subjects No. 4. HMSO, London.

29

Services for Physically Handicapped People

The significance of physical handicaps is determined much more by their social consequences and by personal and public attitudes to them than by their purely medical classification. Although this implies that the needs of handicapped persons are essentially social in character, it does not mean that they are of no concern to doctors. Without the co-operation of the medical profession, the services provided to help handicapped people cannot function properly: the health services provide treatment and medical rehabilitation; and medical opinion is required about prognosis and any limitations that should be imposed on physical activity.

Definitions of three related terms 'Impairment', 'Disability' and 'Handicap' have been published by the World Health Organization. All three are broad in their meaning and relate to interference with psychological, physiological or anatomical structure or function. *Impairment* is simply a loss of one or more of these. *Disability* stems from an impairment, and is as a consequence of it a restriction or lack of ability to perform an activity in what is accepted as a normal manner. Finally *handicap* is the disadvantage a person suffers because, as a result of his impairment or disability he is unable to play a role which would be considered normal for someone of his or her age, sex and cultural background. Problems presented by physically handicapped children and adults differ, and so does the legislation concerning them. We shall deal with children first.

The significance of handicaps in children depends upon the extent to which they interfere with physical, emotional, social and, perhaps most important educational development. In adults considerations are the restrictions the handicaps impose on ability to lead an independent social life—to work, to marry and to enjoy a normal social and family life.

Physically Handicapped Children

Broadly speaking there are two ways in which a handicap may disturb family life: it may require separation of the affected child from parents, brothers and sisters because of the need for hospital treatment or for educational facilities that can be provided only in a residential school; and it may have an adverse effect upon the mental or physical health of other members of the family.

There are also two ways in which a handicap may influence the course of education. On the one hand it may be of such a nature that the child cannot be educated by normal methods, as, for example, in the case of blind and deaf children and children with gross spastic defects. Here the difficulties are mainly educational. On the other hand a physical handicap, although in no way affecting educability, may make it difficult or impossible for a child to attend an ordinary school. For example a child may be in hospital undergoing protracted surgical treatment or may be unable to meet the physical demands of school life because of congenital heart disease. Such difficulties are essentially medical.

Until the present century, responsibility for the welfare and education of physically handicapped children rested almost entirely with parents. Most of the crippling disabilities of childhood such as those arising from rickets, bone and joint tuberculosis, and blindness and deafness due to infection in infancy were directly related to a low standard of living; a handicapped child, if too disabled to work on the land or in a factory, remained, perhaps neglected, at home or, if abandoned by its family, was admitted to the general mixed workhouse.

In the eighteenth century voluntary effort had begun to prepare the way for a more humane public approach, but the services provided were inevitably local and limited in scope. For the most part they were concerned with the welfare and training of the two groups of children whose handicaps have always aroused sympathy: the blind the first school for whom was established in Liverpool, 1792; and the deaf and dumb whose first school opened in Edinburgh 1760. The needs of children with less appealing handicaps were largely ignored.

With the introduction of compulsory education in 1870 and the subsequent development of school health services, the extent of the need for special educational facilities to help severely handicapped children to compensate for their handicaps was slowly uncovered. Appropriate services developed slowly too and it is only since the Education Act, 1944, that an attempt has been made to ensure that all severely handicapped children receive an education suited to their 'age, ability and aptitude'. Under the act local education authorities were statutorily responsible for 'ascertaining' all the children in their areas likely to need specialized educational facilities and for providing those facilities.

The latest Education Act in 1981 takes a unified approach to all children with learning difficulties. Although the majority of handicapped children are catered for within ordinary schools the Act recognizes that there is a small minority of children who require special arrangements however, and lays an obligation on local authorities to provide for this group. Included are all children with special needs from 2 years of age upwards, and at the request of parents those under 2 years. Special and sensitive procedures in which parents are involved are used to assess handicapped children.

If some concession is made to their special needs, for example a seat at the front of the class for a child with defective sight or hearing, children with moderate handicaps can often attend an ordinary class. This undoubtedly is the best place for them. Unfortunately most severely handicapped children lose a great deal of time from school for medical reasons, and their educational progress tends to be slower than that of other children of their own age. To help them in their unequal struggle they need a great deal of individual attention.

Although the government has decided following the recommendation of the Warnock Committee in 1978 to avoid, as far as possible, the differentiation of educational approaches to handicapped children from those to their normal peers, the impairments they suffer raise differing issues which are worth brief mention.

Blind and partially sighted children

Blind children are considered to be those with no sight or whose sight is, or is likely to become, so defective that they require education by methods not involving the use of sight. Partially sighted children are those who by reason of defective vision cannot follow the ordinary curriculum without detriment to their sight or to their educational development, but can be educated by special methods involving sight. At the present time about 3,000 children of school age (5 per 10,000) have such poor vision that they are unable to read ordinary school books; 2,000 of them can be taught by visual methods with the help of magnifying glasses and specially printed books, but the education of the rest depends upon non-visual methods. It is the practice to meet the needs of the partially sighted so far as possible in ordinary schools, reserving special residential schools for the blind. When the defect is stable, for instance, congenital cataract, dislocated lens, corneal scarring after injury or infection, educational classification can be based on tests of visual acuity after full correction. When the defect is progressive medical assessment for appropriate education is more difficult, and rests upon a medical estimate of whether or not the sight is likely to deteriorate beyond the point at which education by visual methods will become impossible. For example the commonest cause of progressive visual deterioration in childhood is now myopia and in the great majority of cases this is progressive only until growth is complete; in a small proportion of cases with choroidal and retinal degeneration the visual defect progresses to blindness and if these children are to come to terms with their tragic disability the sooner they are taught to read by touch the better.

Deaf and partially hearing children

Deaf children are defined as those whose hearing is so defective that they require education by methods used for pupils with little or no naturally acquired speech or language. Partially hearing children are those whose hearing is so defective that they require for their education special arrangements or facilities, but not all the educational methods used for deaf pupils. Modern electronic procedures have been of great benefit in teaching deaf children to speak clearly.

The introduction of audiometry into routine preschool and school examinations has uncovered a great deal of previously unsuspected deafness-about 1 in 25 children tested has an appreciable auditory impairment in both ears. With a little extra attention in the classroom, tuition in lip reading, the provision of suitable hearing aids and the treatment of chronic ear infection, the needs of the great majority of these children can be met in ordinary schools. However, 9 in every 10,000 school children have an auditory defect serious enough to need special educational facilities. Auditory handicap is therefore twice as common as visual handicap although it excites considerably less public sympathy. Today most children classified as deaf are born with their handicap. It must be remembered, however, that congenital deafness is not necessarily or indeed usually genetic in origin; in some cases it is attributable to environmental influences such as maternal rubella, birth injury, anoxia and rhesus incompatibility.

The education of deaf children presents formidable problems, and their long and difficult training must begin very early in life if they are to be taught to speak intelligibly. Early ascertainment is therefore of the utmost importance.

Epileptic children

Epilepsy is a common condition—about 4 per 1000 children of school age are known to be under treatment for it. Fortunately, the great majority of these children are able to attend and make satisfactory progress in ordinary schools. Less than 1 in 10,000 of the school population require special educational arrangements on account of epilepsy; the majority of those who do attend residential schools. Frequency and severity of fits, marked behavioural difficulties and lack of educational progress determine the need for special schooling.

Maladjusted children

Maladjustment has been the term applied to pupils who show evidence of emotional instability or psychological disturbance, and who require special educational treatment in order to effect their personal, social or educational readjustment. The causes of maladjustment are complex and imperfectly understood. The tense emotional atmosphere in homes with marital difficulties, the antipathy that sometimes develops between parent and child and the overcrowding and lack of playing space in the poorer parts of industrial towns are a few of the many influences thought to lie behind the antisocial behaviour (destructiveness, lying, stealing, etc.) of some children. Children with physical handicaps, with chronic or recurrent illness or with a poor intellectual endowment may also present behaviour problems which can become serious if handled impatiently or with lack of understanding by parents, teachers and doctors.

A child guidance service is now provided in most districts by a team consisting of a psychiatrist, an educational psychologist and a psychiatric social worker. But the service is time consuming and costly, the demands upon it are heavy and waiting lists tend to be long. There are also special residential schools to which the most seriously disturbed children can be sent for a period of observation and treatment, although bringing together children of very different types and often with conflicting needs has obvious dangers.

Physically handicapped children

These are pupils who are not suffering from a defect of sight or hearing but who by reason of disease or crippling defect cannot, without detriment to their health or educational development, be satisfactorily educated under the normal regime of ordinary schools.

About 10,000 pupils have physical handicaps as a result of which they need special educational arrangements.

The types of children included under this broad heading are so diverse and their needs so varied that it is difficult to make any worthwhile generalization about them.

In recent years cerebral palsy has been the commonest cause of severe physical handicap, but since about 1970 the number of children with spina bifida in many special schools has equalled or exceeded the number with cerebral palsy. Neonatal surgery has improved the chances of survival of infants with meningomyelocele but the quality of survival is often a matter for regret, and for parents a cause of great distress. Assessment of the medical, social and educational needs of the survivors presents a difficult interdisciplinary problem as it can involve neurosurgeon, urologist, orthopaedic surgeon, paediatrician, general practitioner, school health physician, social worker, health visitor, educational psychologist and teacher.

In the past children most seriously affected with cerebral palsy were regarded as ineducable, and from poorer homes they often found their way into institutions for the mentally defective. Since 1940 many special schools, training centres and clinics have been opened for these unfortunate children, with encouraging results. Other crippling handicaps which also present special problems are muscular dystrophy, congenital heart disease and limb deformities, and rheumatic heart disease, but surgical techniques and the design of surgical appliances have advanced so rapidly in recent years that many of even the more serverely handicapped children eventually become self supporting.

Children with speech defects

Speech defects are very common in childhood—it has been stated that 2 per cent of school children would benefit from treatment by a speech therapist. However, the number of children with such defects who require special schooling is extremely small; the great majority are able to continue with their ordinary schooling while their disability is being assessed and treated. There continues to be such a serious shortage of speech therapists that few health or local education authorities are able to meet the demand for their services.

Delicate children

Delicate children are those children who do not fall into any of the previous categories but who by reason of impaired physical condition need a change of environment or cannot, without risk to their health and educational progress, be educated in ordinary schools. They include children in poor health from many causes including bad home conditions such as lack of sleep and faulty feeding, and children debilitated from asthma and other illnesses or operations. What is usually needed is a period of convalescence under medical supervision, with good food, fresh air and plenty of rest, and a programme of teaching which enables them to progress for a while at a slower educational pace. To meet those needs an extensive system of open air schools has been developed over the past 50 years. The demand for such accommodation is declining but is still substantial. About three quarters of the accommodation is provided in day schools to which the children are taken in special buses. On the average children are kept on the register of a day school for from 18 months to 2 years. The rest of the accommodation is provided in residential schools in which the children rarely stay for more than 6 months.

Appraisal of Services for Physically Handicapped Children

Effective planning must take into account past trends as well as current needs if future requirements are to be met, and like the pattern of mortality, the pattern of disability in childhood has undergone a remarkable change during the 60 years since the school health services began. As we have seen, this change has been characterized by a decline in the incidence of disability due to adverse postnatal environmental influences, in particular malnutrition and infection, with the result that disability due to natal and prenatal, including genetic, influences has become increasingly prominent. This is particularly obvious in the case of blindness and physical disability.

At the beginning of the nineteenth century two-thirds of those applying for relief at the Liverpool School for the Indigent Blind were thought to have lost their sight because of smallpox. By the end of the century smallpox had virtually disappeared, and the Ophthalmological Society of the United Kingdom estimated that a third or more of the inmates of blind schools had lost their sight because of ophthalmia neonatorum. Nowadays the contribution of infection to the amount of blindness in school children is negligible, and congenital defects, myopia, diseases of the central nervous system and tumours together account for more than 80 per cent of all cases. Associated with this change in the pattern of causes of blindness has been a steady decline in the number of children requiring special educational facilities. Between 1923 and 1983 the number of school children registered as blind in England fell from 2,723 to 929. After 1955 there was a sharp but temporary increase as a cohort of children with retrolental fibroplasia moved through the blind schools. This condition was caused by intensive administration of oxygen to premature infants from about 1947 to 1958.

The causes and the incidence of physically crippling disease in childhood have changed in much the same way. At the beginning of the present century rickets, bone and joint tuberculosis, rheumatic heart disease and osteomyelitis were the principal causes of disablement. Rickets as a cause of deformity is now confined to some immigrant children, osteomyelitis and bone and joint tuberculosis are no longer of any importance, and rheumatic heart disease is rare. In the immediate post war period there was a temporary increase in the amount of disablement due to poliomyelitis. The number of cases notified between 1945 and 1956 was between 2,000 and 8,000 a year. But with the introduction of effective vaccines, the numbers have declined sharply and since 1969 the annual number of notifications has often been zero. With the decline of infections, there has been a substantial reduction in the overall incidence of severe disablement; cerebral palsy, spina bifida, congenital heart disease and asthma are now the major causes of crippling in childhood.

Paradoxically, therefore, as special services for handicapped children have developed the need for them has declined. With the rising standard of living and even more effective control of the common infections of childhood and their complications, it seems fairly certain that the incidence of serious disablement in childhood will decline still further. At the same time with smaller classes and more modern buildings and equipment many more handicapped children can be given the benefit of an education in an ordinary school. Although more refined, elaborate and expensive educational services are likely to be introduced to deal with the hard core of serious disablement which will remain, it seems likely that the demand for and cost of special education will be further reduced before the end of the century.

The classification of handicapped children into mutually exclusive categories has had its uses but it is no longer very acceptable. Many children, whatever their main physical disability, have multiple handicaps. The assessment and fostering of each child's physical, emotional, intellectual and social assets is more important than the definition of a leading disability. Many more multidisciplinary assessement centres are needed, but there is a danger that the fragmentation of hospital paediatrics into an increasing number of sub-specialties may tend to work against this trend.

Physically Handicapped Adults

Adults with a handicap which interferes with their ability to work may be grouped as follows:

(*a*) Those handicapped since childhood (e.g. the congenitally blind). For this group special educational facilities and expert guidance during the transition from school to work are of outstanding importance.
(*b*) Those with a temporary handicap (e.g. multiple fractures after a road accident). Here the need is for efficient and well coordinated medical rehabilitation services to reduce the period of incapacity and to enable the worker to return, if possible, to his previous occupation.
(*c*) Those who acquire a permanent handicap (e.g. the loss of a limb) but are still capable of employment in open industry. In this group industrial rehabilitation is the paramount need. A change of occupation is often necessary, so retraining and help in finding suitable employment may be called for.
(*d*) Those with a permanent handicap so incapacitating that although capable of some work they may never be fit for ordinary employment (for example gross rheumatoid arthritis). The need of this group is for work under sheltered and supervised conditions.
(*e*) Those with a permanent, and often progressive handicap (e.g. multiple sclerosis) which for practical purposes eventually makes them

unsuitable for any employment. In this group the first need may be for adequate medical and nursing care, preferably at home, but if this is not possible, in an institution. Occupations will become mainly diversional.

In general the prevalence of handicap increases exponentially with age. Far and away the most important source of information and distribution is a sample survey by Amelia Harris of the adult population not confined to institutions. It was commissioned by the Office of Population Censuses and Surveys and published in 1971 under the title National Survey of Impaired and Handicapped People in Great Britain. She estimated that outside institutions there were about 3 million handicapped people in the country, rather more of them women than men, and that about 10 per cent were under 45, 30 per cent were 45 to 64 and 70 per cent 65 years of age and over. Subsequent research has shown that about 35 per cent of these suffer from arthritis and rheumatism, and about 25 per cent from diseases of the cardio-vascular or respiratory systems including stroke.

Evolution of services

Except under the Poor Law, there were no public services for handicapped adults before the end of the nineteenth century. In 1897 the Workman's Compensation Act recognized some financial obligation to persons injured at work, and in 1911 the National Health Insurance Act offered general practitioner care for sick and disabled workers in the lower wage ranges. But it is only recently that an attempt has been made to provide comprehensive services to help seriously disabled persons to find and keep suitable employment.

The two World Wars played a significant part in arousing public interest and compelling national action. In 1914-18 an attempt was made to reduce the serious loss of manpower due to badly treated gunshot wounds, and in particular those associated with fractures, by setting up rehabilitation centres in military hospitals. Immediately after the war public sympathy for permanently disabled ex-service men, notably for the blind, led to the establishment of Government Instructional Factories to retrain them and to the introduction of the King's National Roll scheme to encourage firms to employ them. The idea of medical rehabilitation for the injured took root and became an accepted, if inadequate, part of hospital practice. But the feelings of urgency about the need to find employment for the disabled was soon dissipated, and apart from some improvement in services for the blind, no further progress was made until the Second World War. Then the acute shortage of manpower, both in the armed forces and in industry, led to a considerable expansion of medical rehabilitation services in hospitals and to the introduction of a national service for non-medical rehabilitation and resettlement under the Disabled Persons (Employment) Acts of 1944 and 1958, and the Chronically Sick and Disabled Persons Act of 1970.

Contemporary services

Medical responsibility for the care of a patient incapacitated by illness or injury extends far beyond the immediate problem of diagnosis and treatment and can be said to end only when that patient is once more able to lead a reasonably independent social life. This demands from the doctor an appreciation of the effects of pathology upon function, and in particular upon ability to work and to perform such personal activities of daily life as washing, dressing, eating, getting up and down stairs, etc. It requires from the hospitals a medical rehabilitation service that will minimize disability.

For the patient, rehabilitation should be a continuous process. But present day services for the disabled have such complex ramifications that we shall attempt to clarify their pattern by describing them under four headings: medical rehabilitation; industrial rehabilitation; welfare services; and services for young persons.

Medical rehabilitation

At most large hospitals a senior member of the medical staff is now responsible for co-ordinating rehabilitation services, which include physiotherapy, remedial gymnastics and occupational therapy. Therapy may be directed towards the strengthening of a particular function, or it may have the more general purpose of restoring physical and mental confidence after illness or injury. As we have indicated, such services were in the first place designed to meet the needs of the war injured; they are now used to great advantage in a wide range of medical and surgical conditions, including diseases and injuries of the central nervous system, for instance poliomyelitis, paraplegia, hemiplegia, chest conditions such as asthma, bronchitis and after thoracic and abdominal operations.

The aim of medical rehabilitation is to shorten the period between serious accident or illness and return to independent life in the community. For most men and many women this means return to employment; but for many other women it means return to domestic responsibilities, and a number of hospitals now provide special rehabilitation services for disabled housewives.

For hospital rehabilitation services to be fully effective, regular conferences between medical staff, social workers and disablement resettlement officers (see below) are essential. Inadequately supervised and badly co-ordinated services can delay or even prevent an eventual return to work by unnecessarily prolonging the need for attendance at hospital.

Industrial rehabilitation

Public responsibility for helping a disabled person to overcome the difficulty experienced in 'obtaining or keeping employment of a kind which apart from his injury, disease or deformity would be suited to his age, experience and qualifications' is now accepted by the Department of Employment under the Acts of 1944 and 1958 and 1970 listed on the previous page.

The legislation is therefore extensive, and much of it though excellent, is not relevant here. A great deal of the responsibility and control of policy for disabled people is exercised centrally. The services fall under six headings:

(*a*) *Disablement resettlement officer*

Resettlement is managed in each employment exchange and a specialist placing service is operated through a disablement resettlement officer (DRO) who advises disabled persons about the disabled persons' register and helps them to find suitable employment or, if necessary, arranges for them to attend courses of rehabilitation or vocational training. The DRO has detailed knowledge of local working conditions and occupational opportunities and of the physical and mental demands that particular jobs make. He also keeps in close touch with employers and hospitals in his area. Some 500 to 600 DROs are employed throughout the United Kingdom.

(*b*) *Disabled persons' register*

Application for registration, which is voluntary, is made at the local employment exchange through the DRO When the disability is obvious as is the case with the loss of a limb no medical certificate is required; in other cases confirmation from hospital or general practitioner may be asked for. There is an obligation on employers with 20 or more employees to employ 3 per cent of registered disabled, and certain occupations such as lift operator and car park attendant are 'designated' or reserved for the disabled. Not all people entitled to register do so—many because they are able and prefer to compete openly for employment; about half a million are currently registered compared with almost twice that number in 1950 (See table 29.1). About half a million people are now registered on the general register of disabled persons, and there are special registers for the blind.

Table 29.1 All persons registered in Great Britain under the Disabled Persons (Employment) Acts, with the percentage distribution of underlying medical conditions 1950-1976

	Year			
	1950	1960	1970	1976
Number of persons in thousands	936.2	691.7	643.3	543.1
Underlying medical condition	Percentage distribution			
Amputations	8.1	7.9	6.8	6.1
Arthritis and rheumatism	4.2	4.2	4.2	4.4
Diseases of digestive system	8.1	5.5	3.2	2.7
Diseases of heart and circulatory system	6.3	7.4	9.8	11.0
Diseases of lungs	7.9	7.9	9.2	8.2
Ear defects	4.6	4.6	4.4	4.4
Eye defects	6.6	7.2	7.1	6.7
Injuries of head, face, neck, thorax, abodomen, pelvis and trunk	5.1	4.3	3.9	3.4
Injuries and diseases of lower limb	13.9	11.9	12.9	12.5
Injuries and diseases of upper limb	9.4	8.9	8.6	8.0
Injuries and diseases of spine	3.0	4.4	8.5	10.4
Nervous and mental disorders	9.1	10.1	12.6	14.3
Tuberculosis	6.3	8.2	4.2	3.0
Congenital malformations	1.6	1.9	—	—
Other conditions	5.8	5.6	4.6	4.9
All conditions	100	100	100	100

(*c*) *Employment rehabilitation centres*

There are now 27 employment rehabilitation centres in the country. One unit is fully residential and two others have some residential accommodation for men. At non-residential units, persons who are unable to travel daily from home are found accommodation in lodgings or hostels. Employment rehabilitation centres do not offer training for specific occupations: their purpose is to provide individual rehabilitation under conditions approximating to those at work for disabled persons who, although no longer requiring medical treatment, are not yet fit to stand the strain of normal full-time employment. Table 29.2 shows a rising trend in attendances over 20 years from the mid nineteen-fifties and also the changing nature of the disabilities of entrants, with mental illness and spinal problems replacing tuberculosis as the principal causes of disability. During 1981 over 15,000 men and women attended the centres. Unfortunately, only about a quarter of those completing the courses were in employment or training 3 months after the end of their course, compared with about half in 1978, the fall being caused largely by a huge fall in job vacancies which occurred in that short period.

Each unit is directed by a Rehabilitation Officer, and the staff consists of a Vocational Officer who is an occupational psychologist responsible for assessing occupational aptitudes, a Social Worker to help the disabled with personal problems, a Chief Occupational Supervisor in charge of the workshop and a Disablement Resettlement Officer who is responsible for finding suitable employment at the end of the course. Medical advice and supervision are provided by the Employment Medical Advisory Service (Chapter 18).

(*d*) *Government training centres*

Intensive training courses of from 6 to 12 months are provided by the Department of Employment in more than 50 skilled and semiskilled occupations at 30 government training centres. Although now mainly concerned with retraining the able-bodied these courses are also available for disabled persons, and some of the centres are situated alongside or are in the same building as employment rehabilitation centres. The training is costly, so applicants are not accepted unless there is a reasonable prospect that at the end of their course they will be fit to enter the trade for which they have been trained and to stand up to normal working conditions.

Table 29.2 Changes in the percentage distribution of entrants to Employment Rehabilitation Centres by main disability category between 1956 and 1976

Disability	1956	1961	1966	1971	1976
Amputations	2.3	2.1	2.4	2.0	1.7
Arthritis and Rheumatism	3.6	3.2	2.4	2.6	3.6
Diseases of digestive system	3.6	3.4	3.2	2.5	2.5
Diseases of heart and circulatory systems	7.0	8.5	8.2	9.4	9.1
Diseases of respiratory system other than TB	5.9	6.6	5.9	6.5	5.1
Ear defects	0.9	} 2.9	} 3.4	1.4	2.2
Eye defects	1.3			2.5	2.6
Injuries of head and trunk		2.4	2.4	2.2	2.2
Injuries, disease or deformity, lower limb	4.8	6.2	8.2	7.7	7.0
Injuries, diseases or deformity, upper limb	3.9	3.6	5.2	4.6	5.0
Injuries, disease or deformity of spine	5.1	7.7	10.7	12.4	13.8
Psychoneurosis	11.3	13.5	13.5	12.9	12.3
Psychosis	4.2	8.9	8.0	6.1	6.6
Mental subnormality	1.8	2.3	2.4	2.7	3.3
Epilepsy	3.6	4.3	4.5	4.5	5.6
Other organic nervous diseases	5.0	7.0	6.7	6.0	5.2
Respiratory TB	22.4	6.6	2.4	1.2	0.4
Other TB	2.4	1.2	0.5	0.4	0.2
Other diseases	9.6	7.7	4.9	5.5	5.7
Diagnosis not made or not confirmed	0.7	0.7	1.4	0.5	—
No obvious disability	0.6	1.2	3.7	6.4	5.9
Totals	100.0	100.0	100.0	100.00	100.0
Number of clients	9,608	10,714	11,807	14,025	13,959

(*e*) *Sheltered employment*

Some disabled persons are so severely handicapped that they are unlikely ever to obtain employment in open industry. To meet their needs a non-profit distributing, and also, it must be admitted, non-profit making company, Remploy, was set up by the Ministry of Labour in 1945 under the Disabled Persons (Employment) Act. The first Remploy factory was opened at Bridgend, Glamorgan. Today about 8,200 severely disabled men and women are employed in 89 Remploy factories. Their disabilities are due to such conditions as advanced rheumatoid arthritis, multiple sclerosis and to a decreasing extent chronic bronchitis. Remploy products are very varied, and include furniture, books (printing and binding), knitwear and orthopaedic equipment. In addition to the Department of Employment's Remploy factories, there are also sheltered workshops run by the major local authorities, and by voluntary organizations such as the Royal National Institute for the Blind.

(f) *Designated jobs*

The DRO retains legal control over the posts of operator of a passenger lift and car park attendant. In neither case may a person who does not appear on the disabled persons register be appointed without a permit from the DRO.

Welfare services and residential arrangements

With the help of rehabilitation and resettlement services many disabled adults are now able to find work which gives them economic independence. However, there are some so severely handicapped that they can never become economically self supporting, and a few need almost continuous care and attention. Responsibility for their welfare rests largely with the major local authorities under Part II of the National Assistance Act, 1948 (Part I is concerned with financial assistance for those whose needs are not met by National Insurance or other sources). Their responsibilities begin with ascertainment 'of persons who are blind, deaf or dumb, and other persons who are substantially and permanently handicapped by illness, injury or congenital deformity' with the purpose of assessing their social and welfare needs and making arrangements to meet those needs. The services include home visiting, clubs, outings, holiday homes, transport to and from home, sheltered workshops, day centres and home employment. The standard and range of services vary a great deal from authority to authority and although the welfare needs of the blind are now well catered for, in general services for other categories of severely handicapped people are still inadequate.

In the late 1960s it was found that large numbers of physically handicapped adults—many of them quite young—were being accommodated with elderly people on long stay geriatric wards and with little expectation of ever finding a suitable alternative. The social concern which followed this finding led to the construction of specially designed units. Currently there are about 80 such units run by the NHS, and others provided by social services. In turn, the place of such units has come to be questioned, as attention has been drawn to the unsuitably institutionalized social environment which most provide. Current policy is to maintain people in their own homes to the greatest possible extent, adapting the home environment, and providing support and relief to them and their family carers. Where this is insufficient homely residential accommodation should be provided.

Services for school leavers

Services for disabled school leavers merit special mention. Disabled adolescents need extra care and attention if they are to be found suitable employment and helped to keep it. Their placing can be very difficult, particularly when their educational attainment is low, as it often is. The main source of help is the Youth Employment Service of the local authority. Careers officers visit schools to give talks on choice of employment and to interview all children nearing school leaving age. Careers officers often need to see disabled young people several times. Their difficulties have to be discussed with teachers, parents and the school doctor, and the local Employment Medical Adviser has to be kept informed about their placement in employment to ensure a measure of continuing supervision. Some authorities now provide specialist careers officers to carry out this important task.

Appraisal of Services for Physically Handicapped Adults

The medical, social, educational and occupational needs of handicapped adults are complex and inter-related and to meet them calls for the coordination of many different services. Medical rehabilitation is provided through the hospital services; occupational rehabilitation, vocational training and resettlement services are the responsibility of the Department of Employment, while social, welfare and youth employment services are provided by local authorities. Taken together these services give a reasonably comprehensive cover, but because of failures in communication between different sectors some seriously handicapped adolescents and adults do not use to the best advantage the facilities which are available to them.

The main hindrance to the development of rehabilitation services is the low level of interest shown by hospital consultants and general practitioners in the rehabilitation and occupational needs of their patients. What is needed is a reorientation of medical thought rather than the introduction of novel techniques. A study in 1971 showed that only 30 per cent of hospitals with more than 200 beds had made a named consultant responsible for rehabilitation, and there were only 131 consultants in physical medicine and rheumatology in the whole of England and Wales, 89 were in the London Metropolitan area. The position has subsequently improved, but in many hospitals physiotherapy and occupational therapy are still physically separated and quite often they act as independant units and there is need for the development of assessment clinics, as described in the report of the Sub-Committee on Rehabilitation, (1972), to provide: focal points to bring together all services concerned in a patient's rehabilitation, both inside and outside hospital; assessment reports for the Department of Employment and the local authorities; and a safeguard against patients becoming 'lost' and failing to get the rehabilitation services they need.

In addition the long-term disabled and their families require timely and comprehensive information about services available, support in their homes from statutory and voluntary organizations, appropriate aids and domestic adaptations and brief but regular periods of care away from the home. Also, in the case of a tiny minority, long-term residential accommodation should be available which meets the needs of the physically handicapped person for privacy and the optimal degree of independence.

Further Reading

Deakin J. J. (1974) *Joey. An Unforgettable Story of Human Courage*. Charles Scribners & Sons, New York.

Rehabilitation (1972) Report of a Sub-Committee of the Standing Medical Advisory Committee, DHSS and Welsh Office. HMSO.

30

Services for Mentally Handicapped People

When the Intelligence Quotients of children in a random sample of the population are measured, the results form a continuous distribution, and they range from the low scores of grossly subnormal children at one end to the high scores of exceptionally gifted children at the other. Although a small proportion of children with low scores are identified by physical stigmata such as those with Down's syndrome, microcephaly, or hypothyroidism, the great majority have no distinguishing features. There is therefore no biological or statistical justification for drawing a line between persons of 'normal' intelligence and the mentally subnormal. The grounds for division are social, determined by the extent to which the mental handicap interferes with the ability to lead a normal life. In particular they depend on educability and amount of care and protection required.

The Intelligence Quotient is by no means an exact or constant measure of 'intelligence'. When children in a group are tested and later retested, the average IQ of the group remains much the same but the IQs of individual children may vary by as much as 10 points. This is because test results are influenced by physical health, home conditions, willingness to cooperate with the examiner and many other factors. Broadly speaking, however, it can be said that most children with a score below about 70, who amount to about 3 per cent of all children in the country, are unlikely to be able to cope with a standard school education; they therefore require special educational facilities.

Most children and adults with an IQ below about 50 are unable to lead independent lives. Whether the less severely handicapped among them have been looked after at home, with or without outside help, or whether they have required some form of institutional care, has depended on their social behaviour, home circumstances, and the supporting and training services available. Current policy is directed towards closing down long stay institutions and housing mentally handicapped people in the community. These are not primarily medical matters, but, as in the case of physically handicapped children, the doctor has an important part to play in relation to ascertainment, classification and, where possible, prevention and treatment.

The Mental Health Act, 1959, brought together under a single legal code all forms of mental disorder, a term which is stated to mean 'mental illness, arrested or incomplete development of mind, psychopathic disorder and any other disorder or disability of mind'. The term mental disorder and the legal statement of its meaning was retained without amendment in the Mental Health Act, 1983. No further definition of mental illness was provided and no clear distinction drawn between it and mental handicap. Moreover, the words 'mental handicap' do not appear in the Act at all, though there is a reference to the combination of arrested or incomplete development of the mind with impairment of intelligence and impairment of social functioning; this would currently conform with most people's definition of mental handicap.

In this Chapter we are concerned with the needs of the services for persons with mental handicap.

Evolution of Services

Although for more than 400 years it has been recognized in a general and confused way that a 'born fool' is different from a lunatic who 'hath had understanding, but by disease, grief or other accident hath lost the use of his reason', it is only during the present century that there has been any clear understanding of the distinct needs of the mentally handicapped and the mentally ill. A few asylums for idiots were established by voluntary organizations during the nineteenth century, but for the most part severely subnormal children and adults who were abandoned or could not be cared for at home were placed in lunatic asylums and the only refuge for those with less severe degrees of subnormality who were unable to support themselves and could get no help from relatives or charitable sources was the general mixed workhouse.

The social inadequacy of the severely handicapped is evident and their needs are much the same in any type of society. But the difficulties and limitations of handicap become more obvious as the complexities of life multiply with advancing industrialization, and choice of occupation becomes increasingly dependent upon educational attainment. In

England and Wales the introduction of compulsory education quickly drew attention to the fact that, apart altogether from the question of gross and unmistakable mental defect, there were many children who appeared to be too dull to derive much benefit from the teaching provided by ordinary schools. Gradually, special educational services developed to meet their needs, and these were codified in regulations made under the Education Act, 1944. Over the same period it became accepted that 'ineducable defectives' deserved and had the right to help outside the walls of the workhouse and the mental hospital. Under the Mental Deficiency Act, 1913, local authorities were made 'mental deficiency authorities'. They became responsible for home visiting, guardianship and supervision of the subnormal in the community and for the provision of 'colonies' for the severely handicapped who for one reason or another could not be cared for at home. With the National Health Service Act, 1946, these colonies became 'mental deficiency hospitals' under the new hospital boards, but responsibility for domiciliary care and supporting services remained with the local authorities. The Mental Health Act, 1959, greatly enlarged the local authorities' responsibilities for community care of mentally handicapped children and adults and a system of training centres and workshops was developed. With the Education (Handicapped Children) Act 1971 education authorities were required to provide education for all children regardless of mental ability, and the former old Junior Training Centres became special schools under the aegis of local education authorities who were also required to provide educational facilities in hospitals for the mentally handicapped. Responsibility for the welfare of older mentally handicapped persons now lies with the Social Services Departments of the local authorities, but to the greatest extent possible they and their families should always be involved in decision-making about their care.

Contemporary Services

Educational services

Educationally subnormal children are defined as those 'who by reason of limited ability or other conditions resulting in educational retardation, require some specialized form of education wholly or partly in substitution for that normally given in ordinary schools'. They form by far the largest group of handicapped children with special educational needs. It should be noted that the definition of educational subnormality is based upon the practical consideration of educational difficulty rather than upon the theoretical concept of innate ability. Children may become educationally retarded as the result of many influences, for example lack of parental interest or ability, emotional disturbance, irregular school attendance and frequent change of school as well as because of limited intellectual ability. A few children are educationally retarded in relation only to certain subjects, such as mathematics or reading, and have an average or above average grasp of the rest of the school curriculum. The provision of educational services to meet such varied needs is clearly a complex matter and includes individual attention and special classes in ordinary schools as well as special schools.

The special schools, about one-third of which are residential, have the great advantage of classes small enough to permit an individual as well as a group approach. The teaching is focused upon the need to help the mentally handicapped to acquire the minimum amount of knowledge and basic skills necessary to cope with some of the complexities of modern life. The decision to send a child to a special school is not taken lightly. In an ordinary school a dull child may become duller and perhaps even drift into delinquency as a result of frustration and boredom, but attending a special school unfortunately still carries some stigma. For the border-line case it is only when there are serious behaviour or home difficulties that admission to a special school is considered, a contingency the chance of which is enhanced by the fact that children with an intellectual handicap tend to receive less sympathy and understanding both at school and at home than children with almost any other type of disability. The decision rests upon consultation between educational psychologist, school medical officer, teacher and parents and on general assessment of social adjustment and abilities, as well as on standard intelligence and performance tests. The more seriously retarded child is no problem to recognize and early admission to a special school is usually called for.

All but the most grossly affected children have some abilities and aptitudes which, with patience and understanding, can be developed, and many who at one time would have been declared untrainable are now being helped to develop fully their limited abilities in preparation for fairly independent adult life in the community. These children are given training in personal cleanliness, drawing, painting, music and expressive crafts. The aim is also to teach them to grasp the essentials for ordinary living: the rudiments of road safety; the handling of money; the buying of clothing and food; and the use of public transport, the post office, and health services.

Adult training centres, workshops and hostels

Young people from schools for the educationally subnormal require a continuing educational programme to adapt them to the social needs and demands of adult life and to prepare them for work in a sheltered workshop, or, possibly, for a place in open industry. Older people need sheltered work in an environment where attention can be paid to their social requirements. Local authorities are responsible for providing these facilities. The purpose is to get away from the traditional occupational therapy at one time provided in hospitals for the mentally handicapped and to provide in its place productive work and in children realistic preparation for life in the community. Many centres undertake contract work for the local authority, for example a laundry service for homes, and day nurseries, or for private firms in the district. It has become clear that because few mentally handicapped people require medical supervision or professional nursing care it is inappropriate to base management on hospitals. If parents and relatives are able with the help of local authority services to provide the social support they need, the best place for them is at home. To meet the needs of those who have no homes or whose homes are unsuitable many local authorities provide residential accommodation. About 11,500 mentally handicapped children and adults now live in local authority hostels and homes. The demand for such accommodation still greatly exceeds the supply. Current policy is to replace hostel accommodation with ordinary flats and houses.

Hospitals for the mentally handicapped

In England and Wales in 1976 there were about 47,000 mentally handicapped persons under statutory care and protection. For every admission there are 10 readmissions. The vast majority of patients are living in the community under local authority supervision or guardianship. Supervision involves regular visits from the social services department; guardianship has a legal meaning and implies stricter supervision by an approved person who acts *in loco parentis*. Despite the development of local authority services hospital care has continued to be needed for some mentally handicapped children and adults. In the past the isolation of these hospitals and their separation from the main stream of medicine and nursing could be held responsible for their low standards of care, overcrowding, lack of equipment and shortage of staff. For the first 20 years of the National Health Service little was done to improve the situation; mental subnormality hospitals as they were called remained neglected, overcrowded and under-financed. Since about 1970, partly as the result of public disclosures of the deplorable conditions in some of the hospitals, there has been a move to remedy the worst of the deficiencies created by years of neglect. More capital has been invested in the services. New buildings have been erected, old buildings have been closed down or renovated to make them more suitable for patient care and improved opportunities for staff training have been provided. The move towards informal admissions, outpatient clinics, day patient facilities, industrial therapy units and hospital schools provided by local authorities has also helped to raise the standards of care.

Appraisal of Services

Out of date buildings and shortage of trained personnel, equipment and accommodation are complaints that can be made about many medical and social services. They can be made with particular force about services for mentally handicapped people. At the present time 12,000 mentally handicapped children under 5 in Britain are waiting for special education. In spite of the emphasis now placed on community care, and the increasing provision by local authorities of training centres, workshops and hostels, the position is equally serious with regard to accommodation for the more severely handicapped in need of care and protection.

The pressure on facilities for special education reflects in part the general shortage of ordinary teachers and classrooms; were there smaller classes, and more teachers, it is possible that fewer border-line children would need to be referred to special teachers. But pressure on special accommodation comes from below as well as from above. Although the incidence of mental subnormality at birth is almost constant, with the decline of perinatal, infant and preschool death rates many more subnormal children are now living to school age. At the same time, as local authorities have extended and strengthened their community services, the need for hospital accommodation has been reduced.

In conclusion we may ask if the prospect of advances in understanding of the aetiology of mental handicap offers any hope for a reduction of its incidence by prevention or treatment. For the most part mental handicap is no more than an expression of man's biological variability which is due to the interaction between genotype and environment, but in a proportion of cases biochemical or chromosomal abnormalities underly gross mental defect. Knowledge of some of these causes, for example phenylketonuria, already permits the application of preventive or curative measures; and of a few others it is sufficient to sustain the hope that sooner or later it may be possible to do so. On present knowledge, however, it seems unlikely that medical intervention will have a significant effect on more than a small proportion of all cases of mental handicap and the problem will remain at almost its present size. Indeed, medical advances may to some extent exacerbate it. Handicapped children, especially those in institutions, are particularly vulnerable to infectious disease. With the introduction of chemotherapy, antibiotics and effective preventive inoculation, handicapped individuals who at one time would have died in infancy now survive into adult life. This is strikingly evident in relation to Down's syndrome. And as the chances of survival improve, an increasing number of mentally handicapped adults in the community will outlive the parents and relatives who have looked after them and will need life long support. It is now policy not to admit mentally handicapped children to hospital, to discharge the remaining in-patients into houses in the community, and to attempt to re-integrate the great majority of adult residents into their own communities. If successful, these policies will bring to an end more than a century of hospital provision for mentally handicapped people.

31

Services for Mentally Ill People

In the preceding chapter we discussed the medical and social needs of persons with mental handicap, which is incomplete development of the intellect manifested before adult life. We now turn to the needs of patients with mental illness namely temporary or permanent disturbance of the mind, characterized by behaviour and reasoning disorders and usually occurring in adult life. Some indication of the magnitude of the problem is provided by the fact that in 1980 nearly a quarter of the hospital beds in England and Wales were occupied by such patients.

It is often difficult to draw a line between health and somatic disease. It is even more difficult to decide where mental health ends and mental illness begins. A person whose behaviour deviates substantially from some generally recognized but ill-defined pattern regarded as normal is thought to be mentally ill. But in the general population the range of behaviour extends from strict adherence to the locally accepted norms, through eccentricity and the hinterland of psychoneurosis, to the extremity of gross psychosis. Moreover, standards of acceptable social behaviour vary enormously from one civilization to another, from one community to another and even from group to group within the same community; so that behaviour which in one society would be accepted as no more than amiable eccentricity, in another may be considered to require medical treatment or even compulsory detention. Dostoevsky describes an uncle who used to shoot a gun from his window at passers-by he did not like, and who sometimes opened a trapdoor to spit on a sleeping relative who also had incurred his displeasure. In Pre-Revolution Russia these practices were not apparently regarded as particularly remarkable. What determines the significance of abnormal behaviour is the extent to which it interferes with ability to lead a life acceptable as tolerably normal in the context of its social surroundings. This is also true of physical handicap; but in the case of mental illness there is the added complication that some degree of control or physical restraint may be needed, either for the affected person's own sake or for the sake of others, and it may have to be imposed without the person's full understanding or consent.

The custodial aspect of care for mentally ill people has largely determined the nature of the services which have evolved to meet their needs, and in spite of the advances of the past 40 or 50 years it is still of some importance. For the sake of the patient, and sometimes of the family and the community, the more severe forms of psychiatric illness usually require hospital admission. In general, however, whether a patient can be cared for at home depends to a considerable extent on social circumstances. This is hardly less true today, when very effective forms of therapy can be given in outpatient clinics or day hospitals, than it was when George III at Windsor Castle endured treatment by beating, purging and strait-jacket restraint.

Evolution of Services

The history of services for the mentally ill is long and complicated. Three broad phases are discernible.

Until about the end of the eighteenth century the public attitude towards madness was one of superstitious fear, engendered by the belief that it was due to demonic possession. Lunatics were treated with deliberate brutality. The rich were incarcerated in private mad houses, the poor died in jails and workhouses.

It has been said that the devil himself helped the first reforms along by moving into Royalty. Certainly George III's death saw the beginning of a more humane approach, and during the nineteenth century many public lunatic asylums were built. Although by modern standards patients were still cruelly treated, the cruelty was not malicious, but was due to ignorance. Throughout the century the main concern of reformers was to provide legal safeguards against the dangers of wrongful compulsory detention.

Since the beginning of the twentieth century advances in psychological medicine have resulted in a change in attitude towards mental illness, and the emphasis has shifted from compulsory segregation to early diagnosis, active treatment and where necessary social rehabilitation.

The nineteenth century preoccupation with the legal aspects of admission to lunatic asylums culminated in the Lunacy Act, 1890. Under this Act certification was so hemmed in with legal safeguards that a patient was likely to be admitted to an asylum only as a last resort when the illness had reached an advanced stage. So long as both the general public and the medical profession regarded lunacy as irreversible, this was of little consequence. But from the end of the nineteenth century the work of Charcot, Freud, Jung, Adler, and others suggested that at least some forms of mental illness were treatable, an impression substantially reinforced by the study of psychoneurotic behaviour (shell shock) during the First World War. Society began to treat lunatics as sick persons not dangerous animals; but most people still regarded with fear and repugnance the legal formality of certification and the locked doors of the lunatic asylums. The Mental Treatment Act, 1930, introduced the idea of voluntary and temporary admission for treatment; it emphasized the need for psychiatric outpatient clinics, and underlined the new approach by using the expressions 'mental hospital' and 'mental illness' in place of 'lunatic asylums' and 'lunacy'. Movement in the direction of early treatment and social rehabilitation was carried several stages further by the Mental Health Act, 1959, with its emphasis on community services. It insisted that the great majority of patients suffering from mental illness should be admitted to and treated in hospitals in the same way as patients with any other illness, and that compulsory admission and detection should be a last resort. The Mental Health Act, 1983, has further enhanced the protection of patients.

Contemporary Services

Mentally ill patients, or their relatives, usually seek advice in the first instance from their general practitioners. If a doctor considers one of his patients to be in need of specialized treatment he seeks the opinion of a consultant psychiatrist, who sees the patient at a psychiatric clinic or, if the illness is severe, in the patient's home. If the psychiatrist thinks that hospital treatment is advisable, he can arrange for the patient to be admitted to a mental hospital or the psychiatric ward of a general hospital or to attend a psychiatric clinic or a day hospital. Occasionally the general practitioner is faced with a psychiatric emergency. In this case, he can call on the help of a social worker of the local authority to arrange compulsory admission to hospital.

The Mental Health Act, 1959, greatly simplified the machinery for compulsory admission. An application is founded on the written recommendations of two medical practitioners that detention in hospital is necessary in the patient's own interests or for the protection of others. One of the recommending practitioners must be approved as having special experience in mental disorders. The application is made by the nearest relative of the patient or by the Social Services Department. Compulsory admission and detention may not normally exceed 28 days; the rights of the patient have been further extended by the Mental Health Act of 1983 which allows him to appeal to a Mental Health Review Tribunal if he is dissatisfied with his admission, detention or treatment. No treatment may now be given without consent unless the case is an emergency or falls into certain categories of severe illness. A Mental Health Commission has been established which has been charged with keeping under review all aspects of care of detained patients.

In–patient care

Between 1954 and 1978 the average number of psychiatric patients resident in hospital in England and Wales fell from 152,000 to 79,000 a decline of 48 per cent. Over the same period the number of patients admitted to mental hospitals rose from 77,000 to 172,000 an increase of 123 per cent. These trends provide a striking illustration of the way in which the pattern of care in mental hospitals is changing. On the one hand many long-stay patients are being rehabilitated and returned to the community; on the other while 51,500 patients are admitted each year in the early stages of mental illness the number of previous patients who are readmitted has risen to 120,500.

So far as possible first admissions are accommodated in new or modernized admission wards with access to the wide range of facilities demanded by present day methods of investigation and treatment. At the same time a growing tendency has been to admit patients with less severe forms of mental illness to psychiatric wards in district general hospitals.

Most recently there has been increased interest in reducing admissions in the first place through the provision of appropriate day hospitals, day care centres and domiciliary support. Standards of care and treatment for the long stay patient are also rapidly improving. There are still some aggressive and difficult patients who receive heavy sedation and close supervision; but in all hospitals most doors, and in some hospitals all doors, have been unlocked, and patients have much greater freedom of movement in and about the buildings, which are consequently less prison-like. It is now clear that modern drugs and an imaginative programme of recreation and occupational rehabilitation can produce so much improvement in the behaviour of long stay patients that many of them are able to return to their homes, sometimes to work if it is available.

This improvement is not achieved merely by providing work on the wards. Day rooms and dining rooms are more cheerful and more homely; facilities are provided for physical training, for watching and playing games, for dances and entertainment of various kinds; and more realistic occupational rehabilitation is being offered in workshops inside and outside the hospital buildings. Patients who improve are able to go home for the day or the weekend, and relatives are encouraged to accept them back. A period in an employment rehabilitation centre if there is one in the area can sometimes hasten the slow process of return to the community.

Psychiatric clinics and day hospitals

Psychiatric clinics, providing full facilities for diagnosis and treatment by both physical and psychological methods, are now generally available, and many day hospitals have been established. Their purpose is to enable patients to maintain family and social ties while undergoing investigation and treatment. In this way admission to hospital can often be avoided to the patient's benefit and that of the community; clinics and day hospitals are easier to run and less expensive than residential institutions and the process of institutionalization, from which some do not recover, is avoided.

After–care services

In 1980 over 180,000 patients were discharged from mental hospitals in England and Wales and another 200,000 attended psychiatric clinics and day hospitals for the first time. Total attendances were almost 1¾ million, over four-fold more than in the immediate post-war years. The problem of providing after-care services for such a large population is formidable. It is not made easier by the division of responsibility between District Health Authorities, local authorities and the Department of Employment, or by the acute shortage of social workers. Social workers attempt to ensure that patients fit to leave hospital have a suitable home to go to before they are discharged and to help patients discharged from hospital to adjust to family life and employment. Rehabilitation and vocational training services are available for them through the Department of Employment. But co-ordination of these varied services is difficult to achieve and the results are still far from satisfactory. In particular there is need for many more sheltered workshops and for more hostels in which patients who have no homes can live under supervision and from which they can go out to work.

Since 1974 health authorities have increasingly undertaken joint planning of mental health services with their matching social service and housing departments and the problems caused by the dispersal of administrative and financial responsibility are slowly being overcome.

The Incidence of Mental Illness

In view of the difficulty of defining mental illness, it is not surprising that knowledge of the amount of illness in the community is very incomplete. In England and Wales at the present time there are as we have seen about 80,000 patients in mental hospitals, and 200,000 new cases and about three times as many old cases attending psychiatric clinics every year. This suggests that the prevalence of mental illness severe enough to warrant detention in hospital or out-patient investigation and treatment is at least 18 per 1,000 of the population. This estimate takes no account of the large number of patients with mental illness who are under the care of their general practitioners nor of the large number of old people with severe mental infirmity who are in long-stay and geriatric hospitals or are being cared for at home. In addition there is an unknown but certainly a large amount of mental ill health in the population which never comes to medical attention but causes a great deal of sickness, absence from work, and personal and family distress. Estimates of the proportion of patients seen by general practitioners who are found to be suffering from some form of psychiatric disorder like dementia, psychosis, neurosis, psychosomatic conditions, organic illnesses with a psychological overlay and personality disorder have been estimated at between 20 and 25 per cent and it has been suggested that as much as one third of all long-term absence from work is due to psychoneurotic conditions.

It is hardly necessary to point out that if knowledge of present day incidence of mental illness is incomplete, estimates of past and future trends are even less reliable. A few general observations are permissible. The incidence of mental illness attributable to systemic causes such as acute and chronic infection, malnutrition, alcohol and toxic hazards in industry is considerably less today than it was 100 or even 50 years ago. For example, in the mental hospitals in England and Wales during the present century the proportion of male admissions due to syphilis has declined from about 1 in 5 to less than 1 in 200. On the other hand mental illness associated with drug dependence is increasing and in recent years there has been a marked upturn in the incidence of alcohol-related disorders. We can be less confident about the trend of those forms of mental illness whose aetiology is still obscure: schizophrenia, manic-depressive psychosis and psycho-neurosis. It is possible that there has been some reduction in the incidence of overt schizophrenia which is still responsible for one-twelfth of first admissions to hospital (and 1 in 6 of all admissions) as the result of social improvements, for breakdown from this condition is commoner in poor than in favourable social circumstances. There is some evidence, however, that manic-depressive psychosis is becoming more frequent, particularly among women, and it is certain that in the ageing population the amount of mental disease associated with advanced age is rising. It is also said that the stresses of urban and industrial life have been responsible for an increase in the amount of psychoneurotic and psychosomatic illness in the community, but there is as yet little evidence to support this view.

Appraisal of Services

The continuing low standard of care in many mental hospitals is one of the most unsatisfactory features of the contemporary medical services. This deficiency has its origin in the historical circumstances which divided mental from other hospitals. Almost all of them were built more than 50 years ago, many more than a century ago, and they were designed not to treat illness, but to protect society from the embarrassing and occasionally dangerous behaviour of the insane. Lunatic asylums, built as detention barracks, serve now in part as hospitals, in part as hostels and in part as rehabilitation centres. Their wards are badly designed, inadequately equipped and are far too large for modern methods of treatment. Their separation from other hospitals has isolated them and often adds to the difficulty of attracting doctors and nurses.

Some hope for the future is offered by the striking decline in the number of occupied mental hospital beds, due to the discharge of many long-stay patients and the shorter average duration of stay among new admissions and re-admissions. There is some prospect that with the help of modern therapy, an expansion of still inadequate community services, day hospitals, hostels, sheltered workshops and local and health authority domiciliary services and day centres, there will be a further decline in the demand for psychiatric beds.

In the past treatment has been less effective in mental illness than in almost any other branch of medicine. The value of modern therapy is difficult to assess, but it is undoubtedly more effective in the control of symptoms than ever before. It remains difficult to say how often psychotherapy is effective, but it may be time consuming so that only some of the large number of psychoneurotic persons in the population can be treated by this method. The contribution of those with scarce skills such as psychotherapists and clinical psychologists can however be increased many fold by what they can offer to the professional development of colleagues, particularly psychiatric nurses in the hospital and community and social workers. There is reason to believe that these skills can be optimally used when therapists work with groups of patients rather than with single individuals. Improved care is promised by the prospect of a planned and balanced expansion of the still inadequate community services. The achievements of modern therapy in the control of psychosis are more concrete. In selected cases, particularly in patients with manic depressive psychosis, electro-convulsive therapy, lithium and the tricyclic antidepressants often produce an immediate and sometimes a dramatic improvement although relapse is not uncommon. There are now many drugs which have valuable sedative effects on patients in a state of psychotic distress and chemical sedation has replaced the padded cell and the strait-jacket. In spite of these therapeutic advances, it seems likely that for some time to come services for the mentally ill will depend for the most part on maintainance therapy, care, protection and social rehabilitation rather than on cure.

32

Services for Elderly People

The twentieth century has seen a great increase in the number and proportion of old people in the population. Eighty to 90 years ago the high birth rates and high death rates of the nineteenth century produced a population with a concentration in the younger age groups. The decline in the birth rate from 1870 until just before the Second World War and the reduction of mortality from infectious disease and malnutrition in childhood and young adult life have subsequently modified population structure to produce a smaller proportion of infants and children and a much greater proportion of old people (figure 3.1). In Britain in 1901 there were 1,600,000 people aged 65 or more (4.7 per cent of the population). At the 1981 census the number was 7,985,000 (14.9 per cent of the population); 5 million were over 70 years of age and nearly a million and a half over 80 years of age (at this age there were more than 2 women to every man). The expectation of life at birth in 1981 was 70.8 for males and 76.9 for females and now nearly three-quarters of all our live born infants can expect to live through to retirement. Although there have always been old people, senescence as a normal feature of life is new.

Injury, mental illness, neoplasm, arthritis and degenerative vascular states are common in the elderly, although they are not peculiar to old age. It is not because of special pathology that health and social services for old people need special consideration, although multiple pathology is certainly much commoner in old people than in young and middle aged adults. It is because the pathology of old age is associated with retirement from work, failing physical and mental powers, social isolation and a terminal illness, often preceeded by a long period of incapacity. Against this background we shall look briefly at the history of services for old people and describe in more detail the services now available to them.

Evolution of Services

Public provision of personal medical and social services for old people is of very recent origin. In the nineteenth century except for a few homes provided by charitable and religious organizations, the only refuge for destitute old people and sick old people with no one to look after them was the general mixed workhouse along with the destitute of all ages. Many workers subscribed to friendly societies which provided them with small weekly payments during sickness or disablement while they were of working age and their relatives with a death grant when they died, but medical attention in old age was very rarely included among the benefits. The introduction in 1908 of a noncontributory pension of 25p per week for needy persons over 70 years of age and in 1911 (National Health Insurance Act) of general practitioner care for old people who had paid the necessary insurance contributions during their working lives helped a small proportion of those in need. But the great majority of old people who were urgently in need of medical and nursing attention and had no children or other relatives to look after them were admitted to Poor Law Hospitals, notorious for their low standard of care. The transfer of the Poor Law Institutions to local authorities in 1929 had less effect on the low standards of hospital care than might have been expected. However, progressive authorities, following the example of charitable organizations, began to provide accommodation for well old people in residential houses and to convert the best of the hospital accommodation into general hospitals.

The less satisfactory Poor Law Institutions although transferred to local authorities remained unchanged until in 1948 when under the National Health Service Act they became the responsibility of the newly created Regional Hospital Boards as hospitals for the chronic sick. At the same time, also under the National Health Service Act, old people, like all other members of the population, became entitled to the services of a general practitioner free of charge and, at the discretion of their general practitioner, to specialist advice and hospital care as required. Under the same Act the home nursing, domestic help, health visitor and other care and after care services which local authorities were empowered to provide became available for old persons who needed them. Post war social security legislation has provided retirement pensions for all, with supplementary benefits if resources are insufficient to meet basic needs. This has removed from old people's lives the threat of financial destitution although many still have an unacceptably low standard of living.

Finally under the Local Authorities Social Services Act, 1970, local authorities have been made responsible for providing comprehensive social services for the care of the elderly (and other persons in need of help and support). This is implemented through their Social Services Committees and the Directors of Social Services.

Contemporary Services

For a number of reasons the provision of services for the elderly presents a difficult and confusing problem. First, it is now usual to define the elderly as those aged 65 years and over and geriatrics as the branch of medicine dealing with persons of this age group. But there is nothing physiologically or medically significant about the 65th birthday. At one time old age was defined physiologically—men and women were old when they were no longer able to work. Today it is defined chronologically in terms of the age at which insured men become entitled to draw their retirement pensions. (For even less clear biological reasons, women may draw theirs when they are 60.) But many men and women remain physically fit and mentally alert until long past their seventieth birthdays. And on the other hand about 40 per cent of patients in the medical wards of general hospitals and in mental hospitals are over 65, while about 10 per cent of patients admitted to geriatric assessment and long-stay units are under 65. Second, whether old people who are ill or have become severely disabled are admitted to hospital or remain at home is determined more by their social circumstances and the availability of supporting services than by medical diagnosis. Third, the type of hospital to which an old person is admitted (general hospital, mental hospital, long-stay hospital, geriatric assessment unit or psychogeriatric unit) tends to depend as much on the availability of beds in the area and on the attitudes of the general practitioners and their relationship with local consultants as on medical and nursing needs. Finally the administrative separation of health services from local authority services gives rise to difficulties in what, so far as old people are concerned, is a continuum of medical and social needs.

District Health Authority services

District Health Authorities are responsible under the National Health Service Act for providing domiciliary medical and nursing services and out-patient and in-patient hospital services for old people as for all other members of the community. However, there are certain features of these services that deserve special mention.

Domiciliary health services

Less than 5 per cent of people over 65 years of age are in geriatric units, mental hospitals and old peoples' homes. Of the 95 per cent of the elderly living in their own homes or the homes of relatives or friends, many are ill and disabled. This places a great burden on relatives and makes heavy demands on domiciliary health and social services. General practitioners provide medical attention and can obtain domiciliary or out-patient consultant advice when they think it is needed. They can call on community nurses, usually attached to group practices, for skilled and semi-skilled nursing services and on a wide range of local authority and voluntary welfare services (see below), although these still vary greatly in quality and availability from area to area. In the past, domiciliary medical services were concerned with medical crises, with acute illnesses and exacerbations of chronic illnesses as they arose. Old people are sometimes reluctant to seek medical advice through fear of hospital admission, and they may be ignorant of the welfare services that they can call on for support. General practitioners are now well aware that early mobilization of medical, nursing and social services can delay the onset of dependency in old age and health visitors with their open access to the homes of practitioners' patients are in a key position to detect and draw attention to old peoples' medical and social needs.

Hospital services

Many sick old people are admitted to and treated in the medical and surgical wards of general hospitals and in mental hospitals. But most teaching and district general hospitals now also have geriatric departments or geriatric assessment units. The diseases of old age are in themselves no different from the diseases of middle life, but old people much more often have multiple pathology, in their illnesses social complications are the rule rather than the exception, and they need special facilities for rehabilitation if they are to be returned to their homes. A domiciliary visit by the geriatrician can sometimes avert hospital admission with the help of outpatient rehabilitation, day hospital care and supporting social services. Day hospitals, attached to and usually within the grounds of the main hospital, permit physically and sometimes mentally infirm old people to continue to live at home while receiving hospital care during the day time. Patients are brought to the day hospital by ambulance in the morning and returned home in the evening for one or more days a week. In the unit they are under medical supervision and can be given nursing attention, physiotherapy and occupational therapy. Geriatric departments also enable relief to be given to relatives when the burden of home care has become too heavy by arranging for elderly people to be admitted temporarily or intermittently to the wards. However, despite all these improved facilities, there are still many old people who require long-stay care. Attempts are being made to improve the quality of care in long-stay hospitals. Large overcrowded wards have been divided into smaller units and buildings have been modernized, so far as this is possible in nineteenth century hospitals and Poor Law buildings. But the Health Advisory Service, set up by the Department of Health and Social Security in 1969 and given as its first task the examination of long-stay hospitals, continues to report that the care of patients in them is still far from satisfactory. The separation of long-stay hospitals from the mainstream of medicine and their out of date and unsuitable buildings makes them unattractive places to work in and, often therefore, difficult to staff. And although the patients in long-stay hospitals are not nearly so ill assorted as the patients in the old Poor Law Institutions, they are still very mixed in respect of their need for medical and nursing care.

Local authority and voluntary services

Local authorities, through their social services committees, have under the National Assistance Act of 1948 statutory responsibility for providing comprehensive social services, and as part of their remit they are responsible for the care of the elderly. Many of the services they now provide were originally introduced by voluntary agencies, and voluntary organizations continue to provide services to supplement those of the local authorities and to pioneer new methods of meeting unsatisfied needs. The voluntary services are provided by many different organizations.

Old people's homes

Residential accommodation is available for elderly people who are in need of hospital care but are unable to live independent lives in the community because of frailty and increasing infirmity. This was required under Part III of the Act of 1948, and is known as 'Part III accommodation'. Residents make a contribution to the cost, a general practitioner provides medical attention and a resident matron and her staff look after residents with short term illnesses. An increasing number of these homes are new buildings, specially designed with separate or twin bedrooms, several small lounges and television, washing and ironing rooms. Other homes have been established by adapting large old houses, but these may be inconvenient and difficult to run even after extensive structural alterations have been made. Some homes are still in buildings constructed under the nineteenth century Poor Law and these are usually very unsatisfactory. The demand for places in old people's homes greatly exceeds the supply and with the shortage of suitable building sites, the rising cost of building, and the shortage of money to pay trained staff, it is likely to continue so.

Housing for old people

The demand for places in old people's homes and for geriatric day-hospital and in-patient care is augmented by the inadequate housing in which so many old people live, houses with dangerous staircases, insufficient heating and awkwardly placed cupboards, sinks, baths and lavatories, so that all local authorities now provide some special housing for elderly people who are more or less self sufficient; this is generally known as sheltered housing. It varies in type from area to area—for example in large towns flatlets may be built with central heating, all accommodation on one floor and specially designed kitchens, lavatories and sitting baths, and in less populous areas small bungalows may be grouped near a shopping centre and other amenities. Some authorities are experimenting with groups of flats or bungalows with a restaurant and a resident warden, and this is often called warden controlled sheltered housing.

Supporting services in the home

The most valuable of these is the Home Help Service. This enables many elderly people to continue to live at home who otherwise would have to be admitted to an old people's home or even to a geriatric hospital. The home help visits the home 2 or 3 times a week for about 4 hours at a time. She helps with the housework, does the shopping and prepares a meal. Another useful service, pioneered by the Women's Royal Voluntary Service and now organized, with voluntary help, by the local authority is 'Meals-on-Wheels'. Clinical manifestations of malnutrition are quite common among very old people, especially those living alone. This is due to a combination of factors including poverty, lack of facilities for storing, preparing and cooking food and, sometimes, indifference. Hot cooked meals are delivered from insulated containers direct to the homes of such old people for a very modest charge. Other services are: laundry services and provision of incontinence pads, both invaluable where an incontinent old person is being nursed at home; night sitters who undertake to sit up all night with sick old people to give exhausted relatives a night's rest (these are in very short supply); and 'good neighbour' schemes whereby someone living near an isolated and infirm old person agrees to help with the shopping, cooking and housework.

Other services

Various voluntary organizations and some local authorities help old people in other ways. For example there are: luncheon clubs where hot meals are brought from a central kitchen to a suitable building in the neighbourhood; old people's clubs, day centres, handicraft centres and rest centres to combat social isolation; free transport for visiting friends and relatives; and day outings and special holiday arrangements.

Appraisal of Services

The purpose of most of the services we have described is to attempt to maintain the independence of elderly people by trying to ensure that no old person enters hospital or fails to return home after completion of treatment for lack of any service which the community can reasonably be expected to provide. This is both a humane and a sensible objective—humane because, understandably, most old people want to live in their own homes, and sensible because the problem of caring for the aged sick and infirm would become unmanageable if the whole responsibility were placed on public institutions. But inadequacies in day hospital, outpatient and supporting domiciliary services are already imposing a very heavy burden on those looking after the extremely old at home. For example surveys show that a large number of bedfast incontinent old people are being cared for by middle aged and elderly relatives with no help from district nurse, laundry or other services. Sometimes this is because of ignorance about the existence of supporting services, but more often it is because the local services are inadequate. The number of people reaching extreme old age, however it is defined, is increasing year by year, and among the very old the prevalence of causes of dependency which are immobility, incontinence, dementia, deafness and blindness is high. Local authority and voluntary services are already overburdened and even if they are greatly expanded it will still be impossible to keep many dependent old people at home. It is clear that to provide them with a reasonable standard of care there will need to be a considerable increase in the number of hospital beds and places in local authority, voluntary and private residential homes and sheltered housing. For example, over the age of 75 the prevalence of people with a degree of mental frailty requiring constant attention is about 15 per cent. This will mean at least an additional 75,000 cases in the population in 10 years' time and to cater for only 10 per cent of them in hospital will require-7,500 more beds. Indeed, a substantial increase in the number of long stay beds is required now if even the present level of need is to be met.

Against this should be set the increasing proportion of elderly people who have their own homes, and are able to provide resources to contribute towards improved arrangements for their ease in extreme old age.

Index